Bone Marrow Failure

Editor

COLIN A. SIEFF

HEMATOLOGY/ONCOLOGY
CLINICS OF NORTH AMERICA

www.hemonc.theclinics.com

Consulting Editors
GEORGE P. CANELLOS
H. FRANKLIN BUNN

August 2018 • Volume 32 • Number 4

ELSEVIER

1600 John F. Kennedy Boulevard • Suite 1800 • Philadelphia, Pennsylvania, 19103-2899

http://www.theclinics.com

HEMATOLOGY/ONCOLOGY CLINICS OF NORTH AMERICA Volume 32, Number 4
August 2018 ISSN 0889-8588, ISBN 13: 978-0-323-61390-3

Editor: Stacy Eastman
Developmental Editor: Kristen Helm

Hematology/Oncology Clinics (ISSN 0889-8588) is published bimonthly by Elsevier Inc., 360 Park Avenue South, New York, NY 10010-1710. Months of issue are February, April, June, August, October, and December. Business and Editorial Offices: 1600 John F. Kennedy Blvd., Ste. 1800, Philadelphia, PA 19103–2899. Customer Service Office: 3251 Riverport Lane, Maryland Heights, MO 63043. Periodicals postage paid at New York, NY and at additional mailing offices. Subscription prices are $413.00 per year (domestic individuals), $787.00 per year (domestic institutions), $100.00 per year (domestic students/residents), $471.00 per year (Canadian individuals), $974.00 per year (Canadian institutions) $536.00 per year (international individuals), $974.00 per year (international institutions), and $255.00 per year (international and Canadian students/residents). International air speed delivery is included in all *Clinics* subscription prices. All prices are subject to change without notice. **POSTMASTER:** Send address changes to *Hematology/Oncology Clinics of North America*, Elsevier Health Sciences Division, Subscription Customer Service, 3251 Riverport Lane, Maryland Heights, MO 63043. Customer Service (orders, claims, online, change of address): Elsevier Health Sciences Division, Subscription **Customer Service, 3251 Riverport Lane, Maryland Heights, MO 63043. Tel: 1-800-654-2452 (U.S. and Canada); 314-447-8871 (outside U.S. and Canada). Fax: 314-447-8029. E-mail: journalscustomerservice-usa@elsevier.com (for print support); journalsonlinesupport-usa@elsevier.com (for online support).**

Reprints. For copies of 100 or more, of articles in this publication, please contact the Commercial Reprints Department, Elsevier Inc., 360 Park Avenue South, New York, New York 10010-1710; Tel.: 212-633-3874, Fax: 212-633-3820, E-mail: reprints@elsevier.com.

Hematology/Oncology Clinics of North America is covered in *MEDLINE/PubMed (Index Medicus), EMBASE/ Excerpta Medica, and BIOSIS.*

Contributors

CONSULTING EDITORS

GEORGE P. CANELLOS, MD
William Rosenberg Professor of Medicine, Department of Medical Oncology, Dana-Farber
Cancer Institute, Boston, Massachusetts, USA

H. FRANKLIN BUNN, MD
Professor of Medicine, Division of Hematology, Brigham and Women's Hospital, Harvard
Medical School, Boston, Massachusetts, USA

EDITOR

COLIN A. SIEFF, MB,BCh, FRCPath
Associate Professor of Pediatrics, Harvard Medical School, Senior Associate in Medicine,
Dana-Farber and Boston Children's Cancer and Blood Disorders Center, Boston,
Massachusetts, USA

AUTHORS

SUNEET AGARWAL, MD, PhD
Assistant Professor of Pediatrics, Division of Hematology/Oncology, Harvard Medical
School, Staff Physician, Dana-Farber Boston Children's Cancer and Blood Disorders
Center, Boston Children's Hospital, Boston, Massachusetts, USA

ROBERT A. BRODSKY, MD
Professor of Medicine and Oncology, Director, Division of Hematology, The Johns
Hopkins University School of Medicine, Baltimore, Maryland, USA

KATHERINE R. CALVO, MD, PhD
Hematology Section, Department of Laboratory Medicine, Clinical Center, National
Institutes of Health, Bethesda, Maryland, USA

KATHERINE CLESHAM, MD
Hematology Registrar, Department of Pediatric Hematology, Camelia Botnar
Laboratories, UCL Great Ormond Street Hospital, London, United Kingdom

AMY E. DeZERN, MD, MHS
Associate Professor of Oncology and Medicine, Division of Hematologic Malignancies,
The Johns Hopkins University School of Medicine, Baltimore, Maryland, USA

ROBIN DOWSE, MD
Hematology Registrar, Department of Pediatric Hematology, Camelia Botnar
Laboratories, UCL Great Ormond Street Hospital, London, United Kingdom

STEVEN M. HOLLAND, MD
Laboratory of Clinical Immunology and Microbiology, National Institute of Allergy and Infectious Diseases, National Institutes of Health, Bethesda, Maryland, USA

HOJUN LI, MD, PhD
Assistant Professor, Division of Hematology/Oncology, Dana-Farber and Boston Children's Cancer and Blood Disorders Center, Boston, Massachusetts, USA

R. COLEMAN LINDSLEY, MD, PhD
Assistant Professor of Medicine, Department of Medical Oncology, Dana-Farber Cancer Institute, Boston, Massachusetts, USA

HARVEY F. LODISH, PhD
Professor, Whitehead Institute for Biomedical Research, Cambridge, Massachusetts, USA

JUDITH C.W. MARSH, MB ChB, MD
Professor of Clinical Haematology, Department of Haematological Medicine, King's College Hospital, King's College London, London, United Kingdom

LISA J. McREYNOLDS, MD, PhD
Clinical Genetics Branch, Division of Cancer Epidemiology and Genetics, National Cancer Institute, National Institutes of Health, Bethesda, Maryland, USA

GHULAM J. MUFTI, MB BS, DM
Professor of Haemato Oncology, Head of Haematology, Department of Haematological Medicine, King's College Hospital, King's College London, London, United Kingdom

KASIANI C. MYERS, MD
Division of Bone Marrow Transplantation and Immune Deficiency, Cincinnati Children's Hospital Medical Center, Cincinnati, Ohio, USA

DAVID G. NATHAN, MD
President Emeritus, Robert A. Stranahan Distinguished Professor of Pediatrics and Professor of Medicine, Department of Pediatric Oncology, Dana-Farber Cancer Institute, Division of Hematology/Oncology, Boston Children's Hospital, Department of Pediatrics, Harvard Medical School, Boston, Massachusetts, USA

ADAM S. NELSON, MBBS, FRACP
Division of Bone Marrow Transplantation and Immune Deficiency, Cincinnati Children's Hospital Medical Center, Cincinnati, Ohio, USA

CHARLOTTE M. NIEMEYER, MD
Department of Pediatrics and Adolescent Medicine, Division of Pediatric Hematology and Oncology, Medical Center, University of Freiburg, German Cancer Consortium (DKTK), Freiburg, Germany

SUSHREE S. SAHOO, MSc
Department of Pediatrics and Adolescent Medicine, Division of Pediatric Hematology and Oncology, Faculty of Medicine, Medical Center, University of Freiburg, Faculty of Biology, University of Freiburg, Spemann Graduate School of Biology and Medicine, University of Freiburg, Freiburg, Germany

SUJITH SAMARASINGHE, MD, PhD
Consultant Hematologist, Department of Pediatric Hematology, Camelia Botnar Laboratories, UCL Great Ormond Street Hospital, London, United Kingdom

SHARON A. SAVAGE, MD
Chief, Clinical Genetics Branch, Division of Cancer Epidemiology and Genetics, National Cancer Institute, Bethesda, Maryland, USA

EVA J. SCHAEFER, MD
Department of Medical Oncology, Dana-Farber Cancer Institute, Boston, Massachusetts, USA

PHILLIP SCHEINBERG, MD
Head, Division of Hematology, Hospital A Beneficência Portuguesa, São Paulo, Brazil

MICHELLE L. SCHOETTLER, MD
Pediatric Hematology/Oncology/Stem Cell Transplant Fellow, Department of Pediatric Oncology, Dana-Farber Cancer Institute, Division of Hematology/Oncology, Boston Children's Hospital, Department of Pediatrics, Harvard Medical School, Boston, Massachusetts, USA

COLIN A. SIEFF, MB,BCh, FRCPath
Associate Professor of Pediatrics, Harvard Medical School, Senior Associate in Medicine, Dana-Farber and Boston Children's Cancer and Blood Disorders Center, Boston, Massachusetts, USA

MICHAEL F. WALSH, MD
Assistant Member, Departments of Medicine and Pediatrics, Divisions of Solid Tumor and Clinical Cancer Genetics, Memorial Sloan Kettering Cancer Center, New York, New York, USA

MARCIN W. WLODARSKI, MD
Department of Pediatrics and Adolescent Medicine, Division of Pediatric Hematology and Oncology, Faculty of Medicine, Medical Center, University of Freiburg, German Cancer Consortium (DKTK), Freiburg, Germany; Department of Hematology, St. Jude Children's Research Hospital, Memphis, Tennessee, USA

Contents

Acquired aplastic anemia and inherited bone marrow failure syndromes both present with pancytopenia and must be distinguished because they have differences in treatment decisions and continued monitoring requirements. Advances in the genetic interrogation of patient samples have led to the identification of inherited germline diseases and appreciation that patients with inherited bone marrow failure disorders may be normal in appearance with few expected clinical clues. Somatic mutations in aplastic anemia may have prognostic value. Hematopoietic stem cells from inherited marrow failure diseases can correct the proliferative defect and may develop further somatic mutations that progress to myelodysplastic syndrome or acute myeloid leukemia.

Idiopathic acquired aplastic anemia is a rare, life-threatening bone marrow failure syndrome characterized by cytopenias and hypocellular bone marrow. The pathophysiology is unknown; the most favored model is of a dysregulated immune system leading to autoreactive T-cell destruction of hematopoietic stem and progenitor cells in a genetically susceptible host. The authors review the literature and propose that the major driver of acquired aplastic anemia is a combination of hematopoietic stem and progenitor cells intrinsic defects and an inappropriately activated immune response in the setting of a viral infection. Alterations in bone marrow microenvironment may also contribute to the disease process.

Aplastic anemia (AA) is an immune-mediated disorder that overlaps closely with clonal disorders, such as myelodysplastic syndrome and paroxysmal nocturnal hemoglobinuria (PNH). PIGA mutations in PNH clones and functional loss of HLA, including structural HLA mutations, likely represent immune escape clones and correlate with response to immunosuppressive therapy (IST). Somatic mutations typical for myeloid malignancies and age-related clonal hematopoiesis are detected in a proportion of patients with AA, but their significance is unclear and seems to depend on whether patients are tested at diagnosis or after IST, patient age and ethnicity, and the methodology of molecular testing used.

Horse antithymocyte globulin plus cyclosporine remains standard immunosuppressive therapy in severe aplastic anemia, with hematologic response rates of 60% to 70%. In those refractory to this regimen, a second course of therapy with rabbit antithymocyte globulin plus cyclosporine or alemtuzumab produces responses in 30% to 40%. Eltrombopag, a thrombopoietin receptor agonist, showed activity as a single agent in those refractory to initial immunosuppression, with hematologic response rates of 40% to 50%. When combined with immunosuppression as frontline therapy, eltrombopag increased the rate of overall and complete response rates. Longer follow-up is needed to better define these outcomes.

This article summarizes the recent development in the field of front-line unrelated donor transplantation for idiopathic aplastic anemia. The role of unrelated donor transplant in the algorithm of pediatric aplastic anemia is reviewed and incorporates upfront unrelated donor transplant. Newer strategies to delineate which children should receive immune suppression or transplant are also discussed.

Hematopoietic stem cell transplantation (bone marrow transplantation [BMT]) is the only curative treatment of severe aplastic anemia. BMT from a human leukocyte antigen (HLA)-matched sibling donor is the standard of care for young patients; immunosuppressive therapy is used for older patients or those lacking matched sibling donors. Patients with refractory or relapsed disease are increasingly treated with HLA haploidentical BMT. Historically, haploidentical BMT led to high rates of graft rejection and graft-versus-host disease. High-dose posttransplant cyclophosphamide, which mitigates the risk of graft-versus-host disease, is a major advance. This article provides an overview of the haploidentical BMT approach in severe aplastic anemia.

Clonal hematopoiesis as a hallmark of myelodysplastic syndrome (MDS) is mediated by the selective advantage of clonal hematopoietic stem cells in a context-specific manner. Although primary MDS emerges without known predisposing cause and is associated with advanced age, secondary MDS may develop in younger patients with bone marrow failure syndromes or after exposure to chemotherapy. This article discusses recent advances in the understanding of context-dependent clonal hematopoiesis in

MDS, with focus on clonal evolution in inherited and acquired bone marrow failure syndromes.

Fanconi anemia (FA) is a DNA repair disorder associated with a high risk of cancer and bone marrow failure. Patients with FA may present with certain dysmorphic features, such as radial ray abnormalities, short stature, typical facies, bone marrow failure, or certain solid malignancies. Some patients may be recognized owing to exquisite sensitivity after exposure to cancer therapy. FA is diagnosed by increased chromosomal breakage after exposure to clastogenic agents. It follows autosomal recessive and X-linked inheritance depending on the underlying genomic alterations. Recognizing patients with FA is important for therapeutic decisions, genetic counseling, and optimal clinical management.

Dyskeratosis congenita (DC) is a rare, inherited bone marrow failure (BMF) syndrome characterized by variable manifestations and ages of onset and predisposition to cancer. DC is one of a spectrum of diseases caused by mutations in genes regulating telomere maintenance, collectively referred to as telomere biology disorders (TBDs). Hematologic disease is common in children with DC/TBD. Timely diagnosis of underlying TBD in patients with BMF affects treatment and has been facilitated by increased awareness and availability of diagnostic tests in recent years. This article summarizes the pathophysiology, evaluation, and management of hematopoietic failure in patients with DC and other TBDs.

Shwachman-Diamond syndrome (SDS) is an inherited bone marrow failure syndrome classically associated with exocrine pancreatic dysfunction and neutropenia, with a predisposition toward progressive marrow failure, risk of myelodysplastic syndrome, and leukemia. Most patients carry biallelic mutations in the Shwachman-Bodian-Diamond syndrome gene, which is an integral component of ribosome maturation and biogenesis. This article reviews the diagnosis, clinical characteristics, and treatment modalities of SDS and reports advances in the understanding of the molecular pathophysiology of SDS.

Diamond-Blackfan anemia (DBA) is a severe congenital hypoplastic anemia caused by mutation in a ribosomal protein gene. Major clinical issues concern the optimal management of patients resistant to steroids, the first-line therapy. Hematopoietic stem cell transplant is indicated in young patients with an HLA-matched unaffected sibling donor, and recent results with matched unrelated donor transplants indicate that these patients also do well. When neither steroids nor a transplant is possible, red cell transfusions are required, and iron loading is rapid in some patients with DBA, so effective chelation is vital. Also discussed are novel treatments under investigation for DBA.

GATA2 deficiency is an immunodeficiency and bone marrow failure disorder caused by pathogenic variants in *GATA2*. It is inherited in an autosomal-dominant pattern or can be due to de novo sporadic germline mutation. Patients commonly have B-cell, dendritic cell, natural killer cell, and monocytopenias and are predisposed to myelodysplastic syndrome, acute myeloid leukemia, and chronic myelomonocytic leukemia. Patients may suffer from disseminated human papilloma virus and mycobacterial infections, pulmonary alveolar proteinosis, and lymphedema. The bone marrow eventually takes on a characteristic hypocellular myelodysplasia with loss of monocytes and hematogones, megakaryocytes with separated nuclear lobes, micromegakaryocytes, and megakaryocytes with hypolobated nuclei.

Myelodysplastic syndromes (MDS) in children and adolescents are a rare heterogeneous group of clonal stem cell disorders. Complete or partial loss of chromosome 7 constitutes the most common cytogenetic abnormality encountered in any type of childhood MDS, is associated with more advanced disease, and usually requires a timely allogeneic stem cell transplantation. This article provides insights into the current understanding of the genotype, phenotype, and clonal evolution patterns in pediatric MDS associated with the loss of chromosome 7.

HEMATOLOGY/ONCOLOGY CLINICS OF NORTH AMERICA

ISSUE OF RELATED INTEREST

Medical Clinics of North America, March 2017 (Vol. 101, Issue 2)
Anemia
Thomas G. DeLoughery, *Editor*
Available at: http://www.medical.theclinics.com/

THE CLINICS ARE AVAILABLE ONLINE!
Access your subscription at:
www.theclinics.com

Preface

Acquired and Inherited Bone Marrow Failure Syndromes

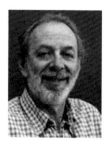

Colin A. Sieff, MB,BCh, FRCPath
Editor

Acquired aplastic anemia (AA) and inherited bone marrow failure syndromes (IBMFS) are rare disorders characterized by the failure of production of mature erythrocytes, leukocytes, and platelets by the bone marrow. Pancytopenia is the usual presentation of acquired AA, while the inherited diseases may predominantly affect one or more lineages and variably evolve into broad hematopoietic failure. AA has usually been considered a consequence of an abnormal immune response to infectious or toxic agents such as drugs or chemicals. In contrast, the IBMFS are due to inherited or de novo mutations in genes that have important cellular housekeeping functions, such as DNA repair (Fanconi anemia), telomere maintenance (dyskeratosis congenita), ribosomal function (Shwachman-Diamond syndrome and Diamond-Blackfan anemia), or transcriptional regulation. Both AA and the IBMFS are characterized by an increased risk of clonal evolution and progression to myelodysplastic syndrome (MDS) and acute myeloid leukemia (AML). The somatic mutations involved in clonal evolution of both AA and IBMFS provide fascinating insights into how immune escape in AA and correction of a proliferative defect in IBMFS can improve hematopoiesis but are not necessarily linked to progression to MDS and acute leukemia.

In recent years, the advances in our ability to interrogate the genome have revealed that there is considerable overlap of AA with the IBMFS; many AA patients likely harbor a genetic susceptibility that may drive a dysregulated immune response. IBMFS were previously thought to affect mainly children, but it has become apparent that low penetrance and variable expressivity result in presentation in adults as well, while novel recently described genetic mutations such as MECOM (MDS1 and EVI1 complex locus) can lead to profound aplasia in young children. These advances emphasize the importance of accurate diagnosis at first presentation, since the management of acquired AA and the IBMFS are very different. IBMFS often involve congenital defects and extrahematopoietic manifestations that require an interdisciplinary approach

Hematol Oncol Clin N Am 32 (2018) xiii–xiv
https://doi.org/10.1016/j.hoc.2018.05.001
0889-8588/18/© 2018 Published by Elsevier Inc.

hemonc.theclinics.com

to management to provide guidance for anticipated complications, genetic counseling for families, as well as avoidance of treatment-related toxicity.

In the following articles, we discuss the pathogenesis and advances in the optimal medical management as well as different hematopoietic stem cell transplant approaches to management. The pathogenesis and management of the major classical IBMFS are discussed along with newer syndromes such as germline GATA2 mutations and novel insights into the role of monosomy 7 in pediatric MDS/AML. Study of this rare but fascinating group of diseases continues to provide important insights into the biology of not only marrow failure but also steps in the progression to malignancy.

Colin A. Sieff, MB,BCh, FRCPath
Harvard Medical School
Dana-Farber and Boston Children's
Cancer and Blood Disorders Center, D3104
450 Brookline Avenue
Boston, MA 02215, USA

E-mail address:
colin.sieff@childrens.harvard.edu

Dedication

The publishers and authors of this issue of *Hematology/Oncology Clinics of North America* wish to express our collective gratitude to our editor, Dr. Colin A. Sieff. Despite perilous distractions he has conceived, organized, edited and shepherded all of our efforts into an issue of which we can be very proud. We all wish the Sieff family good health and well-deserved happiness.

Hematol Oncol Clin N Am 32 (2018) xv
https://doi.org/10.1016/j.hoc.2018.05.002
0889-8588/18/© 2018 Published by Elsevier Inc.

hemonc.theclinics.com

Introduction to Acquired and Inherited Bone Marrow Failure

Colin A. Sieff, MB,BCh, FRCPath

KEYWORDS

- Aplastic anemia • Inherited bone marrow failure • Germline mutations
- Somatic mutations

KEY POINTS

- Acquired aplastic anemia and inherited bone marrow failure syndromes both can present with pancytopenia and must be distinguished at presentation because they have important differences with respect to critical treatment decisions as well as specific continued monitoring requirements.
- The rapid recent advances in the genetic interrogation of patient samples have led to the identification of new inherited germline diseases and the appreciation that patients with classic inherited bone marrow failure disorders may be normal in appearance with few if any of the expected clinical clues.
- Somatic mutations in aplastic anemia may have prognostic value although there is considerable variation at the individual level.
- Hematopoietic stem cells from several inherited marrow failure diseases can correct the proliferative defect and may then still develop further somatic mutations that can progress to myelodysplastic syndrome or acute myeloid leukemia.

INTRODUCTION

Bone marrow failure (BMF) disorders are characterized by presentation with pancytopenia or single-lineage cytopenias. Although acquired aplastic anemia (AA) is the most common BMF disease at all ages, children and adults may have an inherited BMF (IBMF) disease that must be diagnosed if present, because this is critically important not only for treatment choices but also to monitor for progression to myelodysplastic syndrome (MDS) or acute myeloid leukemia (AML). MDS and AML occur with increased frequency through acquisition of somatic mutations in medically treated patients with acquired AA but have a much greater likelihood in patients with germline

Disclosure Statement: No disclosures to report.
Division of Hematology/Oncology, Dana-Farber and Boston Children's Cancer and Blood Disorders Center, Dana 3104, 450 Brookline Avenue, Boston, MA 02215, USA
E-mail address: Colin.Sieff@childrens.harvard.edu

Hematol Oncol Clin N Am 32 (2018) 569–580
https://doi.org/10.1016/j.hoc.2018.04.008
0889-8588/18/© 2018 Elsevier Inc. All rights reserved.

hemonc.theclinics.com

IBMF.[1] Many of the germline mutations diagnostic of IBMF set the stage for additional somatic mutations and cytogenetic changes that account for this increased risk. In this article and other articles in this issue, acquired AA and IBMF are discussed with respect to management challenges and to the recent exciting wealth of genetic information that has accrued with the advances in the ability to interrogate the genome by next-generation techniques in the clinic, at an ever-declining cost.

ACQUIRED APLASTIC ANEMIA

AA is the most frequent cause of pancytopenia at all ages but still rare, with an annual incidence of 2 cases per million in developed countries to 4 cases per million to 7 cases per million in Asia. There are 2 age peaks, 15 to 25 years and greater than 60 years,[2] which may suggest differences in etiology between these 2 groups, because germline IBMF syndromes are more frequently diagnosed in younger patients. AA is usually idiopathic but sometimes secondary to infection (eg, hepatitis and Epstein-Barr virus), drugs (chloramphenicol and others), or toxins (benzene, insecticides). Although acquired AA usually occurs in normal children and adults with no previous history of growth failure or congenital abnormalities that suggest an IBMF syndrome, recent genetic studies have shown that IBMF disorders can present without any of these telling clinical clues and, therefore, must be excluded. As might be expected, AA that occurs in infants and young children is more likely due germline mutations.[3,4]

Pathophysiology

Although the pathophysiology of AA is unknown, several lines of evidence support a role for the immune system (see Schoettler and Nathan's article, "The Pathophysiology of Acquired Aplastic Anemia: Current Concepts Revisited," in this issue). Evidence supporting this mechanism comes from identical twin transplants, two-thirds of whom require immunosuppressive pretransplant conditioning for sustained engraftment. These data could also indicate, however, an underlying stem cell defect, because a significant proportion of twin transplants require no conditioning, suggesting that replacement of stem cells is sufficient to cure the disease. Other lines of evidence for an immune mechanism include the greater likelihood of developing AA in individuals with certain HLA alleles and the body of evidence that demonstrates an activated immune system (see Schoettler and Nathan's article, "The Pathophysiology of Acquired Aplastic Anemia: Current Concepts Revisited," and Mufti and Marsh's article, "Somatic Mutations in Aplastic Anemia," in this issue). Immunological evidence includes the oft-cited data of response to treatment with antithymocyte globulin (ATG) and cyclosporine (CsA), but it should borne in mind that the mechanism by which these medications work is unknown. The observation that AA patients with short telomeres respond as well to treatment with ATG and CsA as patients with normal-length telomeres emphasizes that how precisely these agents work is still unknown; ATG has stimulatory (low-concentration) as well as inhibitory (high-concentration) effects on colony formation of $CD34^+$ bone marrow cells from normal, AA, and MDS individuals,[5,6] which raises questions about the conclusion that their use supports an immunosuppressive mechanism of action. Furthermore, more intense and specific immunosuppression, such as rabbit ATG and alemtuzumab, does not improve the results. In addition, one of the hallmarks of autoimmune disease is the identification of self-antigens to which the immune attack is directed, and such an antigen expressed on hematopoietic stem cells (HSCs) has never been identified.

The presence of a dysregulated activated immune system is important to the pathophysiology of acquired AA, and the finding of HLA loss of heterozygosity (6pLOH) is a convincing indication of how somatic mutations might lead to the escape of AA HSCs from immune attack.[7] Specifically, a recent study of 312 Japanese 6pLOH patients revealed *HLA-B*40:02* as one of the most frequent lost alleles.[8] Furthermore, using a monoclonal antibody to the B4002 allele in 28 patients, B4002-granulocytes were present not only all 12 6pLOH-positive patients but also in 9 of 16 6pLOH-negative patients due to mutations in *HLA-B*40:02*. This is consistent with HLA loss allowing the escape of HSCs that present an antigen to cytotoxic T cells in the context of B4002. Clonal escape has also been postulated as a mechanism for the increased incidence and survival of paroxysmal nocturnal hemoglobinuria (PNH) clones in AA. The *PIGA* gene is required for the synthesis of the glycosylphosphatidylinositol (GPI) anchor of proteins, such as CD55 and CD59, whose absence confers the increase in complement sensitivity and hemolysis characteristic of PNH. Approximately 50% of AA patients have GPI-negative cells at diagnosis, suggesting the hypothesis that a dysregulated immune system recognizes an antigen expressed on GPI itself. A recent report showed that 13 of 17 AA patients have T cells that bind to synthetic GPI dimers loaded onto CD1d, a nonpolymorphic HLA antigen expressed on a subset of CD34$^+$ cells.[9] This increase in binding was comparable to PNH cells and significantly greater than in normal controls.

Although these data support a role of a dysregulated immune system, the recent discovery of somatic mutations in AA and new germline mutations suggests that mutations in HSCs may underlie the dysregulated immune response (**Fig. 1**). Perhaps these mutant cells also instigate an aberrant immune response in AA, which, in an attempt to rid the body of these malcontents, eliminates normal stem cells as well.

Clonal Hematopoiesis of Indeterminate Potential

HSCs, through random aging-associated mutations, may acquire a proliferative advantage by clonal dominance of their progeny. Clonal hematopoiesis of indeterminate potential (CHIP) occurs in 10% of 70-year-old to 79-year-old and 20% of greater than 90-year-old normal individuals that confers an increased but low risk of progression to MDS and AML (0.5%–1.0% per year) and is also associated with an increased all-cause mortality due to cardiovascular disease.[10]

Somatic Mutations

It has long been known that AA patients who are in remission after ATG and CsA have an approximately 15% risk of clonal progression to MDS or AML. Several studies have now shown that clonality is due to acquisition of somatic mutations in surviving stem cells and that the genes involved have differing impacts on progression to MDS or AML.[11,12] As discussed in detail by Drs. Mufti and Marsh's article, "Somatic Mutations in Aplastic Anemia," in this issue, somatic mutations in ASXLI, DNMT3A, BCOR/BCORL1, and PIGA are the most frequently reported affected genes in several large AA studies, with a reported incidence of one-fifth to one-third of AA patients. ASXL1 and DNMT3A along with TP53, RUNX1, CSMD1, and NOTCH1 are unfavorable mutations associated with worse overall survival and response after treatment with ATG/CsA, increasing clone size, and increased risk of progression to MDS or AML. In contrast, BCOR/BCORL1 and PIGA mutations are not observed in CHIP, may decline in expression over time, and do not confer an increased risk of MDS and AML. Mutations in these genes have to be evaluated in the context of CHIP. In addition to the increasing incidence with age, there may also be ethnic differences in the genes affected and the influence of telomere attrition in approximately 30% of patients in the absence of

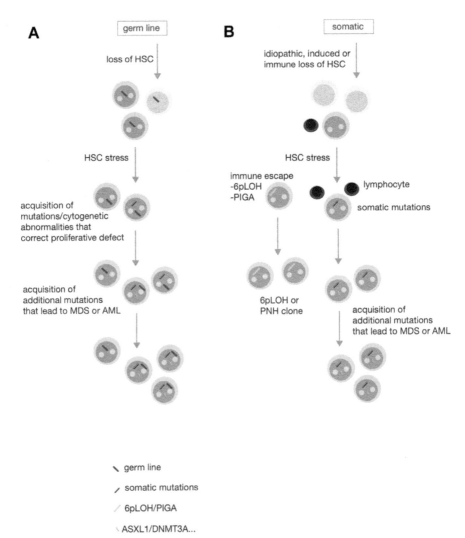

Fig. 1. (*A*) Germline: mutations of IBMF diseases lead to stem cell failure and stress in surviving HSC. These cells can acquire cytogenetic changes or mutations that partially correct the proliferative defect (eg, somatic reversion in FA or isochromosome 7 in SDS.) Further mutations, however, can inactivate these pathways and lead to MDS/AML. (*B*) Somatic: HSCs lost through toxic damage, immune dysregulation, or possibly a mutation that incites an immune response. Stress in surviving stem cells may select for somatic mutations that improve growth, and additional mutations result in MDS or AML.

genetic mutations that are diagnostic of a telomeropathy. What is needed are detailed studies of evolving clonal architecture before and at intervals after treatment with ATG/CsA.

Treatment

Without treatment, the prognosis for patients with severe AA is poor, with only approximately 10% survival at a year after diagnosis. Advances in immunosuppressive treatment with horse ATG and CsA as well as improvements in supportive care have led to a markedly better outlook with many long-term survivors, and Dr. Scheinberg discusses in his article on "Recent Advances and Long-Term Results of Medical Treatment of Acquired Aplastic Anemia: Are Patients Cured?," in this issue, whether patients who have survived 15 years can be considered cured. Also discussed are the recent studies that have shown an improvement in response rates when the thrombopoietin mimetic eltrombopag is started early with ATG and CsA.[13,14]

HSC transplantation (HSCT) is the only definitive curative treatment of AA, and, after IBMF syndromes have been excluded (**Fig. 2**), most centers offer HSCT at diagnosis for children and young adults who have an HLA-matched sibling donor, with approximately 90% long-term survival and cure. Patients without a matched sibling donor and older individuals usually receive ATG and CsA. Although overall survival is excellent, disease-free survival is not as good and patients may relapse or acquire somatic mutations that increase the risk of progression to MDS or AML. In recent years the results of matched unrelated donor (MUD) transplants have markedly improved in patients who do not respond to or relapse after ATG/CsA. These patients have a longer red cell and platelet transfusion history than those treated immediately after diagnosis with possible HLA sensitization and hemosiderosis and/or infections, all factors that adversely affect prognosis after HSCT. The major unanswered question now is whether even better results might be obtained if MUD transplants are carried out at diagnosis, before a significant number of transfusions or infection. In the article on "Upfront Matched Unrelated Donor Transplantation in Aplastic Anaemia," in this issue, Drs. Clesham, Dowse, and Samarasinghe discuss MUD transplantation in detail and reported excellent results in a retrospective report of MUD transplants,[15] due to improved donor selection with high-resolution typing, advances in supportive care, and improved conditioning regimens. A US-wide prospective randomized study to address this question in children is under way (TransIT, clinicaltrials.gov NCT02845596).

Are there other transplant approaches in patients who do not have matched related or unrelated donors? Haploidentical transplantation has the advantage that many more patients have parent or sibling donors, and Drs. DeZern and Brodsky discuss, in their article on "Haploidentical Donor Bone Marrow Transplantation for Severe Aplastic Anemia," in this issue, the exciting results they have obtained using high-dose cyclophosphamide post-transplantation to prevent graft-versus-host disease. Together with cord blood as a stem cell source, the options for transplantation are expanding.

INHERITED BONE MARROW FAILURE SYNDROMES
Classic

In children, it has long been recognized that although acquired AA is still the most common cause of BMF, germline inheritance of mutations that cause classic IBMF syndromes have to be excluded in all new patients (see **Fig. 2**). Fanconi anemia (FA), dyskeratosis congenita (DC), Shwachman-Diamond syndrome (SDS), and amegakaryocytic thrombocytopenia can present with growth retardation, congenital abnormalities, or cytopenias at birth but often show evidence of BMF only as older children or adults. The clinical presentation and diagnostic criteria for the classic IBMF syndromes are summarized in **Table 1**, with features that should alert physicians to possibility of an inherited syndrome. IBMF should be suspected in any child with poor growth, a telling feature of many conditions. In addition, congenital malformations, presentation of cytopenia at a young age, and/or a family history of other affected individuals are important clues to their diagnosis.

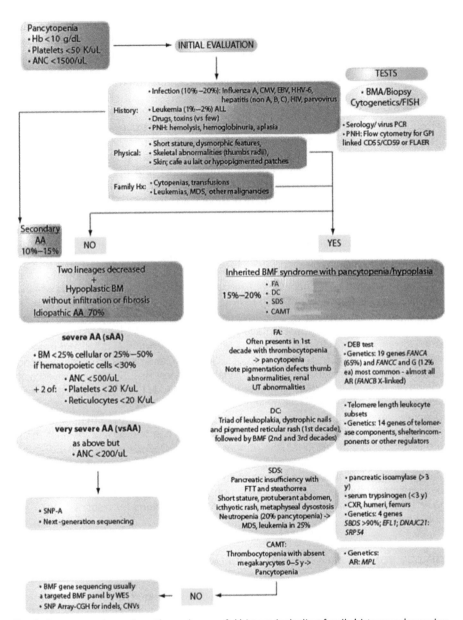

Fig. 2. Pancytopenia work-up through a careful history, including family history and examination for growth and congenital anomalies. This leads to further testing, including bone marrow aspiration, biopsy, and cytogenetics/fluorescence in situ hybridization, as well as the indicated test to exclude inherited disorders. It is now part of the work-up to include sequencing of blood and skin fibroblasts, which can easily be obtained at the time of the bone marrow.

FA patients are at high risk of BMF, MDS, leukemia, head and neck squamous cell carcinoma, and other malignancies. Careful monitoring is required (see Savage and Walsh's article, "Myelodysplastic Syndrome, Acute Myeloid Leukemia, and Cancer Surveillance in Fanconi Anemia," in this issue). DC is associated with a spectrum of

Table 1
Inherited bone marrow failure syndromes

Disorder	Major Physical Features	Hematology	Laboratory Tests
FA	Short stature, skin hyperpigmentation/ hypopigmentation; limb or hand, skeletal, facial dysmorphologies; renal, gonadal, neurocognitive/ central nervous system, cardiopulmonary, gastrointestinal anomalies	Thrombocytopenia in first decade, progressing later to pancytopenia	Chromosomal breakage or cell-cycle arrest induced by mitomycin C or diepoxybutane
DC or telomere biology disorders	Nail dystrophy; lacey or reticular skin pigmentation; oral leukoplakia; liver cirrhosis; short stature; pulmonary fibrosis; vascular anomalies; hyperhidrosis; and ophthalmologic, hair (early graying, early hair loss) dental, central nervous system, gastrointestinal, facial cardiac, genitourinary anomalies	Cytopenia of 1 or more lineages; thrombocytopenia with macrocytic anemia progressing to pancytopenia	Telomere lengths less than first percentile
Shwachman-Diamond syndrome	Steatorrhea, thoracic dysplasias, Jeune syndrome, metaphyseal dysostosis, short stature	Neutropenia in majority, intermittent in 2/3 or chronic in 1/3; anemia and/or thrombocytopenia in 1/2	Low serum trypsinogen (age <3 y), low serum pancreatic isoamylase (age >3 y)
Amegakaryocytic thrombocytopenia	May be present but nonspecific	Thrombocytopenia at birth or later and moderate or transient. Progression to severe AA	BM shows paucity or absence of megakaryocytes; MPL mutations
Diamond-Blackfan anemia	Thumb anomalies, short stature, cleft lip or palate, Pierre Robin syndrome, facial dysmorphologies, and cardiac and genitourinary anomalies	Severe hypoplastic anemia during first few months of life; hydrops fetalis and later presentations occur	BM erythroid hypoplasia; elevated erythrocyte adenosine deaminase

clinical presentations that are frequently underappreciated, leading to missed diagnoses, and Dr. Agarwal discusses, in the article on "Evaluation and Management of Hematopoietic Failure in Dyskeratosis Congenital," in this issue, clinical phenotypes along with diagnosis, genetics and management of hematopoietic failure. SDS is discussed by Drs. Nelson and Myers in the article on "Diagnosis, Treatment and Molecular Pathology of Shwachman-Diamond Syndrome," in this issue; they review the broad clinical features and diagnosis, including new SDS genes that account for patients who do not have SBDS mutations, as well as clinical management and pathogenesis of BMF.

New Inherited Bone Marrow Failure Syndromes

With respect to IBMF syndromes, next-generation whole-exome sequencing of germline tissue, such as skin fibroblasts in pancytopenic patients, has led to the identification of several novel genes that are characterized by distinct clinical phenotypes (**Table 2**). In addition, it has become clear that patients with classic IBMFs may not present with the expected clinical phenotype.

HSCs are at a proliferative disadvantage in individuals with IBMF diseases and can acquire mutations specific to each disease that for a time improve or correct proliferation in the impaired cells; frequently, however, further somatic mutations or cytogenetic abnormalities are acquired that lead to MDS and or AML (see **Fig. 1**).

The spectrum of cytogenetic or clonal mutations in IBMF diseases is discussed in detail by Drs. Schaefer and Lindsley in the article on "Significance of Clonal Mutations in Bone Marrow Failure and Inherited Myelodysplastic Syndrome/Acute Myeloid Predisposition Syndromes," in this issue, for example

- In SDS, an isochromosome 7 always affects the functional rather than the null allele in this autosomally inherited condition and increases expression of the SBDS-encoded protein.
- In SDS and Diamond Blackfan anemia, ribosomal stress leads to p53 stabilization and cell-cycle arrest or apoptosis. TP53 mutations allow escape from apoptosis in mutant cells and may improve function, although this mutation increases the risk of leukemia.
- Monosomy 7 in patients with acquired AA or IBMF has always raised alarms of disease progression to leukemia and been a strong indication for HSCT in individuals with GATA2 or RUNX1 mutations. The context, however, may be important. For example, patients with SAMD9 or SMAD9L mutations, which are on chromosome 7q21, frequently develop monosomy 7 that can be transiently correct the defect (discussed later). The complexity of monosomy 7 or deletions of 7q are discussed by Drs. Wlodarski, Sahoo, and Niemeyer in the article on "Monosomy 7 In Pediatric Myelodysplastic Syndromes," in this issue.

The recent rapid advances in the genetic interrogation of clinical material by next-generation sequencing has led to novel insights into the role of germline and somatic mutations in patients who present with acquired AA. The finding of short telomeres in a small proportion of AA patients led to the discovery of mutations in the telomerase complex genes TERT, TERC, DKC1, RTEL, and TINF2.[16,17]

Next-generation sequencing and conventional genetic sequencing have recently brought to light new germline mutations showing that defective HSCs may underlie more acquired AA cases than previously suspected. In some instances, these mutations lead to HSC loss, whereas in others aberrant HSCs could induce an immune response that might eliminate them (see **Table 2**). These rare BMF disorders often have a broad range of clinical manifestations that make diagnosis difficult:

Table 2
Other gene mutations associated with bone marrow failure and myelodysplastic syndrome/acute myeloid leukemia

Disorder	Major Physical Features	Hematology	Laboratory	References
GATA2 • AD	Warts, atypical mycobacterial infections, lymphedema, deafness, pulmonary alveolar proteinosis	AA, MDS, or AML BM with dysplastic megakaryocytes with monocyte and hematogone loss	Low B cells, T cells, and natural killer cells; low immunoglobulin levels	Hsu et al,[22] 2011; Kazenwadel et al,[23] 2012
MECOM/EVI1 • AD	Radioulnar synostosis, other skeletal and cardiac abnormalities	Amegakaryocytic thrombocytopenia Severe neonatal AA without dysplasia		Germeshausenet al,[19] 2018
HOXA11	Radioulnar synostosis and thrombocytopenia	Amegakaryocytic thrombocytopenia		Thompson and Nguyen,[21] 2000
SAMD9 • AD	MIRAGE = MDS, infection, restriction of growth, adrenal hypoplasia, genital, enteropathy	Severe BMF Some patients improve through somatic genetic correction.	Monosomy 7 common, low Igs	Narumi et al,[24] 2016
SAMD9L	Ataxia-pancytopenia syndrome	Improvement in some		Chen et al,[4] 2016
ERCC6L2 • AR	Neurologic learning problems, developmental delay, intracranial vascular abnormality	BMF ± dysplasia with monosomy 7		Tummala et al,[25] 2014
RUNX1	Familial platelet disorder/AML	Thrombocytopenia		Song et al,[26] 1999; Keel et al,[27] 2016
SRP72 • AD	2 unrelated pedigrees with familial AA/MDS	Pancytopenia		Kirwan et al,[28] 2012

Abbreviations: AD, autosomal dominant; AR, autosomal recessive; Igs, immunoglobulins.

- GATA2 haploinsufficiency can lead to a broad spectrum of clinical presentations, including BMF, immunodeficiency, and lymphatic manifestations, often with a high risk of MDS and AML (discussed in detail by Drs Lisa J. McReynolds and colleagues' article, "Germline *GATA2* Mutation and Bone Marrow Failure," in this issue).
- Mutations in *MECOM* (MDS1 and EVI1 complex) account for patients with radio-ulnar synostosis (congenital fusion of the radius and ulna) who can also present with hematological features that include amegakaryocytic thrombocytopenia that progresses to pancytopenia and severe BMF.[18–20] Radioulnar synostosis with amegakaryocytic thrombocytopenia may also be due to mutations in *HOXA11*,[21] again with variable presentation. Fathers of both index cases had normal platelet counts.
- *SAMD9*, located at 7q21.2. Gain-of-function mutations in this tumor suppressor act as a growth restriction protein and manifest as the MIRAGE syndrome (see **Table 1**) or a more subtle mild BMF phenotype. Monosomy 7 or deletions of 7q can lead to MDS. Alternatively, in some patients somatic reversion events such as loss of the monosomy 7 or 7q- clone by uniparental disomy (UPD), or additional in cis *SAMD9* mutations can result in improvement in hematopoiesis through genetic correction.
- *SAMD9L* mutation can present as thrombocytopenia and a hypocellular bone marrow (BM) with features of MDS. Similar genetic correction events were observed that led to improved hematopiesis and prolonged survival.[3]

In conclusion, the reviews in this issue cover a broad-spectrum BMF disorders, with focus on the important aspects of diagnosis, pathophysiology, and clinical management. The wealth of recent molecular data in patients with acquired and IBMF show that there is an area of overlap that must be defined carefully to select the most appropriate treatment.

REFERENCES

1. Shimamura A. Aplastic anemia and clonal evolution: germ line and somatic genetics. Hematology Am Soc Hematol Educ Program 2016;2016(1):74–82.
2. Shimamura A, Nathan DG. Acquired aplastic anemia and pure red cell aplasia. In: Orkin SO, Nathan DG, Ginsburg D, et al, editors. Hematology of infancy and childhood, vol. 1, 7th edition. Philadelphia: Saunders Elsevier; 2009. p. 276–305.
3. Bluteau O, Sebert M, Leblanc T, et al. A landscape of germ line mutations in a cohort of inherited bone marrow failure patients. Blood 2018;131(7):717–32.
4. Chen D-H, Below JE, Shimamura A, et al. Ataxia-pancytopenia syndrome is caused by missense mutations in SAMD9L. Am J Hum Genet 2016;98(6):1146–58.
5. Killick SB, Marsh JC, Gordon-Smith EC, et al. Effects of antithymocyte globulin on bone marrow CD34+ cells in aplastic anaemia and myelodysplasia. Br J Haematol 2000;108(3):582–91.
6. Chen G, Kook H, Zeng W, et al. Is there a direct effect of antithymocyte globulin on hematopoiesis? Hematol J 2004;5(3):255–61.
7. Katagiri T, Sato-Otsubo A, Kashiwase K, et al. Frequent loss of HLA alleles associated with copy number-neutral 6pLOH in acquired aplastic anemia. Blood 2011;118(25):6601–9.
8. Zaimoku Y, Takamatsu H, Hosomichi K, et al. Identification of an HLA class I allele closely involved in the autoantigen presentation in acquired aplastic anemia. Blood 2017;129(21):2908–16.

9. Gargiulo L, Zaimoku Y, Scappini B, et al. Glycosylphosphatidylinositol-specific T cells, IFN-γ-producing T cells, and pathogenesis of idiopathic aplastic anemia. Blood 2017;129(3):388–92.

10. Jan M, Ebert BL, Jaiswal S. Clonal hematopoiesis. Semin Hematol 2017;54(1): 43–50.

11. Kulasekararaj AG, Jiang J, Smith AE, et al. Somatic mutations identify a subgroup of aplastic anemia patients who progress to myelodysplastic syndrome. Blood 2014;124(17):2698–704.

12. Yoshizato T, Dumitriu B, Hosokawa K, et al. Somatic mutations and clonal hematopoiesis in aplastic anemia. N Engl J Med 2015;373(1):35–47.

13. Townsley DM, Scheinberg P, Winkler T, et al. Eltrombopag added to standard immunosuppression for aplastic anemia. N Engl J Med 2017;376(16):1540–50.

14. Desmond R, Townsley DM, Dumitriu B, et al. Eltrombopag restores trilineage hematopoiesis in refractory severe aplastic anemia that can be sustained on discontinuation of drug. Blood 2014;123(12):1818–25.

15. Dufour C, Veys P, Carraro E, et al. Similar outcome of upfront-unrelated and matched sibling stem cell transplantation in idiopathic paediatric aplastic anaemia. A study on behalf of the UK Paediatric BMT working party, paediatric diseases working party and severe aplastic anaemia working party of EBMT. Br J Haematol 2015;171(4):585–94.

16. Yamaguchi H, Calado RT, Ly H, et al. Mutations in TERT, the gene for telomerase reverse transcriptase, in aplastic anemia. N Engl J Med 2005;352(14):1413–24.

17. Yamaguchi H, Baerlocher GM, Lansdorp PM, et al. Mutations of the human telomerase RNA gene (TERC) in aplastic anemia and myelodysplastic syndrome. Blood 2003;102(3):916–8.

18. Niihori T, Ouchi-Uchiyama M, Sasahara Y, et al. Mutations in MECOM, encoding oncoprotein EVI1, cause radioulnar synostosis with amegakaryocytic thrombocytopenia. Am J Hum Genet 2015;97(6):848–54.

19. Germeshausen M, Ancliff P, Estrada J, et al. MECOM-associated syndrome: a heterogeneous inherited bone marrow failure syndrome with amegakaryocytic thrombocytopenia. Blood Adv 2018;2(6):586–96.

20. Walne A, Tummala H, Ellison A, et al. Expanding the phenotypic and genetic spectrum of radioulnar synostosis associated hematological disease. Haematologica 2018. [Epub ahead of print].

21. Thompson AA, Nguyen LT. Amegakaryocytic thrombocytopenia and radio-ulnar synostosis are associated with HOXA11 mutation. Nat Genet 2000;26(4):397–8.

22. Hsu AP, Sampaio EP, Khan J, et al. Mutations in GATA2 are associated with the autosomal dominant and sporadic monocytopenia and mycobacterial infection (MonoMAC) syndrome. Blood 2011;118(10):2653–5.

23. Kazenwadel J, Secker GA, Liu YJ, et al. Loss-of-function germline GATA2 mutations in patients with MDS/AML or MonoMAC syndrome and primary lymphedema reveal a key role for GATA2 in the lymphatic vasculature. Blood 2012; 119(5):1283–91.

24. Narumi S, Amano N, Ishii T, et al. SAMD9 mutations cause a novel multisystem disorder, MIRAGE syndrome, and are associated with loss of chromosome 7. Nat Genet 2016;48(7):792–7.

25. Tummala H, Kirwan M, Walne AJ, et al. ERCC6L2 mutations link a distinct bone-marrow-failure syndrome to DNA repair and mitochondrial function. Am J Hum Genet 2014;94(2):246–56.

26. Song WJ, Sullivan MG, Legare RD, et al. Haploinsufficiency of CBFA2 causes familial thrombocytopenia with propensity to develop acute myelogenous leukaemia. Nat Genet 1999;23(2):166–75.
27. Keel SBB, Scott A, Sanchez-Bonilla M, et al. Genetic features of myelodysplastic syndrome and aplastic anemia in pediatric and young adult patients. Haematologica 2016;101(11):1343–50.
28. Kirwan M, Walne AJ, Plagnol V, et al. Exome sequencing identifies autosomal-dominant SRP72 mutations associated with familial aplasia and myelodysplasia. Am J Hum Genet 2012;90(5):888–92.

The Pathophysiology of Acquired Aplastic Anemia
Current Concepts Revisited

Michelle L. Schoettler, MD[a,b,c], David G. Nathan, MD[a,b,c],*

KEYWORDS

- Acquired aplastic anemia • Pathophysiology • PNH • Clonal hematopoiesis
- Immune suppressive therapy

KEY POINTS

- The pathophysiology of acquired aplastic anemia is unknown. The leading hypothesis is cytotoxic T-cell destruction of hematopoietic stem cells, but no inciting autoantigen has been identified.
- The most striking evidence supporting the role of auto-reactive T cells in acquired aplastic anemia is the presence of leukocytes with acquired copy number neutral loss of heterozygosity (6pLOH).
- Clonal hematopoiesis is common in acquired aplastic anemia. The most frequent somatic mutations are *BCOR/BCOR1*, *PIG-A*, and 6pLOH.
- That hematopoietic stem cells have other non–immune-related genetic defects is further evidenced by shortened telomeres in leukocytes and germline mutations in patients with acquired aplastic anemia.
- Although equine ATG, cyclosporine, and eltrombopag have improved acquired aplastic anemia clinical outcomes, we do not understand their mechanisms.

INTRODUCTION

Idiopathic acquired aplastic anemia (aAA) is a rare, life-threatening bone marrow failure syndrome characterized by cytopenias and a hypocellular bone marrow. Aplastic anemia (AA) is classified as either inherited or acquired. Inherited bone marrow failure syndromes (IBMFS) are rare genetic diseases that are well-characterized clinically and usually associated with an identified germline mutation. They typically present in childhood, although they can be diagnosed later in life and are associated with an

Disclosure Statement: No disclosures from either author.
[a] Department of Pediatric Oncology, Dana-Farber Cancer Institute, 450 Brookline Avenue, Boston, MA 02215-5450, USA; [b] Division of Hematology/Oncology, Boston Children's Hospital, 450 Brookline Avenue, Boston, MA 02215, USA; [c] Department of Pediatrics, Harvard Medical School, 450 Brookline Avenue, Boston, MA 02215, USA
* Corresponding author. 450 Brookline Avenue, Boston, MA 02215-5450.
E-mail address: David_Nathan@dfci.harvard.edu

Hematol Oncol Clin N Am 32 (2018) 581–594
https://doi.org/10.1016/j.hoc.2018.03.001
0889-8588/18/© 2018 Elsevier Inc. All rights reserved.

increased risk of developing malignancy. AA is considered acquired (aAA) if no inherited syndrome is identified. The incidence of aAA is low, ranging from 2 to 14 per million per year, with higher incidences reported in Asia than Europe.[1–3] There is a bimodal age of peak presentation, with the first occurring in patients aged 15 to 25 years and the second in patients over 60 years old.[4] The prognosis for severe or very severe aAA with supportive care only is dismal, with mortality rates exceeding 80% at 2 years.[5] Overall survival rates at 2 years after treatment with immune suppressive therapy (IST) with cyclosporine and antithymocyte globulin (ATG) are typically greater than 80%.[6,7] However, event-free survival, with events defined as death or requirement for a subsequent therapy, decreases over time and is as low as 58% at 60 months in a recent pediatric study.[8]

The pathophysiology of aAA is unknown, although the most favored model is that of a dysregulated immune system leading to autoreactive T-cell destruction of hematopoietic stem and progenitor cells (HSPC) in a genetically susceptible host. In addition to the immune component, HSPC intrinsic defects and bone marrow microenvironment dysfunction are thought to contribute to the disease process. Herein we summarize the current concepts regarding the pathophysiology of aAA and propose that destruction of HSPCs by a combination of intrinsic HSPC genetic defects and an inappropriately activated immune response, perhaps to a viral infection to viral infection is the major driver of aAA.

DYSREGULATED IMMUNE SYSTEM

An immunologic mechanism in aAA was suspected when lymphocyte infusions in mice resulted in a hypocellular bone marrow.[9] It was further supported in humans when identical twin bone marrow transplantation without conditioning was initially unsuccessful in 15 of 23 patients, but hematopoiesis was restored with conditioning and repeat transplantation.[10] And finally, this model is largely accepted given favorable responses to IST with equine ATG and cyclosporine, 2 entirely nonspecific agents.[11]

Destruction or dysfunction of HSPC by activated cytotoxic T cells in the setting of infection, drug, or another unidentified environmental trigger is thought to occur via recognition of an autoantigen(s) presented via class I or II HLA molecules.[11] However, there is no definitive evidence of this mechanism because an inciting autoantigen has not been identified. Furthermore, there have been very few demonstrations of HSPC specific in vivo cytotoxic T-cell repertoires. There are many studies delineating immunologic changes seen at diagnosis and during treatment. It is unclear if these immunologic changes result in the disease process of aAA, or are secondary to other concurrent, unidentified processes such as a preceding hepatitis, Epstein-Barr virus, or another viral infection.

T Cells

A number of studies have demonstrated increased percentages of activated CD8[+] cytotoxic T cells in patients with aAA in both peripheral blood and bone marrow.[8–10] In vitro coculture of CD8[+] T cells from untreated patients with AA enhances apoptosis of CD3[-]bone marrow cells from normal individuals[12] and inhibits colony formation of CD34[+] cells.[13] Putative HSPC death from T cells expanded in vivo has been demonstrated in 2 patients. In 1 patient, CD8[+] cells induced cell death in 75% of autologous bone marrow mononuclear cells,[14] and in the second patient, a CD4[+] T-cell clone demonstrated cytotoxicity against autologous CD34[+] cells in an HLA-DRB1 restricted manner.[13]

Abnormalities in the number and/or function of all types of CD4[+] cells are reported, with increased T helper (Th)1 and Th2 cells, and decreased T regulatory (Treg) cells.[15]

Treg cells play an important role in suppressing autoreactive T cells, and are thus believed to influence autoimmune diseases. Treg cells present in aAA are functionally impaired and unable to suppress normal effector T cells.[15,16] A decrease in the number of Treg cells in aAA correlates with disease severity, and conversely increased numbers of Treg cells predict better response to IST.[15,17] Because Treg depletion and dysfunction are regularly observed after viral infections[18] and in our experience, viral infection often precedes aAA, the Treg findings in aAA are of unclear pathophysiological significance. However, in general Treg cells tend to be depressed in autoimmunity.

A subset of patients with aAA at diagnosis have restricted CD8+ and CD4+ cytotoxic cell receptor diversity, that is, oligoclonal expansion identified by flow cytometry analysis for T-cell receptor subfamilies.[14,19–21] The presence and degree of oligoclonal T-cell expansion predicts response to IST, with strongly skewed T-cell receptor repertoires predicting good or partial response to IST in children.[20] Oligoclonal expansion is also quantitatively related to the disease course. Patients with good response to IST typically have waning or resolution of their immune dominant clones and restoration of T-cell receptor variability.[22] At the time of relapse, patients may have recurrence of original clones or expansion, perhaps indicating further putative antigen presentation.[23]

Limited heterogeneity of the T-cell repertoire in aAA supports the hypothesis that an antigen (presumably on an HSPC) may be driving a pathologic lymphocyte response. However, controls derived from patients with recent viral infections are needed to determine the clinical significance of any these findings, because T-cell clonal expansion is characteristic of such infections.[24] Furthermore in vitro growth of T cells may artificially skew representation of clones, and perfectly healthy individuals of all ages may exhibit skewing and nonpathologic expansion of T-cell clones.[24]

Myelosuppressive Cytokines

T cells likely play a role in the pathogenesis of aAA via the release of myelosuppressive cytokines. Elevated interferon (IFN)-gamma and tumor necrosis factor (TNF)-alpha levels are found in the serum and bone marrow of patients with aAA.[25,26] Interferon (INF)-gamma alone inhibits murine myeloid progenitors and their differentiation and leads to aplasia.[27] TNF-alpha and INF-gamma induce HSPC death via the Fas/FasL pathway[28] and TRAIL expression.[29] In mice, anti–INF-gamma antibody can partially rescue hematopoiesis in a model of infusion induced bone marrow failure.[30] Thus, T cells, activated by either autoimmune response or viral infection may cause aplasia, particularly in patients with mutated hematopoietic stem cells or overactive immune cells (vide infra).

Immune Cell Dysregulation

That viral infection or other insult may lead to an inappropriate immune response in certain patients is illustrated by hemophagocytic lymphohistiocytosis. Mutations in the perforin gene, *PRF1*, cause some forms of familial hemophagocytic lymphohistiocytosis, and heterozygous mutations have been reported in aAA.[31] Polymorphisms in *TNF2*, the gene forTNF-alpha,[32,33] INF-gamma,[34] and IL-6 genes[33] result in excessive myelosuppressive cytokine gene expression and are associated with an increased immune response and reported in aAA.

HLA Genes

A number of studies have reported the epidemiologic association between certain class I and class II HLA alleles and increased or decreased risk of aAA. These studies are limited by effect size and reporting of statistically significant data that may have little clinical relevance. A recent metaanalysis demonstrated an increased risk of aAA associated with HLA-A and HLA-DRB1 polymorphisms and protective effect of other HLA-DRB polymorphisms.[35] HLA-DRB1*1501 predicts response to cyclosporine therapy.[36] HLA allelic variations are hypothesized to be involved in the pathogenesis of aAA by 2 mechanisms; activation of autoreactive T cells and failure to protect with decreased production of autoregulatory (Treg) cells.[37] However, the mechanistic link of HLA alleles and aAA remains unclear.

Antibodies

As mentioned, T cells, not antibodies, are the usual suspects as the inciters of an autoimmune mechanism of aAA. Therapies including plasmapheresis and anti-CD20 antibodies have been fruitlessly attempted and are rarely effective. Although an autoantigen has not been identified in aAA, multiple antibodies have been observed. Their clinical significance is ill-defined.

Kinectin is an antigen widely expressed and present in all hematopoietic cell lines. Kinectin antibodies are present in many patients with aAA and in vitro are capable of suppressing granulocyte-macrophage colony forming units. However, anti-kinectin–focused T cells were not identified in these patients.[38] Anti-moesin antibodies are also found in patients with aAA. In vitro, they stimulate peripheral mononuclear cells to secrete TNF-alpha and IFN-gamma. However, serum TNF-alpha levels are not influenced by anti-moesin antibody levels observed in patients with aAA.[39] Other antibodies, including heterogenous nuclear ribonucleoprotein antibodies are associated with good response to IST, but their mechanistic link to aAA is unknown.[40]

Surprising Lessons from Clinical Trials

Despite the immune dysfunctions outlined herein, there remain some puzzling results of clinical trials. If cytotoxic T cells play a key role, one would expect further inhibition of T cells to result in improved clinical outcomes. However, alemtuzumab, a humanized CD52 antibody that produces a more profound and durable lymphopenia than ATG, was unsuccessful as a single agent in treatment of naïve patients with aAA. In fact, the response rate was so low in the clinical trial, that the arm was closed for safety concerns. In relapse or refractory settings, there were only modest response rates of approximately 30% to alemtuzumab.[41] Rabbit ATG also more effectively depletes lymphocytes in vivo and is more cytotoxic on a weight basis.[42] However, in a clinical trial, there was an inferior clinical response to rabbit ATG compared with horse ATG (37% versus 68%, respectively).[43]

Perhaps horse ATG (which is really anti-human globulin) and cyclosporine (a drug with protean effects) exert changes beyond immune suppression and thereby may contribute to a clinical response in aAA by mechanisms that are not yet determined. For example, ATG stimulates CD34-dependent colony growth in normal, myelodysplastic, and AA bone marrow[44,45] and it reduces the expression of FAS on aplastic CD34 cells, an antigen that signals apoptosis.[44]

Stem Cell Abnormalities

There is evidence that groups of patients with aAA may have intrinsic abnormalities of their hematopoietic stem cells and progenitors. HSPCs are measured immunophenotypically by the presence of CD34, and progenitors are assayed as myeloid colony-forming cells. Patients with aAA have a decreased number of immature hematopoietic cells at diagnosis, and those that are present demonstrate a poor plating efficiency for colony formation.[46,47] Decreased progenitor cells persist in many patients, even when peripheral blood counts improve with treatment, perhaps suggesting an underlying stem cell abnormality.[47–49] Treatment of aplasia with simple infusion of stem cells from an identical twin donor without conditioning was successful in a small number of patients,[10,50] further supporting a primary stem cell etiology. Finally, there is a growing body of literature identifying germline mutations using next generation and whole exome sequencing in patients with a previously negative work up. This finding suggests that perhaps what is being called aAA, particularly in young people, may be a disease with an unidentified germline mutation in the hematopoietic stem cell.

Telomeres

About one-third of patients with aAA have significantly short telomeres in their leukocytes.[51] Shortened telomeres are associated with poor response to IST.[51,52] Telomeres are structures that stabilize the ends of each chromosome to prevent excessive shortening with replication. Telomeres shorten until they reach a critical length when they signal cessation of division to prevent chromosomal rearrangements. Patients with mutations in the telomere complex (*TERT* or *TERC*) have increased chromosome end-to-end fusions and aneuploidy, suggesting that telomeres play an important role in the prevention of myelodysplasias and leukemias.[53,54]

Dyskeratosis congenita is an IBMFS with genetic mutations that impair telomere length maintenance and is typically associated with other clinical features. A subset of patients with only aAA were found to harbor mutations in some of the same genes found in dyskeratosis congenita, including *TERC*[55,56] and *TERT*.[57] However, the majority of patients with aAA and short telomeres do not share these identifiable mutations. Thus, it is unclear whether telomeres are short secondary to increased stem cell turnover of a few remaining "over-demanded" stem cells or if there are unidentified environmental, genetic or epigenetic modifiers causing erosion of telomeres, which then contribute to disease.

In addition to shortened telomeres, HSPCs from patients with aAA display downregulation of cell cycle check point genes including cyclin-dependent kinase 6 (*CDK6*), *CDK2*, *MYB*, *MYC*, and a Fanconi anemia complementation member (*FANCG*).[37] Taken together, all of these changes in HSPCs in aAA may contribute to the inability of hematopoietic stem cells to compensate and replicate in the setting of insult.

Clonal hematopoiesis

The detection of clonal hematopoiesis in more than 50% of patients with aAA is perhaps the strongest indication that accumulated mutations play an important role in the disorder.[58–62] Early evidence suggesting a link between aAA, paroxysmal nocturnal hemoglobinuria (PNH), myelodysplastic syndrome (MDS), and acute myelogenous leukemia (AML) was noted in the 1960s and has puzzled hematologists for some time.[63] High incidences of subsequent MDS or AML were noted before the use of IST, and are particularly evident after successful treatment with IST. Approximately 10% of patients with aAA will later develop MDS or AML,[64] and as many as 25% will develop PNH.[65–67]

Cytogenetic abnormalities are reported in 4% to 11% patients with of aAA.[68–71] However, given the difficulty of obtaining sufficient numbers of metaphases from a failing marrow, this could be an underestimate. Some common abnormalities are shared with myeloid malignancies including +8, −7, and del(5q). Others, including +6 and + 15, are rarely seen in the AML/MDS.

Somatic Mutations in Aplastic Anemia

In a study of 156 patients by Yoshizato and colleagues,[72] 36% of patients with aAA had a somatic mutation; the most common was *BCOR/BCORL1*. Other clonal expansions of mutated cells fall in several large categories; PNH-like cells or loss of glycophosphotiylinositol-anchored proteins, loss of human leukocyte antigen alleles (6pLOH), and those commonly seen in MDS and/or myeloid malignancies.

Paroxysmal Nocturnal Hemoglobinuria–Like Cells

Paroxysmal nocturnal hemogloblinuria (PNH) is a bone marrow failure syndrome clinically characterized by acquired hemolytic anemia and thrombosis. Such patients have clonal expansion of cells derived from an HSPC carrying a somatic mutation in the *PIGA* gene. PIGA-mutated cells have defective cell surface expression of glycosylphosphatidylinostol (GPI) anchored proteins, including CD55 and CD59, making them vulnerable to complement-mediated hemolysis. PNH and aAA are closely related with multiple reports of the complication of clinically relevant PNH in patients with aAA and vice versa.

Regardless of clinical manifestations of PNH, GPI-deficient, "PNH-like" cells are detectable in more than half of patients with aAA when assessed by sensitive flow cytometry using antibodies to CD55 or CD59 or fluorescence aerolysin in aAA.[73–75] Clonal PNH expansion is strongly linked to HLA-DR2[76] and is a predictor of IST response.[77] This, in combination with an absence of these cell surface proteins in PNH, has led to the hypothesis that the deficient cells have escaped immune destruction. However, there is no direct evidence supporting this particular mechanism. They may have survived for any one of many reasons.

6p Loss of Heterozygosity

An acquired copy number neutral loss of heterozygosity has been identified in approximately 11% to 13% of patients with AA, usually involving the 6p locus, and this finding is the second most common mutation detected in aAA.[36,78] Acquired 6pLOH is characteristic and relatively specific to aAA, because it is exceedingly rare in the general population (prevalence approximately 0.09%).[36] It is also not commonly identified in other bone marrow failure syndromes or MDS. The 6pLOH involves the HLA locus, leading to the loss of expression of one HLA haplotype.[79] Missing HLA alleles were biased to particular alleles including HLA-A*02:01, A*02:06, A*31:01, and B*40:02.[79] The hypothesis is that autoantigens are expressed via these class I HLAs, and that HSPC loss of expression of this HLA via 6pLOH might allow escape from immune attack.[36,79] Thus, clones with PIGA and 6pLOH link clonality in aAA with the model of autodirected cytotoxic T-cell destruction of healthy HSPC (**Fig. 1**).

Myelodysplastic Syndrome/Acute Myelogenous Leukemia

Whole gene sequencing by Yoshizato and colleagues[72] demonstrated that mutations typically found in myeloid leukemias can be found in up to one-third of patients with aAA. *DNMT3A* and *ASXL1* mutations are common to both aAA and MDS. In aAA, these clones tended to increase their clone size over years, although variability was high between individuals. The presence of these mutations is associated with faster progression to MDS/AML, shorter overall survival, and poor response to IST. In contrast, *PIGA* and *BCOR/BCORL1* mutations are underrepresented in MDS and AML compared with patients with aAA, and clone sizes tend to stay stable or decrease over time. Compared with DNMT3A and ASXL2, these "favorable mutations" are associated with decreased mortality.[72] Of note, these data must be interpreted carefully, because somatic *DNMT3A* and *ASXL1* are also found in healthy aged populations and are considered clonal hematopoiesis of indeterminate potential.[80]

These findings suggest a second theoretic model of aAA linking MDS and aAA. The immune surveillance controlling these abnormal clones may result in "bystander" destruction of HSPC. With IST, suppression of the malignant clone is removed; the, clone unchecked may ultimately lead to MDS/AML. Additionally, it is possible that clonal hematopoiesis occurs in the setting of unidentified germline mutations as described elsewhere in this article.

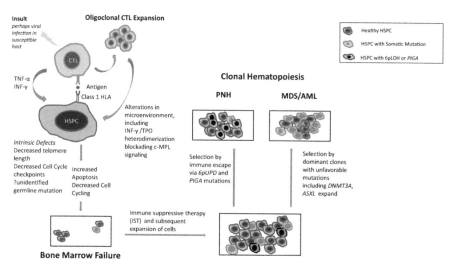

Fig. 1. An unidentified antigen(s) is presented to a cytotoxic T cell (CTL) via a class 1 HLA molecule. Autoreactive CTLs are activated, perhaps by a virus in a susceptible host, and begin to expand. T cells release cytokines including tumor necrosis factor (TNF-α) and interferon (INF-γ), which have direct apoptotic effects on hematopoietic stem and progenitor cells (HSPC) that have intrinsic defects, ultimately resulting in bone marrow failure. After treatment with immune suppressive therapy (IST), cells expand. Clonal hematopoiesis may occur in the setting of immune escape, as evidenced by *PIGA* mutations, which can subsequently lead to clinical paroxysmal nocturnal hemoglobinuria (PNH)or 6p loss of heterozygosity mutations. Alternatively, clonal hematopoiesis may occur via selection of dominant clones with somatic mutations that are identified in both the normal/aging population and those with aAA. Progressive proliferation of these clonal HSPC can then lead to progression of MDS/AML.

Germline Mutations

By definition, aAA may only be diagnosed after exclusion of an IBMFS through a detailed history, physical examination, and functional assays for Fanconi anemia and dyskeratosis congenita or genetic testing for Shwachman Diamond syndrome and congenital amegakaryocytic thrombocytopenia to exclude these classic inherited syndromes. To more rigorously diagnose IBMFS and MDS, a single center study used next generation sequencing–targeted BMF/MDS gene capture on patients diagnosed with aAA who underwent stem cell transplantation from 1990 to 2012. Pathologic mutations in known BMF genes were identified in 5 of 98 patients (5.1%); 3 of these 5 patients had no previous diagnosis, and family history and physical examination failed to distinguish them from other patients with aAA.[81] In a more select population with suspected IBMFS, given family history, congenital abnormalities, and young age but no previously identified mutation, whole exome sequencing identified pathologic mutations in 86 of 179 patients (48%).[82] Mutations included those well-described in IBMFS as well as new mutations rarely described, including *SAMD9/SAMD9L*, *MECOM/EVI1*, and *ERCC6L2*. Mutations in these genes frequently had a distinct clinical phenotype; transient aplasia and monosomy 7 in *SAMD9/SAMD9L*, severe infantile AA in *MECOM/EVI1*, and mild pancytopenia with myelodysplasia in ERCC6L2.

It is well-known that stem cell depletion leads to aplasia and subsequent MDS/AML in IBMFS, just as it does is aAA. These studies as well as those summarized elsewhere in this article support the idea that intrinsic abnormalities of hematopoietic stem cells and progenitors are a key component of aAA. Additionally, a cohort of patients diagnosed with aAA, particularly the young, may have unidentified germline mutations.

ALTERATIONS IN THE HEMATOPOIETIC STEM CELL ENVIRONMENT

Mesenchymal stromal cells from patients with AA are said to fail to form adherent layers in vitro and have reduced ability to sustain hematopoiesis as assessed by total cell proliferation.[83] Alterations in fibroblastic colony forming units and the stromal-derived cytokines ANG1, vascular endothelial growth factor, and vascular cell adhesion molecule-1 have also been reported.[84] Transforming growth factor β is a cytokine implicated in the regulation of hematopoietic stem cell cycling. In vitro and in vivo bone marrow stromal cells of aAA express significantly less transforming growth factor-β than normal stroma.[85] Although these alterations are provocative, they do not establish a clear link to the pathophysiology of AA.

Niches

Bone marrow niches are anatomically distinct spaces in the bone marrow that provide signals that maintain and support HSC. The osteoblastic niche is one of the best studied and is composed of osteoblasts in close proximity to quiescent HSC.[86] The destruction of osteoblasts in mice results in decreased HSC numbers and impaired hematopoiesis.[87] Examination of bone marrow samples in patients with aAA demonstrates fewer endosteal, vascular, and perivascular cells, indicating possible impairment of these niches in patients with aAA.[88]

Hematopoietic Growth Factors

Patients with aAA have markedly elevated serum hematopoietic growth factors including erythropoietin, granulocyte colony stimulating factor, granulocyte macrophage colony stimulating factor, and thrombopoietin (TPO).[89,90] The use of hematopoietic growth factors in bone marrow failure syndromes has a long but frustrating history. Trials have included erythropoietin, granulocyte macrophage colony stimulating factor, granulocyte colony stimulating factor, and interleukins 1, 3, and 6. They demonstrated no effect and except for GCSF, were associated with increased side effects.[91]

TPO is a potent endogenous cytokine that acts via the TPO receptor, also known as MPL, to stimulate platelet production. MPL is present on HSPC and in vitro, TPO has been shown to play an important role in hematopoietic stem cell survival and expansion.[92–94] In vivo patients with *MPL* associated congenital amegakaryocytic thrombocytopenia typically develop AA early in life.[95,96]

Eltrombopag, a small molecule TPO mimetic, was studied initially as monotherapy,[97] and then in combination with ATG and cyclosporine. The addition of eltrombopag improves response rates in aAA.[98] Although eltrombopag is clinically effective, the result gives little insight to the pathophysiology of AA. Eltrombopag binds MPL at a site distinct from that of endogenous TPO, so it may be exerting additional effects. In fact, recent unpublished work (Alvarado and colleagues, ASH abstract 2017) indicates that INF-γ and TPO form heteromeric complexes that hinder binding to the MPL receptor at both high and low affinity.[99] Eltrombopag may evade this process, thus explaining its role on the HSPC and in aAA.

SUMMARY

Acquired aplastic anemia has a complex pathophysiology. Lymphocyte subsets are altered; however, similar alterations are seen in viral infections. Functional assays demonstrate lymphocyte effects on the growth of HSPC, but very few published studies demonstrate T-cell clones expanded in vivo with cytotoxic effects on HSPCs. Immune dysregulation likely occurs in patients with underlying genetic susceptibility in the setting of a second insult. Intrinsic deficits of the hematopoietic stem cell itself are also important in the disease process, as evidenced by shortened telomeres and somatic mutations ultimately leading to clonal hematopoiesis and increased risk of MDS and AML. The hematopoietic stem cell microenvironment may also contribute to disease. While IST with equine ATG, cyclosporine and eltrombopag have improved clinical outcomes, we have much to learn about the underlying mechanisms in aAA and why these agents are effective. The potential role of upfront matched unrelated donor stem cell transplant as first-line treatment for aAA, particularly for younger patients, is currently under investigation.

ACKNOWLEDGMENTS

We thank Drs Joseph Antin, Akiko Shimamura and Blanche Alter for their critical and constructive review of this article.

REFERENCES

1. Incidence of aplastic anemia: the relevance of diagnostic criteria. By the International Agranulocytosis and Aplastic Anemia Study. Blood 1987;70(6):1718–21.
2. McCahon E, Tang K, Rogers PC, et al. The impact of Asian descent on the incidence of acquired severe aplastic anaemia in children. Br J Haemotol 2003; 121(1):170–2.
3. Issaragrisil S, Sriratanasatavorn C, Piankijagum A, et al. Incidence of aplastic anemia in Bangkok. The Aplastic Anemia Study Group. Blood 1991;77(10): 2166–8.
4. Young NS, Kaufman DW. The epidemiology of acquired aplastic anemia. Haematologica 2008;93(4):489 LP–492. Available at: http://www.haematologica.org/content/93/4/489.abstract.
5. Brodsky RA, Jones RJ. Aplastic anaemia. Lancet 2005;365(9471):1647–56.
6. Rosenfeld S, Follmann D, Nunez O, et al. Antithymocyte globulin and cyclosporine for severe aplastic anemia: association between hematologic response and long-term outcome. JAMA 2003;289(9):1130–5.
7. Dufour C, Pillon M, Sociè G, et al. Outcome of aplastic anaemia in children. A study by the severe aplastic anaemia and paediatric disease working parties of the European group blood and bone marrow transplant. Br J Haematol 2015;169(4):565–73.
8. Barnes DW, Mole RH. Aplastic Anaemia in Sublethally Irradiated Mice Given Allogeneic Lymph Node Cells. British Journal of Haematology 1967;13:482–91.
9. Barnes D, Mole RH. Aplastic anaemia in sublethally irradiated mice given allogeneic lymph node cells. Br J Haematol 1967;13(4):482–91.
10. Hinterberger W, Rowlings PA, Hinterberger-Fischer M, et al. Results of transplanting bone marrow from genetically identical twins into patients with aplastic anemia. Ann Intern Med 1997;126(2):116–22.
11. Young NS, Calado RT, Scheinberg P. Review in translational hematology Current concepts in the pathophysiology and treatment of aplastic anemia. Blood 2006; 108(8):2509–19.
12. Xing L, Liu C, Fu R, et al. CD8+HLA-DR+ T cells are increased in patients with severe aplastic anemia. Mol Med Rep 2014;10(3):1252–8.

13. Nakao S, Takami A, Takamatsu H, et al. Isolation of a T-cell clone showing HLA-DRB1*0405-restricted cytotoxicity for hematopoietic cells in a patient with aplastic anemia. Blood 1997;89(10):3691–9.
14. Risitano AM, Maciejewski JP, Green S, et al. In-vivo dominant immune responses in aplastic anaemia: molecular tracking of putatively pathogenetic T-cell clones by TCR β-CDR3 sequencing. Lancet 2004;364(9431):355–64.
15. Kordasti S, Marsh J, Al-khan S, et al. Functional characterization of CD4 + T cells in aplastic anemia. Blood 2012;119(9):2033–43.
16. Solomou EE, Rezvani K, Mielke S, et al. Brief report Deficient CD4 ℮ CD25 ℮ FOXP3 ℮ T regulatory cells in acquired aplastic anemia. Blood 2007;110(5): 1603–6.
17. Sutton KS, Shereck EB, Nemecek ER, et al. Immune markers of disease severity and treatment response in pediatric acquired aplastic anemia. Pediatr Blood Cancer 2013;60(3):455–60.
18. Veiga-Parga T, Sehrawat S, Rouse BT. Role of regulatory T cells during virus infection. Immunol Rev 2013;255(1):182–96.
19. Zeng W, Maciejewski JP, Chen G, et al. Limited heterogeneity of T cell receptor BV usage in aplastic anemia. J Clin Invest 2001;108(5):765–73.
20. Schuster FR, Hubner B, Führer M, et al. Highly skewed T-cell receptor V-beta chain repertoire in the bone marrow is associated with response to immunosuppressive drug therapy in children with very severe aplastic anemia. Blood Cancer J 2011;1(3):e8.
21. Moebius U, Herrmann F, Hercend T, et al. Clonal analysis of CD4+/CD8+ T cells in a patient with aplastic anemia. J Clin Invest 1991;87(5):1567–74.
22. Kochenderfer JN, Kobayashi S, Wieder ED, et al. Loss of T-lymphocyte clonal dominance in patients with myelodysplastic syndrome responsive to immunosuppression. Blood 2002;100(10):3639–45.
23. Wlodarski MW, Gondek LP, Nearman ZP, et al. Molecular strategies for detection and quantitation of clonal cytotoxic T-cell responses in aplastic anemia and myelodysplastic syndrome Molecular strategies for detection and quantitation of clonal cytotoxic T-cell responses in aplastic anemia and myeloid. Blood 2006; 108(8):2632–41.
24. Batliwalla F, Monteiro J, Serrano D, et al. Oligoclonality of CD8 + T cells in health and disease: aging, infection, or immune regulation? Hum Immunol 1996;48(1–2): 68–76.
25. Sloand E, Kim S, Maciejewski JP, et al. Intracellular interferon-gamma in circulating and marrow T cells detected by flow cytometry and the response to immunosuppressive therapy in patients with aplastic anemia. Blood 2002;100(4): 1185–91.
26. Wu Q, Zhang J, Shi J, et al. Increased bone marrow (BM) plasma level of soluble CD30 and correlations with BM plasma level of interferon (IFN)-γ, CD4/CD8 T-cell ratio and disease severity in aplastic anemia. PLoS One 2014;9(11):e110787.
27. Lin F, Karwan M, Saleh B, et al. IFN- g causes aplastic anemia by altering hematopoietic stem/progenitor cell composition and disrupting lineage differentiation. Blood 2015;124(25):3699–709.
28. Liu CY, Fu R, Wang HQ, et al. Fas/FasL in the immune pathogenesis of severe aplastic anemia. Genet Mol Res 2014;13(2):4083–8.
29. Kakagianni T, Giannakoulas NC, Thanopoulou E, et al. A probable role for trail-induced apoptosis in the pathogenesis of marrow failure. Leuk Re 2017;30(6): 713–21.

30. Chen J, Lipovsky K, Ellison FM, et al. Bystander destruction of hematopoietic progenitor and stem cells in a mouse model of infusion-induced bone marrow failure. Blood 2004;104(6):1671–8.

31. Solomou EE, Gibellini F, Stewart B, et al. Perforin gene mutations in patients with acquired aplastic anemia. Blood 2007;109(12):5234–7.

32. Peng J, Liu C, Zhu K, et al. The TNF2 allele is a risk factor to severe aplastic anemia independent of HLA-DR. Hum Immunol 2003;64(9):896–901.

33. Gidvani VK, Ramkissoon SH, Wong EW, et al. Tumor necrosis factor-alpha and interleukin-6 promoter gene polymorphisms in acquired bone marrow failure syndromes. Blood 2004;104(11):3707. Available at: http://www.bloodjournal.org/content/104/11/3707.abstract.

34. Dufour C, Capasso M, Svahn J, et al. Homozygosis for (12) CA repeats in the first intron of the human IFN-gamma gene is significantly associated with the risk of aplastic anaemia in Caucasian population. Br J Haematol 2004;126(5):682–5.

35. Deng XZ, Du M, Peng J, et al. Associations between the HLA-A/B/DRB1 polymorphisms and aplastic anemia: evidence from 17 case-control studies. Hematology 2018;23(3):154–62.

36. Zaimoku Y, Takamatsu H, Hosomichi K, et al. Identification of an HLA class I allele closely involved in the autoantigen presentation in acquired aplastic anemia. Blood 2017;129(21):2908–16.

37. Zeng Y, Katsanis E. The complex pathophysiology of acquired aplastic anaemia. Clin Exp Immunol 2015;180(3):361–70.

38. Hirano N, Butler MO, Von Bergwelt-Baildon MS, et al. Autoantibodies frequently detected in patients with aplastic anemia. Blood 2003;102(13):4567–75.

39. Takamatsu H, Espinoza JL, Lu X, et al. Anti-moesin antibodies in the serum of patients with aplastic anemia stimulate peripheral blood mononuclear cells to secrete TNF-α and IFN-γ. J Immunol 2009;182(1):703–10.

40. Qi Z, Takamatsu H, Espinoza JL, et al. Autoantibodies specific to hnRNP K: a new diagnostic marker for immune pathophysiology in aplastic anemia. Ann Hematol 2010;89(12):1255–63.

41. Scheinberg P, Nunez O, Weinstein B, et al. Activity of alemtuzumab monotherapy in treatment-naive, relapsed, and refractory severe acquired aplastic anemia. Blood 2012;119(2):345–54.

42. Scheinberg P, Fischer SH, Li L, et al. Distinct EBV and CMV reactivation patterns following antibody-based immunosuppressive regimens in patients with severe aplastic anemia. Blood 2007;109(8):3219–24. Available at: http://www.bloodjournal.org/content/109/8/3219.abstract.

43. Scheinberg P, Nunez O, Weinstein B, et al. Horse versus rabbit antithymocyte globulin in acquired aplastic anemia. N Engl J Med 2011;365(5):430–8.

44. Killick SB, Marsh JCW, Gordonsmith EC, et al. Effects of antithymocyte globulin on bone marrow CD34+cells in aplastic anaemia and myelodysplasia [Full text delivery]. Br J Haematol 2000;108:582–91.

45. Flynn J, Cox CV, Rizzo S, et al. Direct binding of antithymoctye globulin to haemopoietic progenitor cells in aplastic anaemia. Br J Haematol 2003;122(2):289–97.

46. Marsh JC, Chang J, Testa NG, et al. In vitro assessment of marrow "stem cell" and stromal cell function in aplastic anaemia. Br J Haematol 1991;78(2):258–67.

47. Manz CY, Nissen C, Wodnar-filipowicz A. Deficiency of CD34+ c-kit+ and CD34+38- hematopoietic precursors in aplastic anemia after immunosuppressive treatment. Am J Hematol 1996;52(4):264–74.

48. Maciejewski JP, Selleri C, Sato T, et al. A severe and consistent deficit in marrow and circulating primitive hematopoietic cells (long-term culture-initiating cells) in acquired aplastic anemia. Blood 1996;88(6):1983–91.
49. Marsh JC, Chang J, Testa NG, et al. The hematopoietic defect in aplastic anemia assessed by long-term marrow culture. Blood 1990;76(9):1748–57.
50. Lu D. Syngeneic bone marrow transplantation for treatment of aplastic anaemia: report of a case and review of the literature. Exp Hematol 1981;9(3):257–63.
51. Brümmendorf TH, Maciejewski JP, Mak J, et al. Telomere length in leukocyte subpopulations of patients with aplastic anemia. Blood 2001;97(4):895–900. Available at: http://www.bloodjournal.org/content/97/4/895.abstract.
52. Sakaguchi H, Nishio N, Hama A, et al. Peripheral blood lymphocyte telomere length as a predictor of response to immunosuppressive therapy in childhood aplastic anemia. Haematologica 2014;99(8):1312–6.
53. Calado RT, Regal JA, Yewdell WT, et al. Constitutional loss-of-function mutations in telomerase are genetic risk factors for acute myeloid leukemia. Blood 2015; 110(11):16. Available at: http://www.bloodjournal.org/content/110/11/16.abstract.
54. Calado RT, Cooper JN, Padilla-Nash HM, et al. Short telomeres result in chromosomal instability in hematopoietic cells and precede malignant evolution in human aplastic anemia. Leukemia 2012;26(4):700–7.
55. Calado RT, Young NS. Review article Telomere maintenance and human bone marrow failure. Bone 2008;111(9):4446–55.
56. Yamaguchi H, Baerlocher GM, Lansdorp PM, et al. Mutations of the human telomerase RNA gene TERC in aplastic anemia and myelodysplastic syndrome. Blood 2003;102(3):916–8. Available at: http://www.bloodjournal.org/content/102/3/916.abstract.
57. Yamaguchi H, Calado RT, Ly H, et al. Mutations in TERT, the gene for telomerase reverse transcriptase, in aplastic anemia. N Engl J Med 2005;352(14):1413–24.
58. Lane AA, Odejide O, Kopp N, et al. Low frequency clonal mutations recoverable by deep sequencing in patients with aplastic anemia. Leukemia 2013;27(4): 968–71.
59. Heuser M, Schlarmann C, Dobbernack V, et al. Genetic characterization of acquired aplastic anemia by targeted sequencing. Haematologica 2014;99(9): e165–7. Available at: http://www.haematologica.org/content/99/9/e165.abstract.
60. Kulasekararaj AG, Jiang J, Smith AE, et al. Somatic mutations identify a subgroup of aplastic anemia patients who progress to myelodysplastic syndrome. Blood 2014;124(17):2698–704. Available at: http://www.bloodjournal.org/content/124/17/2698.abstract.
61. Babushok DV, Perdigones N, Perin JC, et al. Emergence of clonal hematopoiesis in the majority of patients with acquired aplastic anemia. Cancer Genet 2015; 208(4):115–28.
62. Ogawa S. CME article clonal hematopoiesis in acquired aplastic anemia. Blood 2016;128(3):337–48.
63. Dameshek W. Editorial: riddle: what do aplastic anemia, paroxysmal nocturnal hemoglobinuria (PNH) and "hypoplastic" leukemia have in common? Blood 1967;30(2):251–4. Available at: http://www.bloodjournal.org/content/30/2/251.abstract.
64. Tichelli A, Gratwohl A, Würsch A, et al. Late haematological complications in severe aplastic anaemia. Br J Haematol 1988;69:413–8.
65. Narita A, Muramatsu H, Okuno Y, et al. Development of paroxysmal nocturnal hemoglobinuria in children with aplastic anemia. Blood 2016;128(22):1499. Available at: http://www.bloodjournal.org/content/128/22/1499.abstract.

66. Wanachiwanawin W, Siripanyaphinyo U, Piyawattanasakul N, et al. A cohort study of the nature of paroxysmal nocturnal hemoglobinuria clones and PIG-A mutations in patients with aplastic anemia. Eur J Haematol 2006;76(6):502–9.
67. Tichelli A, Gratwohl A, Nissen C, et al. Late clonal complications in severe aplastic anemia. Leuk Lymphoma 1994;12(3–4):167–75.
68. Appelbaum FR, Barrall J, Storb R, et al. Clonal cytogenetic abnormalities in patients with otherwise typical aplastic anemia. Exp Hematol 1987;15(11):1134–9.
69. Socié G, Rosenfeld S, Frickhofen N, et al. Late clonal diseases of treated aplastic anemia. Semin Hematol 2000;37(1):91–101.
70. Keung YK, Pettenati MJ, Cruz JM, et al. Bone marrow cytogenetic abnormalities of aplastic anemia. Am J Hematol 2001;66(3):167–71.
71. Maciejewski JP, Risitano A, Sloand EM, et al. Distinct clinical outcomes for cytogenetic abnormalities evolving from aplastic anemia. Blood 2002;99(9):3129–35. Available at: http://www.bloodjournal.org/content/99/9/3129.abstract.
72. Yoshizato T, Dumitriu B, Hosokawa K, et al. Somatic mutations and clonal hematopoiesis in aplastic anemia. N Engl J Med 2015;373(1):35–47.
73. Schubert J, Vogt HG, Zielinska-Skowronek M, et al. Development of the glycosylphosphatitylinositol-anchoring defect characteristic for paroxysmal nocturnal hemoglobinuria in patients with aplastic anemia. Blood 1994;83(8): 2323–8. Available at: http://www.bloodjournal.org/content/83/8/2323.abstract.
74. Azenishi Y, Ueda E, Machii T, et al. CD59-deficient blood cells and PIG-A gene abnormalities in Japanese patients with aplastic anaemia. Br J Haematol 1999; 104(3):523–9.
75. Kawaguchi K, Wada H, Mori A, et al. Detection of GPI-anchored protein-deficient cells in patients with aplastic anaemia and evidence for clonal expansion during the clinical course. Br J Haematol 1999;105(1):80–4.
76. Maciejewski JP, Follmann D, Nakamura R, et al. Increased frequency of HLA-DR2 in patients with paroxysmal nocturnal hemoglobinuria and the PNH/aplastic anemia syndrome. Blood 2001;98(13):3513–9. Available at: http://www.bloodjournal.org/content/98/13/3513.abstract.
77. Zhao X, Zhang L, Jing L, et al. The role of paroxysmal nocturnal hemoglobinuria clones in response to immunosuppressive therapy of patients with severe aplastic anemia. Ann Hematol 2015;94(7):1105–10.
78. Wlodarski MW, Hirabayashi S, Strahm B, et al. Recurrent 6pLOH is the most common somatic lesion in refractory cytopenia of childhood and occurs very infrequently in severe aplastic anemia. Blood 2012;120(21):644. Available at: http://www.bloodjournal.org/content/120/21/644.abstract.
79. Katagiri T, Sato-Otsubo A, Kashiwase K, et al. Frequent loss of HLA alleles from hematopoietic stem cells in patients with hepatitis-associated aplastic anemia. Blood 2011;118(21):6601–10.
80. Steensma DP, Bejar R, Jaiswal S, et al. Clonal hematopoiesis of indeterminate potential and its distinction from myelodysplastic syndromes. Blood 2015;126(1): 9–16.
81. Keel SB, Scott A, Bonilla MS, et al. Genetic features of myelodysplastic syndrome and aplastic anemia in pediatric and young adult patients. Haematologica 2016; 101(11):1343–50.
82. Bluteau O, Sebert M, Leblanc T, et al. A landscape of germline mutations in a cohort of inherited bone marrow failure patients. Blood 2018;131(7):717–32. Available at: http://www.bloodjournal.org/content/early/2017/11/16/blood-2017-09-806489.abstract.

83. Hamzic E, Whiting K, Gordon Smith E, et al. Characterization of bone marrow mesenchymal stromal cells in aplastic anaemia. Br J Haematol 2015;169(6): 804–13.

84. Shipounova IN, Petrova TV, Svinareva DA, et al. Alterations in hematopoietic microenvironment in patients with aplastic anemia. Clin Transl Sci 2009;2(1): 67–74.

85. Rizzo S, Killick SB, Patel S, et al. Reduced TGF-beta1 in patients with aplastic anaemia in vivo and in vitro. Br J Haematol 1999;107(4):797–803.

86. Wu JY, Scadden DT, Kronenberg HM. Role of the osteoblast lineage in the bone marrow hematopoietic niches. J Bone Miner Res 2009;24(5):759–64.

87. Visnjic D, Kalajzic Z, Rowe DW, et al. Hematopoiesis is severely altered in mice with an induced osteoblast deficiency. Blood 2004;103(9):3258–64.

88. Wu L, Mo W, Zhang Y, et al. Impairment of hematopoietic stem cell niches in patients with aplastic anemia. Int J Hematol 2015;102(6):645–53.

89. Kojima S, Matsuyama T, Kodera Y, et al. Measurement of endogenous plasma granulocyte colony-stimulating factor in patients with acquired aplastic anemia by a sensitive chemiluminescent immunoassay. Blood 1996;87(4):1303–8. Available at: http://www.ncbi.nlm.nih.gov/entrez/query.fcgi?cmd=Retrieve&db=PubMed&dopt=Citation&list_uids=8608218.

90. Schrezenmeier H, Griesshammer M, Hornkohl A, et al. Thrombopoietin serum levels in patients with aplastic anaemia: correlation with platelet count and persistent elevation in remission. Br J Haematol 1998;100(3):571–6.

91. Marsh JC, Ganser A, Stadler M. Hematopoietic growth factors in the treatment of acquired bone marrow failure states. Semin Hematol 2007;44(3):138–47.

92. Kimura S, Roberts AW, Metcalf D, et al. Hematopoietic stem cell deficiencies in mice lacking c-Mpl, the receptor for thrombopoietin. Proc Natl Acad Sci U S A 1998;95(3):1195–200.

93. Zeigler FC, de Sauvage F, Widmer HR, et al. In vitro megakaryocytopoietic and thrombopoietic activity of c-mpl ligand (TPO) on purified murine hematopoietic stem cells. Blood 1994;84(12):4045–52.

94. Yoshihara H, Arai F, Hosokawa K, et al. Thrombopoietin/MPL signaling regulates hematopoietic stem cell quiescence and interaction with the osteoblastic niche. Cell Stem Cell 2007;1(6):685–97.

95. King S, Germeshausen M, Strauss G, et al. Congenital amegakaryocytic thrombocytopenia: a retrospective clinical analysis of 20 patients. Br J Haematol 2005;131(5):636–44.

96. Walne AJ, Dokal A, Plagnol V, et al. Exome sequencing identifies MPL as a causative gene in familial Aplastic anemia. Haematologica 2012;97(4):524–8.

97. Olnes MJ, Scheinberg P, Calvo KR, et al. Eltrombopag and improved hematopoiesis in refractory aplastic anemia. N Engl J Med 2012;367(1):11–9.

98. Townsley DM, Scheinberg P, Winkler T, et al. Eltrombopag added to standard immunosuppression for aplastic anemia. N Engl J Med 2017;376(16):1540–50.

99. Luigi J. Alvarado, Alessio Andreoni, Heather D. Huntsman, Hai Cheng JRK and AL. 4 Heterodimerization of TPO and IFNγ impairs human hematopoietic stem/progenitor cell signaling and survival in chronic inflammation. In: American Society of Hematology. 2017. Available at: https://ash.confex.com/ash/2017/webprogram/Paper10.

Somatic Mutations in Aplastic Anemia

Ghulam J. Mufti, MB BS, DM, Judith C.W. Marsh, MB ChB, MD*

KEYWORDS

- Aplastic anemia • Somatic mutations • Myeloid neoplasms • Treatment

KEY POINTS

- The occurrence and significance of somatic mutations in aplastic anemia (AA) are closely linked to the immune response that occurs in AA.
- Somatic mutations in *PIGA* and HLA genes (and possibly *BCOR/BCORL1*) represent immune escape clones that are associated with response to immunosuppressive therapy and very low risk of progression to myelodysplastic syndrome in adults.
- Myeloid-specific somatic mutations, such as *DNMT3A* and *ASXL1*, are found in a proportion of AA patients. When detected at diagnosis, their significance is unclear and difficult to distinguish from age-related clonal hematopoiesis.

IMMUNE FEATURES OF THE DISEASE THAT IMPACT ON THE SIGNIFICANCE OF SOMATIC MUTATIONS IN APLASTIC ANEMIA

Acquired idiopathic aplastic anemia (AA) is in most cases an immune-mediated bone marrow failure disorder.[1–3] AA is characterized by a proinflammatory environment that occurs after an initial insult (likely viral) to the bone marrow, which is driven initially by the CD4$^+$ T-cell compartment. This immune response is characterized by increased helper T cells—T$_H$1 (clonal) and T$_H$17 cells—and reduced or absent regulatory T cells (Tregs). Tregs in AA are also dysfunctional because they show reduced ability to suppress autologous T effectors proliferation. This results in oligoclonal expansion of CD8$^+$ cytotoxic T cells (CTLs) and apoptosis of hematopoietic stem cells (HSCs) and progenitor cells, respectively.[4–7] Response to immunosuppressive therapy (IST) using antithymocyte globulin with cyclosporine occurs in approximately 70% of AA patients.[8–10] Using high-dimensional immunephenotyping by mass cytometry using cytometry by time-of-flight (CyTOF), 2 identified distinct Treg subpopulations (Treg A and Treg B) differing significantly in number and immune phenotype have been

Conflicts of Interest: The authors have no commercial or financial conflicts of interest.
Department of Haematological Medicine, King's College Hospital, King's College London, Denmark Hill, London SE59RS, UK
* Corresponding author.
E-mail address: Judith.marsh@nhs.net

identified between responders and nonresponders to IST. Treg B population predominates in responders to IST and has a memory/activated phenotype (as shown by high expression of CD95, CCR4, and CD45RO).[11]

Considerable overlap exists between AA and other clonal HSCs disorders. AA may be difficult to distinguish from the hypocellular subtype of myelodysplastic syndrome (MDS), hypocellular MDS,[12] and AA may later transform to MDS/acute myeloid leukemia (AML) in approximately 15% of patients at 10 years after IST.[8–10,13] Immune mechanisms to keep mutations in general under check involve innate and adaptive immune responses, including the expression of mutation-related neoantigens, their binding to HLA, and hence their ability to elicit an immune response.[14] Some disease clones may be kept under control by an effective immune system leading to their elimination, whereas other clones may escape such a response. The significance of somatic mutations in AA, therefore, will depend on the underlying immune pathogenetic mechanisms for clonal transformation. The immune response in AA is mainly due to Treg dysfunction and a T_H17 inflammatory response, leading to a subsequent $CD8^+$ T-cell response. With the development of MDS, however, there is a change from a proinflammatory to an immune-suppressive environment, with an increase in Tregs and decrease in T_H17 cells. The number of Tregs is higher in high-risk MDS compared with low-rick/intermediate-risk MDS. In contrast, T_H17 cells are significantly higher in low-risk MDS compared with high-risk MDS, and the high level of T_H17 correlates with increased bone marrow apoptosis. Thus, the balance between T_H1, T_H7, and Tregs reflects the characteristic immune signature of the bone marrow failure; if the balance is toward T_H1 and T_H17 with low/normal Tregs, as in AA and low-risk MDS, there is a proinflammatory immunosuppressive environment, with autoreactivity of the adaptive immune system. In the presence of increased Tregs, as seen in high-risk MDS, immune surveillance switches to immune subversion and subsequent disease progression.[15,16] From preliminary work by the authors' group, the immune response in AA patients with MDS-related somatic mutations is perhaps directed more toward mutation-related neoantigens.[17] Thus, the immune response plays a key role in modulating the fate of abnormal mutated clones, especially low-level clones during the disease course in AA (discussed later).

The immune-mediated nature of AA has other implications for the interpretation of somatic mutations. Abnormal clones may emerge in AA, escape this immune attack, and proliferate with a survival advantage over normal HSCs. This is a feature not only of specific cytogenetic clones, such as trisomy 8, due to increased expression of WT1 and del(13q) but also paroxysmal nocturnal hemoglobinuria (PNH) clones due to acquired somatic mutations of PIG-A or acquired copy number neutral loss of heterozygosity for 6p (6pLOH) or other structural HLA gene mutations. Such clones are in general associated with a good prognosis and low risk of clonal evolution to MDS/AML in adults.[18–22] In addition to the immune response seen in AA and during disease progression, aging is associated with many changes in the immune system, including a chronic low-grade proinflammatory state (termed, *inflammaging*), driven by intracellular inflammasomes that are important mediators for age-related diseases.[23] This may contribute to clonal transformation particularly in older patients with AA. Of relevance here is the biphasic age distribution for AA with peaks at 15 years to 20 years and greater than 60 years.[24,25] It is this older group of AA patients where the possible impact of age-related clonal hematopoiesis (ARCH) is at its greatest and in whom the likelihood that their bone marrow failure might be due to hypocellular MDS instead of AA is increased compared with younger patients.

INTERPRETATION OF CLONALITY IN APLASTIC ANEMIA

Demonstration of clonality in AA, whether by cytogenetics or somatic mutations, does not necessarily indicate malignant transformation. Monoclonal hematopoiesis in AA may be due to a depleted HSC pool, resulting in increased proliferative pressure on the few remaining stem cells to maintain blood counts. It may also represent emergence of an abnormal stem cell that has a proliferative advantage. A major difficulty using standard metaphase cytogenetics in severe AA (SAA) is that up to 12% patients have an abnormal cytogenetic clone in the absence of morphologic evidence of MDS (as summarized by Stanley and colleagues[2]); furthermore, some abnormal karyotypes confer good prognosis in SAA, such as trisomy 8 and del(13q).[21,22,26] It is frequently difficult to obtain sufficient metaphases from a hypocellular bone marrow, thus further limiting their usefulness in predicting malignant transformation. This problem is overcome using fluorescence in situ hybridization or single-nucleotide polymorphism array (SNP-A) analyses that do not require dividing cells. Compared with metaphase cytogenetics, SNP-A increases the detection of abnormal (unbalanced) chromosomal defects to 19% in AA.[27] Another contribution to later malignant disease is the presence of short telomeres in approximately 30% of AA patients in the absence of an inherited telomeropathy. This may reflect increased proliferative stress on remaining stem cells or the presence of an as-yet unidentified telomere gene mutation. Furthermore, short telomeres are occasionally found in other inherited bone marrow failure syndromes.[28] Increased telomere attrition led to depletion of the HSC pool and genomic instability, an increased risk of monosomy 7, somatic mutations, and malignant transformation to MDS/AML.[29,30]

SOMATIC MUTATIONS IN APLASTIC ANEMIA THAT REPRESENT IMMUNE ESCAPE
PIGA Mutations

PNH clones as quantitated by high-sensitivity flow cytometry can be detected in up to 50% of AA patients at some time during the course of their disease, and they are predictive of response to IST.[31,32] Their presence is also associated with a very low risk of later MDS/AML among patients with hemolytic PNH.[33] In the setting of bone marrow failure, PNH clones represent escape clones. A proposed mechanism for this immune escape of PNH HSCs is that autoreactive CTLs target normal HSC and that PNH HSCs are spared from this immune attack. The likely target is either the Glycosylphosphatidylinositol (GPI) anchor or a GPI-linked protein based on the presence of CD1d-restricted GPI-specific T cells in both PNH and AA patients.[34,35] Flow cytometry is more sensitive than PIGA sequencing to detect small PNH clones, as reported from the first of 2 large studies examining somatic mutations in AA. From the King's College Hospital, London, study, PIGA sequencing revealed PIGA mutations in all AA patients with a PNH clone size greater than 10% but in none of those with clone size of less than 10% by flow cytometry.[36] PIGA mutations were detected in 7.5% of 439 AA patients in the National Institutes of Health (NIH)/Cleveland clinic/ Kanazawa university, Japan study and PIGA mutations accounted for 21% of all somatic mutations detected.[37] An additional feature is the relative frequent finding of double PIGA mutations, seen in 35% of AA patients with PIGA mutations.[36] This has been reported previously in a series of 40 AA patients with PIGA mutations; 11 had more than 1 clone and 5 of the 11 had 3 or 4 mutations.[38] PNH clones can also be detected in healthy individuals at very low levels,[39] but in contrast to ARCH (discussed later), it is not known if the frequency of PNH clones increases with age among healthy individuals. In the setting of AA, the incidence of PIGA mutations does not increase with age.[37]

Functional Loss of HLA and Somatic HLA Mutations

There is over-representation of specific HLA haplotypes (both class I and class II) in patients with AA. Earlier work focused on class II HLA haplotypes, demonstrating an association between HLA-DR15 and AA.[40] More recent focus has been on class I HLA haplotypes and 6pLOH. In a recent study from Japan, the most frequent class 1 haplotypes are HLA-B*4002, HLA-B*1402, HLA-A*3303, and HLA-A*6801 and class II haplotypes are HLA-DRB1*1502 and HLA-DRB1*1501.[41] Up to 19% of AA patients had acquired (6pLOH) that may escape immune attack by CTLs targeting autoantigens presented by the missing HLA alleles. Recent work has shown that 6pLOH is especially common in patients with the HLA-B*4002 allele, suggesting that autoantigens presented by HLA-B*4002 are important in immune escape. Using a monoclonal antibody specific to this HLA allele, B4002- granulocytes were detected in all 6pLOH patients and also more than half of patients lacking 6pLOH. Somatic structural mutations in the HLA-B*4002 gene were detected among all patients with HLA-B*4002 − granulocytes. Patients carrying the HLA-B*4002 showed a high response rate to IST and lack of progression to MDS. Thus, expansion of these clones can escape immune attack through either functional loss of HLA due to 6pLOH or other structural mutations in HLA genes.

A similar over-representation of HLA haplotypes has been reported in whites, from a study involving predominantly children, accounting for 77% of patients studied. Somatic loss of HLA (either 6pLOH or loss of function mutations) was found in 17% of patients. Mutations were found in HLA-B*4002 and HLA-B*1402 alleles and less commonly in HLA-A*3303 and HLA-A*6801. In contrast to studies in adults, the presence of HLA mutations in children with AA was associated with a higher number of courses of treatment and a higher incidence of abnormal cytogenetic clones and MDS-associated somatic mutations (ASXL1, RUNX1, and DNMT3A) and disease progression to MDS compared with children lacking HLA mutations.[42] This group had also previously reported a high incidence of PIGA mutations among younger patients.[43] This study is compounded by heterogeneity of patients with the influence of a smaller group of adult patients but does highlight different effects of somatic HLA mutations in AA according to age. The pathogenesis of AA in children is likely to be different from adults, especially because there is a higher incidence of constitutional AA in this younger age group.

BCOR/BCORL1 Mutations?

Among AA patients, there is a notable increase in BCOR and/or BCORL1 mutations compared with MDS and healthy individuals. BCOR mutations were detected in 4% of patients and BCOR/BCORL1 in 9.3% of patients, from the King's College Hospital and NIH/Japan studies, respectively.[36,37] The clones most often remained at a low level or disappeared, and none progressed to MDS. In the King's College Hospital study all patients had a coexisting PNH clone of similar allele burden to the BCOR clone, suggesting BCOR and PIGA mutations occurred in the same clone.[36] Presence of BCOR/BCORL1 correlated with an improved overall survival and response to IST, suggesting that in AA patients BCOR/BCORL1 mutations may give rise to immune escape clones.[37] Paradoxically, however, BCOR/BCORL1 mutations in MDS are associated with a poor prognosis and high risk of transformation to AML.[44]

AGE-RELATED CLONAL HEMATOPOIESIS

Somatic mutations that drive clonal expansion are common in healthy aged individuals, with a progressive increase in incidence of 10% for individuals ages 70 to

79 years and 20% for those ages greater than or equal to age 90. A majority of mutations are in *TET2, DNMT3A,* and *ASXL1*, genes that are recurrently mutated in myeloid malignancies. Less frequent mutations in spliceosome genes are usually restricted to the greater than or equal to 70-year age group.[45–47] ARCH, or its synonym clonal hematopoiesis of indeterminate potential (CHIP), is defined as a variant allele frequency (VAF) of greater than or equal to age 2% in the absence of hematological malignancy or other clonal disorder at the time of analysis.[48] The number of mutations is usually 1 per individual and the median VAF is low, ranging between 9% and 20%. The presence of a mutation in ARCH is associated with an increased risk of a hematological malignancy (0.5%–1%/y) but this risk is higher if the VAF is greater than or equal to age 10%. There is also an increased risk of cardiovascular deaths and all-cause mortality. The most common nucleotide change in the mutation is a cytosine-to-thymine (C→T) transition that is a mutational feature of aging.

Recent studies have demonstrated through different methodological approaches that clonal hematopoiesis can be detected in an even higher proportion of healthy individuals than previously reported. Buscarlet and colleagues[49] targeted 19 AML-specific genes with increased depth of sequencing in 2530 hematologically normal individuals and demonstrated somatic mutations, notably in *DNMT3A* and *TET2*, with a 2 times to 3 times higher incidence than previously reported (in 14.8% of individuals ages 70–79, 24.5% in ages 80–89%, and 42.9% in ages greater than 90 years). Another study of 11,262 Icelanders used the approach of whole-genome sequencing with barcoding of somatic mutations to detect mutations in 12.5% of individuals, rising to greater than 50% in individuals aged greater than 85 years. Again, the most frequent genes mutated were *TET2, DNMT3A, ASXL1,* and *PPMID*, with low VAF (mean 0.17).[50] Using ultradeep sequencing, a further study detected somatic mutations in the majority of older healthy adults.[51] These recent observations thus need to be taken into account in the interpretation of the earlier findings reported in AA patients. Additionally, among individuals with ARCH, it is not known how many have had bone marrow assessment to determine whether bone marrow hypocellularity causing proliferative stress may be a contributing factor to selection of these mutated clones.

SOMATIC MUTATIONS IN APLASTIC ANEMIA ASSOCIATED WITH MYELOID MALIGNANCIES

Following the initial early studies,[52,53] from large studies in adult AA patients, somatic mutations in MDS-associated genes have been reported in up to 33% of patients, most frequently involving *ASXL1, BCOR/BCORL1,* and *DNMT3A*.[36,37,54,55] In contrast to MDS, the mutant clone size is smaller, with median VAF of 9.3% to 20%, and in 1 study the median VAF was less than 10% in 40% of patients. Differences are also seen in the type of mutations, with under-representation of *TET2, JAK2, RUNX1,* and *TP53* in AA (**Fig. 1**).[36,37,45–47,56,57] The number of mutations per patient is lower in AA than in MDS, typically 1 per patient compared with a median of 3 in MDS. The clones are often stable over time and may sometimes disappear. For example, *DNMT3A* or *ASXL1* mutated clone size may increase over time but not in all cases, whereas *BCOR/BCORL1* or *PIGA* mutated clones are more likely to decrease or remain stable.[37]

Thus far, the impact of somatic mutations in AA on clinical and hematological outcomes is not completely predictable. In Yoshizato and colleagues' study,[37] so-called unfavorable mutations (*DNMT3A, ASXL1, TP53, RUNX1,* and *CSMD1*) treated with IST showed worse response, overall survival, and progression-free survival compared with favorable mutations (*PIGA* and *BCOR/BCORL1*). In those patients studied serially, the same mutations detected at diagnosis were present at 6 months post-IST

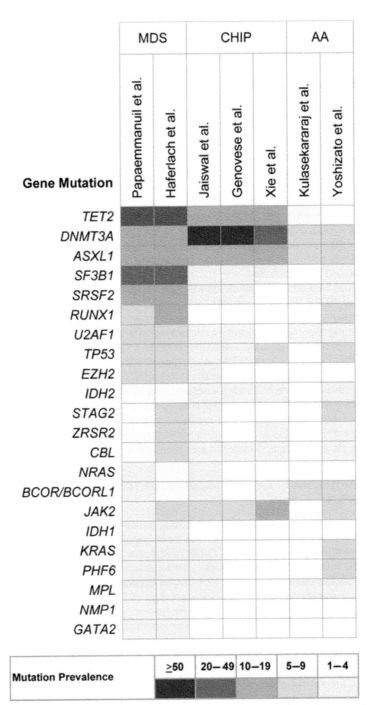

Fig. 1. Frequency of recurrent somatic mutations in MDS, CHIP, and AA. (*From* Malcovati L, Cazzola M. The shadowlands of MDS: idiopathic cytopenias of undetermined significance (ICUS) and clonal hematopoiesis of indeterminate potential (CHIP). Hematology Am Soc Hematol Educ Progam 2015;2015(1):300; with permission.)

although at lower VAF at diagnosis. Unfavorable mutations did not, however, predict later development of MDS/AML but worse survival-free from MDS/AML.[37] In contrast, the study by Kulasekararaj and colleagues[36] examined patients after IST and showed that the presence of a mutation was associated with a significantly increased risk of transformation to MDS/AML, especially in patients with a history of AA for greater than 6 months (40% compared with 4% in patients lacking a mutation), when considering all somatic mutations together. Larger numbers of patients need to be analyzed and with serial sampling, including monitoring of low level clones to determine their true significance.

The impact of age on somatic mutations in AA patients is especially relevant, because, as discussed previously, somatic mutations typical of MDS also occur with increasing frequency in healthy older individuals. The incidence of myeloid-associated mutations in AA, but not *PIGA* or *BCOR/BCORL1* mutations, increases with age.[37] Furthermore, in the older Japanese cohort (median age 60 years), there was a higher incidence of *DNMT3A*, *TET2*, and spliceosome mutations compared with the younger cohort from NIH (median age 29.5 years). Similar to what is seen in AML and normal aging, mutations commonly involved C → T nucleotide transitions at CpG sites.

Ethnicity also seems to have an impact on the type of somatic mutation in AA. Among 210 Korean patients followed-up for at least 8 months after treatment, NGS was performed in 70, of whom 23 (33%) had a mutation. In contrast to the previously described studies of predominantly white patients, the most frequent mutations found were *NOTCH1* in 4 (17.4%), *NF1* in 3 (13%), SCRIB in 3 (13%), and 2 patients each had *BCOR* or *DIS3* or *DNMT3A* (8.7%). There were no cases of *ASXL1* or *TET2*, and 1 case of spliceosome (U2AF1) mutation. For all mutations together, the presence of any mutation did not have an impact on on overall survival or response to IST. In contrast, the presence of either a *NOTCH1* or *DNMT3A* mutations was an independent adverse risk factor for survival.[54] A study from China analyzed 138 AA patients specifically for *ASXL1, TET2, RUNX1, TP53, KRAS*, and *NRAS* mutations by direct sequencing, at some stage of their disease. A mutation was detected in 24 (17.4%) of patients, exclusively involving either *ASXL1* in 14 patients (10%) or *TET2* in 10 (7.3%). *ASXL1* mutations were associated with a higher risk of disease progression to MDS compared with patients who lacked *ASXL1* mutation (33% vs 8%), in contrast to other studies.[55] In addition to ethnicity, some of the differences seen in this study, compared with those from King's College Hospital and NIH/Japan, are that a younger group of patients was analyzed hence raising the possibility that some may have undiagnosed constitutional AA, and the focus was on large clones because Sanger sequencing was used in contrast to next-generation sequencing (NGS) in the other studies.[2]

The relevance of low-level mutations in the setting of AA in terms of whether they are predictive of disease evolution is unclear, especially in light of more recent knowledge concerning ARCH. Furthermore, not infrequently, low-level cytogenetic and PNH clones are detected in AA, some of which may even spontaneously disappear over time.[2,19] It has been proposed that preexisting (low-level) age-related mutations may act as a substrate for clonal selection in the presence of increased proliferative HSC stress in a hypocellular bone marrow.[2] Alternately, or in addition, low-level mutations may later acquire cooperating mutations that result in clonal expansion and malignant transformation to MDS/AML. The lack of cooperating mutations might explain the lack of progression to MDS in white patients with low-level *ASXL* and *DNMT3A*. Serially, characterization of the evolving clonal architecture and mutation hierarchy at the genomic level, and the prognostic significance of specific mutations, size of clone, and multiple clones need to be determined. Furthermore, understanding the role of the immune response in modulating the fate of abnormal clones (in particular low-level clones) during the course of the disease, is of major importance. These questions are being addressed in a multicenter European prospective randomized trial of first-line horse antithymocyte globulin and cyclosporine with or without eltrombopag (ClinicalTrials.gov number, NCT02099747). Serial samples from this trial will be examined for somatic mutations including low-level clones (down to a level of 0.1%–0.5% VAF). Of further importance will be an evaluation of the immune response to these clones, using high-dimensional immune phenotyping by mass cytometry with CyTOF, and the impact of neoantigens.

Short telomeres are found in approximately 30% of AA patients in the absence of a germ-line telomere gene mutation and increase the risk of later MDS/AML after IST [29,39,58] Several studies have shown that the telomere length (TL) is significantly shorter in those AA patients with a somatic mutation compared with patients lacking a mutation.[36,54] Short TL present at diagnosis preceded later acquisition of myeloid-specific somatic mutations, monosomy 7 and subsequent MDS/AML.[59] Accelerated telomere attrition results in genomic instability and represents an important additional risk factor for later clonal transformation.

HYPOCELLULAR MYELODYSPLASTIC SYNDROME AND THE OVERLAP BETWEEN APLASTIC ANEMIA AND MYELODYSPLASTIC SYNDROME

The entity of hypocellular MDS represents a challenging diagnosis and is not included in the World Health Organization classification but accounts for approximately 10% to 20% of MDS patients.[12,60] It has a higher response rate to IST and more favorable prognosis compared with normocellular or hypercellular MDS (n-MDS). Hypocellular MDS is often difficult to distinguish on morphologic and cytogenetic grounds from AA, especially its nonsevere subtype (NSAA) and in older patients. The immune signature of NSAA differs from SAA/very severe AA in that there is a higher number and frequency of Tregs and a lower number of T_H2 and T_H17 cells (and a trend for lower T_H1 cells), indicating a less inflammatory immune response that may favor immune escape of somatic mutations.[4]

In a joint collaboration between King's College Hospital and University of Pavia, an interim analysis on 282 patients with hypocellular MDS, defined by reduced age-adjusted bone marrow cellularity of less than or equal to 25%, has compared the clinical, hematological, cytogenetic, and molecular features with AA and n-MDS. Compared with MDS, hypocellular MDS patients had a higher prevalence of PNH clones but lower than in AA patients. They had a significantly lower risk of leukemic evolution compared with n-MDS but higher than for AA. Targeted sequencing of 24 myeloid-specific genes demonstrated a somatic mutation in 34% of patients. Both the number of mutations per patient and the VAF were significantly lower than n-MDS and significantly higher than in AA. A scoring system was developed based on morphology and immunohistochemistry that predicts for cytogenetic abnormalities, somatic mutations, and risk of leukemic transformation. This enabled the identification of 2 groups of hypocellular MDS patients, 1 with high risk of leukemic evolution and the other with features more closely seen in AA with no evidence of clonal cytogenetic or mutational abnormalities, better overall survival, and low risk of leukemic progression.[61]

STAT3 SOMATIC MUTATIONS IN APLASTIC ANEMIA ASSOCIATED WITH T-CELL LARGE GRANULAR LYMPHOCYTIC LEUKEMIA CLONES

Low-level STAT3 clones can also be detected in a small proportion AA (7%) and MDS (2.5%) patients with unsuspected T-cell large granular lymphocytic leukemia (T-LGL).

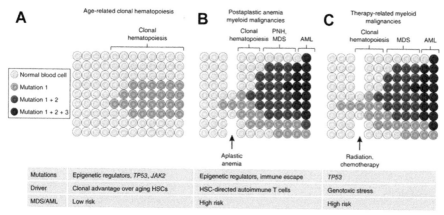

Fig. 2. Clonal hematopoiesis in aging, bone marrow failure, and therapy-related leukemia. (A) In aging, clonal hematopoiesis emerges from mutations in epigenetic regulators (*DNMT3A*, *TET2*, and *ASXL1*), splicing factors (*SF3B1* and *SRSF2*) and other genes, such as *TP53* and *JAK2*. The selection driver is the clonal advantage of mutant cells over aging HSCs, and the risk to progression to MDS and transformation to AML is low. (B) In individuals with AA, clonal hematopoiesis emerges from mutations in epigenetic regulators plus specific cytogenetic abnormalities (MDS) or from genetic events linked with immune escape in patients with PNH. Both MDS and PNH are clonal disorders and represent independent complications that arise during AA evolution, but they rarely coexist. The clonal-selection driver is the autoimmune attack by CTLs of HSCs and the risk of transformation to AML is high. (C) Therapy-related myeloid malignancies are characterized by high prevalence of *TP53* mutations, and the selection driver for clonal hematopoiesis is genotoxic stress. In this case, clonal hematopoiesis increases the risk of therapy-related MDS/AML, but there are cases in which direct clonal evolution does not occur. (*From* Ferrando AA, López-Otín C. Clonal evolution in leukemia. Nat Med 2017;23(10):1138; with permission.)

The *STAT3* somatic mutations are present in the cytotoxic T-lymphocyte (CD3+, CD8+, and CD56+) compartment and in the Vβ expanded population. It has been postulated that the STAT3 T-LGL clone may be the cause of the immune attack by facilitating a persistently dysregulated autoimmune activation leading to marrow failure, although paradoxically such patients showed a trend toward better response to IST and are more likely to be HLADR15 positive. The presence of a *STAT3* mutation does not have an impact on overall survival in AA patients. It is not known if the risk of later MDS/AML is affected by the presence of *STAT3* mutations among AA patients, although a higher frequency of abnormalities of chromosome 7 was observed in MDS patients with a *STAT3* mutation compared with patients lacking a *STAT3* mutation.[62]

SUMMARY

The recent use of NGS to assess clonal hematopoiesis in AA has shown that somatic mutations can be detected in up to 50% of patients, with myeloid-specific mutations in approximately one-third of patients. Similar mutations are associated with aging, where the mutant cells have a clonal advantage over the aging HSCs and the risk of later progression to MDS/AML is low. In contrast in AA, the autoimmune attack on HSCs drives the emergence of somatic mutations and there is a higher risk of progression to MDS/AML in the presence of unfavorable mutations, such as *ASXL1* and *DNMT3A* (Fig. 2).[63] Favorable somatic mutations in *PIGA* and *BCOR/BCORL1* in AA represent clones that have escaped the immune attack process and are associated with response to IST and low risk of MDS/AML progression. Key to the interpretation of myeloid-specific mutations in AA and their potential impact on progression to MDS/AML is the future understanding of the immune mechanism for these mutations, including the role of mutation-related neoantigens. A future goal is to provide a better and more personalized approach to treatment, for example, with the detection of significant somatic mutations prior to the onset of MDS/AML, so that early HSC transplantation might be considered as a possible treatment option instead of IST.[64]

ACKNOWLEDGMENTS

The authors acknowledge the funding from Bloodwise, UK, programme grants 10024 and 14017.

REFERENCES

1. Young NS, Calado RT, Scheinberg P. Current concepts in the pathophysiology and treatment of aplastic anaemia. Blood 2006;108:509–19.
2. Stanley N, Olson TS, Babushok DV. Recent advances in understanding clonal haematopoiesis in aplastic anaemia. Br J Haematol 2017;177:509–25.
3. Shimamura A. Aplastic anemia and clonal evolution: germ line and somatic genetics. Hematology Am Soc Hematol Educ Program 2016;2016:74–82.
4. Kordasti S, Marsh J, Al-Khan S, et al. Functional characterization of CD4+ T-cells in aplastic anemia. Blood 2012;119:2033–43.
5. Solomou EE, Rezvani K, Mielke S, et al. Deficient CD4+ CD25+ FOXP3+ T regulatory cells in acquired aplastic anaemia. Blood 2007;110:1603–6.
6. de Latour RP, Visconte V, Takaku T, et al. Th17 immune responses contribute to the pathophysiology of aplastic anemia. Blood 2010;116:4175–84.
7. Shi J, Lu S, Li X, et al. Intrinsic impairment of CD4+CD25+ regulatory T cells in acquired aplastic anemia. Blood 2012;120:1624–32.
8. Scheinberg P, Nunez O, Weinstein B, et al. Horse versus rabbit antithymocyte globulin in acquired aplastic anemia. N Engl J Med 2011;365:430–8.
9. Rosenfeld S, Follmann D, Nunez O, et al. Antithymocyte globulin and cyclosporine for severe aplastic anemia: association between hematologic response and long-term outcome. JAMA 2003;289:1130–5.
10. Frickhofen N, Heimpel H, Kaltwasser JP, et al, German Aplastic Anemia Study Group. Antithymocyte globulin with or without cyclosporin A: 11-year follow-up of a randomized trial comparing treatments of aplastic anemia. Blood 2003; 101:1236–42.
11. Kordasti S, Costantini B, Seidl T, et al. Deep-phenotyping of Tregs identifies an immune signature for idiopathic aplastic anemia and predicts response to treatment. Blood 2016;128:1193–205.
12. Bennett JM, Orazi A. Diagnostic criteria to distinguish hypocellular acute myeloid leukemia from hypocellular myelodysplastic syndromes and aplastic anemia: recommendations for a standardized approach. Haematologica 2009;94:264–8.
13. Socié G, Henry-Amar M, Bacigalupo A, et al. Malignant tumors occurring after treatment of aplastic anemia. European bone marrow transplantation-severe aplastic anaemia working party. N Engl J Med 1993;329:1152–7.
14. Hackl H, Charoentong P, Finotello F, et al. Computational genomics tools for dissecting tumour-immune cell interactions. Nat Rev Genet 2016;17:441–58.
15. Kordasti SY, Ingram W, Hayden J, et al. CD4+CD25high Foxp3+ regulatory T-cells in myelodysplastic syndrome (MDS). Blood 2007;110(3):847–50.

16. Kordasti SY, Afzali B, Lim Z, et al. IL-17-producing CD4 (+) T-cells, pro-inflammatory cytokines and apoptosis are increased in low-risk myelodysplastic syndrome. Br J Haematol 2009;145:64–72.

17. Coates T, Smith AE, Mourikis A, et al. Neoantigens in MDS are associated with two novel CD4+ T cell subsets and improved overall survival. ASH Annual Scientific Meeting abstract 2017.

18. Sloand EM, Pfannes L, Chen G, et al. CD34 cells from patients with trisomy 8 myelodysplastic syndrome (MDS) express early apoptotic markers but avoid programmed cell death by up-regulation of antiapoptotic proteins. Blood 2007;109:2399–405.

19. Sugimori C, Mochizuki K, Qi Z, et al. Origin and fate of blood cells deficient in glycosylphosphatidylinositol-anchored protein among patients with bone marrow failure. Br J Haematol 2009;147:102–12.

20. Katagiri T, Sato-Otsubo A, Kashiwase K, et al. Frequent loss of HLA alleles associated with copy number-neutral 6pLOH in acquired aplastic anemia. Blood 2011;118:6601–9.

21. Hosokawa K, Katagiri T, Sugimori N, et al. Favorable outcome of patients who have 13q deletion: a suggestion for revision of the WHO 'MDS-U' designation. Haematologica 2012;97:1845–9.

22. Holbro A, Jotterand M, Passweg J, et al. Comment to "Favorable outcome of patients who have 13q deletion: a suggestion for revision of the WHO 'MDS-U' designation" Haematologica. 2012;97(12):1845–9. Haematologica 2013;98(4):e46–7.

23. Furman D, Pascucci B, Parlanti E, et al. Expression of specific inflammasome gene modules stratifies older individuals into two extreme clinical and immunological states. Nat Med 2017;23:174–84.

24. Montané E, Ibáñez L, Vidal X, et al. Epidemiology of aplastic anemia: a prospective multicenter study. Haematologica 2008;93:518–23.

25. Vaht K, Göransson M, Carlson K, et al. Incidence and outcome of acquired aplastic anemia-real-world data from patients diagnosed in Sweden from 2000-2011. Haematologica 2017. https://doi.org/10.3324/haematol.2017.169862.

26. Maciejewski JP, Risitano A, Sloand EM, et al. Distinct clinical outcomes for cytogenetic abnormalities evolving from aplastic anemia. Blood 2002;99:3129–35.

27. Maciejewski JP, Mufti GJ. Whole genome scanning as a cytogenetic tool in hematologic malignancies. Blood 2008;112:965–74.

28. Alter BP, Giri N, Savage SA, et al. Telomere length in inherited bone marrow failure syndromes. Haematologica 2015;100:49–54.

29. Townsley DM, Dimitriu B, Young NS. Bone marrow failure and the telomeropathies. Blood 2014;124:2775–83.

30. Calado RT, Cooper JN, Padilla-Nash HM, et al. Short telomeres result in chromosomal instability in hematopoietic cells and precede malignant evolution in human aplastic anemia. Leukemia 2012;26:700–7.

31. Sugimori C, Chuhjo T, Feng X, et al. Minor population of CD55-CD59- blood cells predicts response to immunosuppressive therapy and prognosis in patients with aplastic anemia. Blood 2006;107:1308–14.

32. Kulagin A, Lisukov I, Ivanova M, et al. Prognostic value of paroxysmal nocturnal haemoglobinuria clone presence in aplastic anaemia patients treated with combined immunosuppression: results of two-centre prospective study. Br J Haematol 2014;164:546–54.

33. Loschi M, Porcher R, Barraco F, et al. Impact of eculizumab treatment on paroxysmal nocturnal hemoglobinuria: a treatment versus no-treatment study. Am J Hematol 2016;91:366–70.

34. Gargiulo L, Papaioannou M, Sica M, et al. Glycosylphosphatidylinositol-specific, CD1d-restricted T cells in paroxysmal nocturnal hemoglobinuria. Blood 2013;121: 2753–61.

35. Gargiulo L, Zaimoku Y, Scappini B, et al. Glycosylphosphatidylinositol-specific T cells, IFN-γ-producing T cells, and pathogenesis of idiopathic aplastic anemia. Blood 2017;129:388–92.

36. Kulasekararaj AG, Jiang J, Smith AE, et al. Somatic mutations identify a subgroup of aplastic anemia patients who progress to myelodysplastic syndrome. Blood 2014;124:2698–704.

37. Yoshizato T, Dumitriu B, Hosokawa K, et al. Somatic mutations and clonal hematopoiesis in aplastic anaemia. N Engl J Med 2015;373:35.

38. Mortazavi Y, Merk B, McIntosh J, et al, for the BIOMED II Pathophysiology and Treatment of Aplastic Anaemia Study Group. The spectrum of PIG-A gene mutations in aplastic anaemia/paroxysmal nocturnal haemoglobinuria (AA/PNH): a high incidence of multiple mutations and evidence of a mutational hotspot. Blood 2003;101:2833–41.

39. Araten DJ, Nafa K, Pakdeesuwan K, et al. Clonal populations of hematopoietic cells with paroxysmal nocturnal hemoglobinuria genotype and phenotype are present in normal individuals. Proc Natl Acad Sci U S A 1999;96:5209–14.

40. Nakao S, Takamatsu H, Chuhjo T, et al. Identification of a specific HLA class II haplotype strongly associated with susceptibility to cyclosporine-dependent aplastic anemia. Blood 1994;84:4257–61.

41. Zaimoku Y, Takamatsu H, Hosomichi K, et al. Identification of an HLA class I allele closely involved in the autoantigen presentation in acquired aplastic anemia. Blood 2017;129:2908–16.

42. Babushok DV, Duke JL, Xie HM, et al. Somatic HLA Mutations expose the role of class I-mediated autoimmunity in aplastic anemia and its clonal complications. Blood Adv 2017;1:1900–10.

43. Babushok DV, Perdigones N, Perin JC, et al. Emergence of clonal hematopoiesis in the majority of patients with acquired aplastic anemia. Cancer Genet 2015;208: 115–28.

44. Damm F, Chesnais V, Nagaata Y, et al. BCOR and BCORL1 mutations in myelodysplastic syndromes and related disorders. Blood 2013;122:3169–77.

45. Jaiswal S, Fontanillas P, Flannick J, et al. Age-related clonal hematopoiesis associated with adverse outcomes. N Engl J Med 2014;371:2488–98.

46. Genovese G, Kahler AK, Handsaker RE, et al. Clonal hematopoiesis and blood-cancer risk Inferred from blood DNA sequence. N Engl J Med 2014;371:2477–87.

47. Xie M, Lu C, Wang J, et al. Age-related mutations associated with clonal hematopoietic expansion and malignancies. Nat Med 2014;20:1472–8.

48. Steensma DP, Bejar R, Jaiswal S, et al. Clonal hematopoiesis of indeterminate potential and its distinction from myelodysplastic syndrome. Blood 2015;126:9–16.

49. Buscarlet M, Provost S, Zada YF, et al. DNMT3A and TET2 dominate clonal hematopoiesis and demonstrate benign phenotypes and different genetic predispositions. Blood 2017;130:753–62.

50. Zink F, Stacey SN, Norddahl GL, et al. Clonal hematopoiesis, with and without candidate driver mutations, is common in the elderly. Blood 2017;130:742–52.

51. Young AL, Challen GA, Birmann BM, et al. Clonal haematopoiesis harbouring AML-associated mutations is ubiquitous in healthy adults. Nat Commun 2016;7: 12484.
52. Lane AA, Odejide O, Kopp N, et al. Low frequency clonal mutations recoverable by deep sequencing in patients with aplastic anemia. Leukemia 2013;27:968–71.
53. Heuser M, Schlarmann C, Dobbernack V, et al. Genetic characterization of acquired aplastic anemia by targeted sequencing. Haematologica 2014;99:e165–7.
54. Park HS, Park SN, Im K, et al. Telomere length and somatic mutations in correlation with response to immunosuppressive treatment in aplastic anaemia. Br J Haematol 2017;178:603–15.
55. Huang J, Ge M, Lu S, et al. Mutations of ASXL1 and TET2 in aplastic anemia. Haematologica 2015;100(5):e172–5.
56. Papaemmanvil E, Gersting M, Malcocati L, et al. Clinical and biological implications of driver mutations in myelodysplastic syndromes. Blood 2013;122(22): 3616–27.
57. Haferlach T, Nagata Y, Grossmann V, et al. Landscape of genetic lesions in 944 patients with myelodysplastic syndromes. Leukemia 2014;28(2):241–7.
58. Scheinberg P, Cooper JN, Sloand EM, et al. Association of telomere length of peripheral blood leukocytes with hematopoietic relapse, malignant transformation, and survival in severe aplastic anemia. JAMA 2010;304:1358–64.
59. Dumitriu B, Feng X, Townsley DM, et al. Telomere attrition and candidate gene mutations preceding monosomy 7 in aplastic anemia. Blood 2015;125:706–9.
60. Tong WG, Quintas-Cardama A, Kadia T, et al. Predicting survival of patients with hypocellular myelodysplastic syndrome: development of a disease-specific prognostic score system. Cancer 2012;118:4462–70.
61. Bono E, McLornan DP, Travaglino E, et al. Hypoplastic myelodysplastic syndrome: combined clinical, histopathological and molecular characterization. Blood 2017, Annual Scientific Meeting of American Society Hematology abstract.
62. Jerez A, Clemente MJ, Makishima H, et al. STAT3 mutations indicate the presence of subclinical T-cell clones in a subset of aplastic anemia and myelodysplastic syndrome patients. Blood 2013;122:2453–9.
63. Ferrando AA, Lopez-Otin C. Clonal evolution in leukemia. Nat Med 2017;23: 1135–45.
64. Ogawa S. Clonal hematopoiesis in acquired aplastic anemia. Blood 2016;128: 337–47.

Recent Advances and Long-Term Results of Medical Treatment of Acquired Aplastic Anemia: Are Patients Cured?

Phillip Scheinberg, MD

KEYWORDS

- Aplastic anemia • Eltrombopag • Immunosuppressive therapy
- Antithymocyte globulin • Cyclosporine • Bone marrow failure

KEY POINTS

- Horse antithymocyte globulin plus cyclosporine remains the current standard immunosuppressive regimen despite many efforts to improve beyond it.
- The thrombopoietin receptor agonist eltrombopag has shown significant activity as a single agent in treatment of refractory patients with hematologic response rates of 40% to 50%.
- When eltrombopag was combined with horse antithymocyte globulin plus cyclosporine in first line (3-drug regimen), overall and complete hematologic response rates were higher than what is observed with immunosuppression alone.
- Late events of relapse and clonal evolution thus far with the 3-drug regimen are in accordance with a vast long-term experience with horse antithymocyte globulin plus cyclosporine alone.
- Longer follow-up will be important to determine durability of response and possible cure rates following the novel regimen, which combines standard immunosuppression with eltrombopag.

INTRODUCTION

For most of the twentieth century, aplastic anemia (AA) was perceived as a disease caused by certain environmental exposures, chemicals (benzene), drugs (chloramphenicol, dipyrone), and/or toxins (pesticides).[1] Several early reports associated the onset of AA to these exposures, but many lacked strong scientific and statistical rigor. The first suggestion that the immune system might be implicated in AA pathogenesis

Disclosures: Advisory, Speaker for Novartis.
Division of Hematology, Hospital A Beneficência Portuguesa, Rua Martiniano de Carvalho, 951, São Paulo 01321-001, Brazil
E-mail address: phillip.scheinberg@bp.org.br

Hematol Oncol Clin N Am 32 (2018) 609–618
https://doi.org/10.1016/j.hoc.2018.03.003
0889-8588/18/© 2018 Elsevier Inc. All rights reserved.

derived from experimental models by Mole in 1964 wherein lymph node cells from C3H/H mice were infused into sublethally irradiated CBA/H mice, which died a few weeks later from pancytopenia.[2] This phenotype resembled AA and suggested that a similar phenomenon could be contributing in humans.

An immune pathogenesis in humans was later inferred in the 1970s when recovery of hematopoiesis was observed in patients who failed to engraft after hematopoietic stem cell transplantation (HSCT).[3] Therapies used in the conditioning, such as antithymocyte globulin (ATG), were credited for the recovery in bone marrow function. Several clinical protocols conducted in Europe, Asia, and the United States in the 1980s and 1990s confirmed the effectiveness of ATG as therapy in severe aplastic anemia (SAA). The addition of cyclosporine (CsA) further increased the hematologic response rate from 40% to 50% (with ATG alone) to 60% to 70% (with the combination of ATG plus CsA). The regimen most studied was based on horse antithymocyte globulin (h-ATG), which has been shown to be the most effective formulation.[4] This combined immunosuppressive therapy (IST) changed the natural history of SAA.

PATHOGENESIS
Immune System

Hematopoiesis is severely reduced in AA, as evidenced by bone marrow specimens, $CD34^+$ cell enumeration, imaging techniques (MRI), or progenitor colony assays. Clinical and laboratory studies suggest that most acquired AA is secondary to immunologically mediated destruction of hematopoietic cells by cytotoxic lymphocytes and their cytokine products, especially interferon-γ (IFN-γ) and tumor necrosis factor-α (TNF-α).

Recognition of hematopoietic stem cells (HSCs) by immune effector cells has been considered to be responsible for the pathogenesis of AA.[5,6] T-helper 1 (Th1)- and Th17-associated inflammatory proteins such as IFN-γ and TNF-α have been shown to be increased and contribute to the destruction of early progenitor cells via a Fas-dependent pathway.[7–12] Skewing of the $CD8^+$ T-cell repertoire in SAA supports an antigen-driven expansion of a few oligoclones, which tends to become more normalized (Gaussian) after successful IST.[13] The target antigens however remain elusive. A reduction of regulatory T cells (Treg) and an increase in Th17-related T cells resulting in a high Th17/Treg ratio at diagnosis tends to normalize in patients responding to IST.[8,10] The genetic loss of one HLA haplotype on chromosome 6p suggests further pressure of the immune system and may provide an escape mechanism of $CD8^+$-mediated HSC destruction and clonal evolution, as seen in certain cases of leukemia relapse.[14,15] Several of these observations have been confirmed in murine models corroborating the important contribution of an aberrant immune system in AA pathogenesis.[1,16,17]

Genetics

Nearly 2 decades ago, shortening of leukocyte telomere lengths (TL) were described in patients with apparent acquired AA.[18,19] This biologic characteristic is recognized in children with the constitutional form of bone marrow failure, dyskeratosis congenita; short TL had not been described in adults without classical physical stigmata of an inherited disorder. Sequencing of genes related to the telomerase complex (TERT, TERC, DKC1, RTEL1, TINF2) were found to be mutated, inferring that in some cases a genetic defect associated with constitutional forms of AA could also be contributing to "acquired" AA pathogenesis.[20–23] Initially, TERC and TERT mutations were identified but later other genes of this complex have also been implicated.[24,25] Telomeres are repeated nucleotide sequences at the ends of chromosomes that protect them from damage. Telomeres erode with cell division; thus, TL maintenance is vital for long-term replicative capacity of lymphocytes and HSCs where expression of the catalytic enzyme telomerase is higher.[26] In telomere diseases, accelerated erosion of the ends of the chromosomes at each cell division leads to a syndrome of marrow failure, pulmonary fibrosis, and cirrhosis.[26] Measurement of the TL can be useful in identifying those with an underlying telomeropathy: very short lengths below the 10th and in particular below the first percentile point toward the possibility of a mutation in a telomerase-related gene.[27,28] Sex hormones increase telomerase activity in vitro by upregulating the *TERT* gene.[29] In a clinical trial, danazol was shown to be highly effective in elongating TL in patients with an underlying telomeropathy, which associated in nearly all patients with hematologic recovery.[30]

Germ-line *GATA2* gene mutations, leading to haploinsufficiency, can also occur in patients with AA. In this syndrome, reduction in monocytes, B, and natural killer cells are characteristic, and the clinical phenotype associates with warts and mycobacterial infections, which are not common in acquired AA.[31] The marrow from patients with *GATA2* deficiency is typically hypocellular and shows varying degrees of dysplasia with atypical megakaryocytes and abnormal cytogenetics.[31]

It is not clear if the identification of a genetic defect defines pathogenesis in AA. Patients with very short TL and/or mutations in genes of the telomerase complex appear to respond to IST, suggesting that in these cases an aberrant immune system still contributes to pathogenesis in conjunction with the genetic defect, which are amenable to immunomodulation.[32,33]

TREATMENT
Immunosuppressive Therapy

The combination of h-ATG/CsA is standard first-line IST in SAA.[34] Prospective studies with this regimen defined its success and limitations. About two-thirds of patients will have a hematologic response to h-ATG/CsA; children do better with a response rate of about 70% to 80%, and older patients fare a little worse with a recovery rate of 50% to 60%.[35–39] Relapses occur in one-third of responding patients, which can usually be treated with more immunosuppression.[40,41] Clonal evolution to myelodysplastic syndrome (MDS) occurs in 10% to 15% of patients long term with monosomy 7, del 13q, and 20q common abnormalities. The explanation for this concerning complication is not well understood, but accelerated telomere attrition rate and molecularly defined preexisting clones have been implicated.[32,42–45] Despite these shortcomings, the advent of the h-ATG/CsA regimen significantly improved survival in SAA with approximately 85% of patients alive long term.[34,38]

The most powerful surrogate for survival in SAA is hematologic response to IST.[46,47] Thus, several efforts to improve the response rate by increasing the intensity of immunosuppression were applied in clinical trials. Unfortunately, none of these efforts yielded a better outcome. The addition of a third immunosuppressant (mycophenolate mofetil, sirolimus) to standard h-ATG/CsA did not improve outcomes, and the use of more potent lymphocytotoxic agents (alemtuzumab, rabbit ATG, cyclophosphamide) either did not improve hematologic recovery rates or were prohibitively toxic.[4,48–53] Using a second course of IST in h-ATG/CsA-refractory patients has been successful in about 30% to 40% of cases with either rabbit ATG/CsA or alemtuzumab.[40,48,54] For those who are refractory to an initial course of rabbit ATG/CsA, the salvage rate appears lower at about 20% with a repeat course of IST, further corroborating the notion that the ATG formulation used as first therapy is critical for the recovery of marrow function in SAA.[48,55,56] Thus, when h-ATG/CsA is used, first hematologic response can be achieved in 75% to 85% of cases with one or 2 courses of IST; conversely, when rabbit ATG/CsA is used, recovery can be expected in only about 50% of cases given the lower response to this regimen in frontline and lower salvage rates. In ATG refractory cases, stem cell transplantation has emerged as a preferred salvage regimen, especially in younger patients with a histocompatible donor.[57–59] In older patients (>40 years), complications of HSCT still occur at a higher rate, making non–transplant options more desirable.[57,58] The improved salvageability along with better supportive care (blood bank, antimicrobials, iron chelation) has resulted in improved survival in initial IST-refractory patients at 5 years of about 50% to 60%, which compares favorably to the 20% survival rate in the 1980s and 1990s in this patient population.[46,60]

Overall, only about one-third of patients who are treated with IST are expected to respond and not experience late events of relapse and/or clonal evolution at 10 years.[34] In this group, survival and quality of life are excellent without the need of continued therapy (CsA, growth factors) to maintain adequate blood counts. Most of these patients are likely cured from their SAA. Among those who relapse, improvement in counts can usually be obtained with more immunosuppression because this event does not correlate with worst survival.[46] CsA dose with time can be tapered, improving the tolerability of long-term use; however, some patients become or remain CsA dependent.[61] In general, a more robust hematologic recovery to IST is associated with better long outcomes and fewer late complications.[34,46] Therefore, in recent years, efforts have been directed to improve the hematologic response rate and robustness of recovery to increase the rate of long-term remissions.

Thrombopoietin Receptor Agonist

Refractory severe aplastic anemia

In 2008, 2 thrombopoietin (THPO) receptor agonists, eltrombopag and romiplostim, were approved for chronic ITP. Soon thereafter, a growing rationale ensued for their use in AA. First, MPL or TPOR, the THPO receptor, is expressed on HSC, and THPO is commonly used in vitro along with other cytokines to stimulate HSCs.[62] Second, reduced numbers of HSCs are observed in *MPL* and *THPO* knockout mouse models.[63,64] Third, TPOR is expressed on early progenitor cells, including stem cells.[62] Fourth, patients with loss of function mutations in *MPL* ultimately develop multilineage marrow failure.[65] These observations strongly support a role of THPO in regulating hematopoiesis at a primitive level. However, the very high endogenous THPO levels in patients with SAA argued against the use of a TPOR agonist in AA.[66,67]

A prospective single-arm study was developed exploring the use of eltrombopag in IST-refractory patients. In this pilot study, 25 SAA patients received a starting eltrombopag dose of 50 mg, which was incremented every 2 weeks by 25 mg up to a total dose of 150 mg.[68] Hematologic response was observed in 11 (44%) patients that was multilineage in 7. The responses tended to occur at a dose of 125 or 150 mg daily, a few weeks after starting the drug. In an extension cohort (total n = 43), the response rate remained at about 40%, and multilineage improvements continued to be seen.[69] The increase in marrow cellularity observed among responders and the more than single lineage count recovery suggested that eltrombopag was having a stimulatory effect on HSC and early progenitor cells. Adverse events were few and comprised mainly upper respiratory infection, fever, and musculoskeletal pain.[68,69] An important observation in follow-up was that the drug could be discontinued in some patients who had a more robust recovery without a negative impact in blood counts.[69] Of the 5 patients who met this study criterion, 4 remained in remission for more than 1 year after its discontinuation.[69] Cytogenetic abnormalities have been observed in this IST-refractory cohort with changes that are commonly seen in AA, such as monosomy 7, trisomy 8, and deletion 13q. The cumulative incidence of clonal evolution of about 15% is also similar to what has been reported historically.[69] On the basis of this experience, eltrombopag was approved in SAA patients who show an insufficient response to IST.

First line

A subsequent trial was conducted using the combination of a marrow-stimulating strategy (eltrombopag) to the optimal IST regimen, h-ATG/CsA.[70] The primary endpoint was a complete response (CR) at 6 months, which has been associated with better long-term outcomes and more durable hematologic recoveries.[34]

A starting eltrombopag dose of 150 mg was chosen based on the dose-response data in the earlier phase 1/2 trial and the extension studies. The combination of h-ATG/CsA and eltrombopag raised some concerns for added hepatotoxicity; thus a 2-week delay in starting eltrombopag was designed into the study after initiation of h-ATG/CsA. Eltrombopag and CsA were given for 6 months and then discontinued. The study was divided into 3 cohorts with approximately 30 patients in each. In cohort 1, the overall hematologic response was 80%, of which 33% were CRs. In cohort 2, eltrombopag duration was shortened to 3 months given that most responses in cohort 1 were observed by 3 months and the desire to abbreviate drug exposure given concerns for clonal evolution. In this group, the response rate at 6 months was overall 87% and complete 26%. A small decline in CRs was noted in cohort 2 at 6 months, which led to the resumption of the 6-month course of eltrombopag in cohort 3. In this latter group, eltrombopag was started on day 1 with h-ATG/CsA given that a significant increase in liver enzymes was not observed with the 3-drug combination in cohorts 1 and 2. The best results were observed in this group, cohort 3, with an overall hematologic response rate of 95% and CR of 58% at 6 months. These results represented a near doubling of the CR rate seen in cohorts 1 and 2 and approximately a six-fold rate increase compared with what has been reported consistently with h-ATG/CsA alone.[34] It is worth noting that most responses following IST alone in SAA are partial, with only about 10% of patients achieving a CR at 6 months.[34] It was not expected that the 3-drug combination would lead to such an increase in efficacy by simply anticipating the eltrombopag start by 2 weeks. The quality of life gain resulted from a more robust and quicker hematologic recovery rate, decreasing transfusion burden and need for hospital visits.[70] Exploratory laboratory studies showed an increase in HSCs defined phenotypically months after h-ATG/CsA/eltrombopag, indicating recovery to a more functional and cellular marrow with adequate stem cell numbers.[70] After a median follow-up of 18 months, the overall survival was greater than 95%.

At 6 months, CsA and eltrombopag were discontinued in cohorts 1 and part of 2, after which a higher relapse rate was observed (54%) than what has been reported (30%–40%) in large trials of hATG/CsA in Europe, Asia, and in the United States.[38] An amendment was made midway into cohort 2 that allowed for continuation of a fixed low dose of CsA after 6 months (2 mg/kg), after which the relapse rate decreased significantly to about 15%.[70] The cumulative incidence of clonal evolution in 2 years was approximately 8%, which is very similar to IST regimens that did not contain eltrombopag.[34,70] In some cases, karyotype abnormalities did not correlate with poor counts or with marrow dysplasia. Pretreatment mutations in telomerase and/or myeloid neoplasm related genes were identified in some cases of patients who clonally evolved, but this was not universal.[42,44]

SUMMARY
Long Term: Are Patients Cured?

With h-ATG/CsA alone, the event-free survival is about one-third in all patients, that is, about half of the 70% who respond. Following IST, one-third of responders do not relapse or demonstrate clonal evolution; they are treatment and transfusion free, without the risks associated with cytopenias (durable response) at 10 years.[34] Most of these patients are likely to be cured given that hematologic relapse and clonal evolution are very unlikely to occur after 10 years of follow-up.[34,38,46,71,72] The combination of h-ATG/CsA/eltrombopag started simultaneously on day 1 has produced the best outcomes of any previous regimen investigated in SAA in decades. Robustness of hematologic recovery to IST has been associated with durability of response and decrease in late complications.[34,46] Thus, the higher and more robust recovery observed with the 3-drug combination is anticipated to result in more durable responses than what has been observed with h-ATG/CsA alone. The survival rate of greater than 95% after a median follow-up of 18 months may indicate that this could occur. The principal cause of death in the first year after SAA diagnosis is the failure to improve marrow function with either IST or HSCT. Persistent and severe neutropenia with associated fungal infections remain important concerns.[60] Given the improvement in marrow function in 80% to 90% of cases with the combination of h-ATG/CsA/eltrombopag, it is anticipated that this will translate into event-free and survival benefits.

Long-term follow-up of the eltrombopag trials will be important to determine the rates of relapse and clonal evolution that can occur years later. The continued low-dose use of CsA permitted a significant reduction in relapse rate, and strategies to wean off CsA by using a very gradual taper regimen or switch to another immunosuppressant with tolerizing properties (sirolimus) are being investigated. The more concerning late complication of MDS to date is in accordance with what has been observed with h-ATG/CsA alone. The appearance of cytogenetic abnormalities of unknown significance early after the treatment course (months) is interesting but is not always associated with worsening blood counts, marrow dysplasia, an increase in blasts, or progression to MDS or leukemia. On occasion, some of these abnormal karyotypes can be transient.[70,73] The interpretation of these findings is still uncertain, but it is possible that eltrombopag might be stimulating abnormal preexisting clones not detected at diagnosis, which does not necessarily correlate with progression to MDS or leukemia. The mechanism and relevance of these detected cytogenetic abnormalities might differ from the clonal evolution that occurs years after diagnosis, usually in patients with a continued inflammatory stimulus due to poorly controlled autoimmunity following IST. These definitions will contribute to the durability of response long term (cure rates) following h-ATG/CsA/eltrombopag and help incorporate this novel 3-drug regimen in the treatment paradigm of SAA.

REFERENCES

1. Scheinberg P, Chen J. Aplastic anemia: what have we learned from animal models and from the clinic. Semin Hematol 2013;50(2):156–64.
2. Barnes DW, Mole RH. Aplastic anaemia in sublethally irradiated mice given allogeneic lymph node cells. Br J Haematol 1967;13(4):482–91.

3. Mathe G, Amiel JL, Schwarzenberg L, et al. Bone marrow graft in man after conditioning by antilymphocytic serum. Br Med J 1970;2(5702):131–6.

4. Scheinberg P, Nunez O, Weinstein B, et al. Horse versus rabbit antithymocyte globulin in acquired aplastic anemia. N Engl J Med 2011;365(5):430–8.

5. Maciejewski JP, Selleri C, Sato T, et al. Increased expression of Fas antigen on bone marrow CD34+ cells of patients with aplastic anaemia. Br J Haematol 1995;91(1):245–52.

6. Nakao S, Takami A, Takamatsu H, et al. Isolation of a T-cell clone showing HLA-DRB1*0405-restricted cytotoxicity for hematopoietic cells in a patient with aplastic anemia. Blood 1997;89(10):3691–9.

7. Zoumbos NC, Gascon P, Djeu JY, et al. Circulating activated suppressor T lymphocytes in aplastic anemia. N Engl J Med 1985;312(5):257–65.

8. Solomou EE, Rezvani K, Mielke S, et al. Deficient CD4+ CD25+ FOXP3+ T regulatory cells in acquired aplastic anemia. Blood 2007;110(5):1603–6.

9. Solomou EE, Keyvanfar K, Young NS. T-bet, a Th1 transcription factor, is up-regulated in T cells from patients with aplastic anemia. Blood 2006;107(10):3983–91.

10. de Latour RP, Visconte V, Takaku T, et al. Th17 immune responses contribute to the pathophysiology of aplastic anemia. Blood 2010;116(20):4175–84.

11. Roderick JE, Gonzalez-Perez G, Kuksin CA, et al. Therapeutic targeting of NOTCH signaling ameliorates immune-mediated bone marrow failure of aplastic anemia. J Exp Med 2013;210(7):1311–29.

12. Gu Y, Hu X, Liu C, et al. Interleukin (IL)-17 promotes macrophages to produce IL-8, IL-6 and tumour necrosis factor-alpha in aplastic anaemia. Br J Haematol 2008;142(1):109–14.

13. Risitano AM, Maciejewski JP, Green S, et al. In-vivo dominant immune responses in aplastic anaemia: molecular tracking of putatively pathogenetic T-cell clones by TCR beta-CDR3 sequencing. Lancet 2004;364(9431):355–64.

14. Ogawa S. Clonal hematopoiesis in acquired aplastic anemia. Blood 2016;128(3):337–47.

15. Katagiri T, Sato-Otsubo A, Kashiwase K, et al. Frequent loss of HLA alleles associated with copy number-neutral 6pLOH in acquired aplastic anemia. Blood 2011;118(25):6601–9.

16. Bloom ML, Wolk AG, Simon-Stoos KL, et al. A mouse model of lymphocyte infusion-induced bone marrow failure. Exp Hematol 2004;32(12):1163–72.

17. Omokaro SO, Desierto MJ, Eckhaus MA, et al. Lymphocytes with aberrant expression of Fas or Fas ligand attenuate immune bone marrow failure in a mouse model. J Immunol 2009;182(6):3414–22.

18. Ball SE, Gibson FM, Rizzo S, et al. Progressive telomere shortening in aplastic anemia. Blood 1998;91(10):3582–92.

19. Brummendorf TH, Maciejewski JP, Mak J, et al. Telomere length in leukocyte subpopulations of patients with aplastic anemia. Blood 2001;97(4):895–900.

20. Savage SA, Giri N, Baerlocher GM, et al. TINF2, a component of the shelterin telomere protection complex, is mutated in dyskeratosis congenita. Am J Hum Genet 2008;82(2):501–9.

21. Yamaguchi H, Calado RT, Ly H, et al. Mutations in TERT, the gene for telomerase reverse transcriptase, in aplastic anemia. N Engl J Med 2005;352(14):1413–24.

22. Yamaguchi H, Baerlocher GM, Lansdorp PM, et al. Mutations of the human telomerase RNA gene (TERC) in aplastic anemia and myelodysplastic syndrome. Blood 2003;102(3):916–8.

23. Fogarty PF, Yamaguchi H, Wiestner A, et al. Late presentation of dyskeratosis congenita as apparently acquired aplastic anaemia due to mutations in telomerase RNA. Lancet 2003;362(9396):1628–30.

24. Jones M, Bisht K, Savage SA, et al. The shelterin complex and hematopoiesis. J Clin Invest 2016;126(5):1621–9.

25. Marsh JCW, Gutierrez-Rodrigues F, Cooper J, et al. Heterozygous RTEL1 variants in bone marrow failure and myeloid neoplasms. Blood Adv 2018;2(1):36–48.

26. Calado RT, Young NS. Telomere diseases. N Engl J Med 2009;361(24):2353–65.

27. Townsley DM, Dumitriu B, Young NS. Bone marrow failure and the telomeropathies. Blood 2014;124(18):2775–83.

28. Vulliamy T, Beswick R, Kirwan MJ, et al. Telomere length measurement can distinguish pathogenic from non-pathogenic variants in the shelterin component, TIN2. Clin Genet 2012;81(1):76–81.

29. Calado RT, Yewdell WT, Wilkerson KL, et al. Sex hormones, acting on the TERT gene, increase telomerase activity in human primary hematopoietic cells. Blood 2009;114(11):2236–43.

30. Townsley DM, Dumitriu B, Young NS. Danazol treatment for telomere diseases. N Engl J Med 2016;375(11):1095–6.

31. Ganapathi KA, Townsley DM, Hsu AP, et al. GATA2 deficiency-associated bone marrow disorder differs from idiopathic aplastic anemia. Blood 2015;125(1):56–70.

32. Scheinberg P, Cooper JN, Sloand EM, et al. Association of telomere length of peripheral blood leukocytes with hematopoietic relapse, malignant transformation, and survival in severe aplastic anemia. JAMA 2010;304(12):1358–64.

33. Townsley DM, Dumitriu B, Kajigaya S, et al. Clinical and genetic heterogeneity of telomere diseases. ASH Annual Meeting Abstracts 2012;120(21):2373.

34. Scheinberg P, Young NS. How I treat acquired aplastic anemia. Blood 2012;120(6):1185–96.

35. Tichelli A, Socie G, Henry-Amar M, et al. Effectiveness of immunosuppressive therapy in older patients with aplastic anemia. European Group for Blood and Marrow Transplantation Severe Aplastic Anaemia Working Party. Ann Intern Med 1999;130(3):193–201.

36. Scheinberg P, Wu CO, Nunez O, et al. Long-term outcome of pediatric patients with severe aplastic anemia treated with antithymocyte globulin and cyclosporine. J Pediatr 2008;153(6):814–9.

37. Scheinberg P, Wu CO, Nunez O, et al. Predicting response to immunosuppressive therapy and survival in severe aplastic anaemia. Br J Haematol 2009;144(2):206–16.

38. Young NS, Calado RT, Scheinberg P. Current concepts in the pathophysiology and treatment of aplastic anemia. Blood 2006;108(8):2509–19.

39. Tichelli A, Marsh JC. Treatment of aplastic anaemia in elderly patients aged >60 years. Bone Marrow Transplant 2013;48(2):180–2.

40. Scheinberg P, Nunez O, Young NS. Retreatment with rabbit anti-thymocyte globulin and ciclosporin for patients with relapsed or refractory severe aplastic anaemia. Br J Haematol 2006;133(6):622–7.

41. Tichelli A, Passweg J, Nissen C, et al. Repeated treatment with horse antilymphocyte globulin for severe aplastic anaemia. Br J Haematol 1998;100(2):393–400.

42. Kulasekararaj AG, Jiang J, Smith AE, et al. Somatic mutations identify a subgroup of aplastic anemia patients who progress to myelodysplastic syndrome. Blood 2014;124(17):2698–704.

43. Dumitriu B, Feng X, Townsley DM, et al. Telomere attrition and candidate gene mutations preceding monosomy 7 in aplastic anemia. Blood 2015;125(4):706–9.

44. Yoshizato T, Dumitriu B, Hosokawa K, et al. Somatic mutations and clonal hematopoiesis in aplastic anemia. N Engl J Med 2015;373(1):35–47.

45. Calado RT, Cooper JN, Padilla-Nash HM, et al. Short telomeres result in chromosomal instability in hematopoietic cells and precede malignant evolution in human aplastic anemia. Leukemia 2012;26(4):700–7.

46. Rosenfeld S, Follmann D, Nunez O, et al. Antithymocyte globulin and cyclosporine for severe aplastic anemia: association between hematologic response and long-term outcome. JAMA 2003;289(9):1130–5.

47. Rosenfeld SJ, Kimball J, Vining D, et al. Intensive immunosuppression with antithymocyte globulin and cyclosporine as treatment for severe acquired aplastic anemia. Blood 1995;85(11):3058–65.

48. Scheinberg P, Nunez O, Weinstein B, et al. Activity of alemtuzumab monotherapy in treatment-naive, relapsed, and refractory severe acquired aplastic anemia. Blood 2012;119(2):345–54.

49. Scheinberg P, Wu CO, Nunez O, et al. Treatment of severe aplastic anemia with a combination of horse antithymocyte globulin and cyclosporine, with or without sirolimus: a prospective randomized study. Haematologica 2009;94(3):348–54.

50. Scheinberg P, Nunez O, Wu C, et al. Treatment of severe aplastic anaemia with combined immunosuppression: anti-thymocyte globulin, ciclosporin and mycophenolate mofetil. Br J Haematol 2006;133(6):606–11.

51. Scheinberg P, Townsley D, Dumitriu B, et al. Moderate-dose cyclophosphamide for severe aplastic anemia has significant toxicity and does not prevent relapse and clonal evolution. Blood 2014;124(18):2820–3.

52. Brodsky RA, Chen AR, Dorr D, et al. High-dose cyclophosphamide for severe aplastic anemia: long-term follow-up. Blood 2010;115(11):2136–41.

53. Tisdale JF, Maciejewski JP, Nunez O, et al. Late complications following treatment for severe aplastic anemia (SAA) with high-dose cyclophosphamide (Cy): follow-up of a randomized trial. Blood 2002;100(13):4668–70.

54. Di Bona E, Rodeghiero F, Bruno B, et al. Rabbit antithymocyte globulin (r-ATG) plus cyclosporine and granulocyte colony stimulating factor is an effective treatment for aplastic anaemia patients unresponsive to a first course of intensive immunosuppressive therapy. Gruppo Italiano Trapianto di Midollo Osseo (GITMO). Br J Haematol 1999;107(2):330–4.

55. Cle DV, Atta EH, Dias DS, et al. Repeat course of rabbit antithymocyte globulin as salvage following initial therapy with rabbit antithymocyte globulin in acquired aplastic anemia. Haematologica 2015;100(9):e345–7.

56. Scheinberg P, Townsley D, Dumitriu B, et al. Horse antithymocyte globulin as salvage therapy after rabbit antithymocyte globulin for severe aplastic anemia. Am J Hematol 2014;89(5):467–9.

57. Gupta V, Eapen M, Brazauskas R, et al. Impact of age on outcomes after transplantation for acquired aplastic anemia using HLA-identical sibling donors. Haematologica 2010;95(12):2119–25.

58. Bacigalupo A, Giammarco S, Sica S. Bone marrow transplantation versus immunosuppressive therapy in patients with acquired severe aplastic anemia. Int J Hematol 2016;104(2):168–74.

59. Bacigalupo A. How I treat acquired aplastic anemia. Blood 2017;129(11): 1428–36.

60. Valdez JM, Scheinberg P, Nunez O, et al. Decreased infection-related mortality and improved survival in severe aplastic anemia in the past two decades. Clin Infect Dis 2011;52(6):726–35.
61. Frickhofen N, Rosenfeld SJ. Immunosuppressive treatment of aplastic anemia with antithymocyte globulin and cyclosporine. Semin Hematol 2000;37(1):56–68.
62. Yoshihara H, Arai F, Hosokawa K, et al. Thrombopoietin/MPL signaling regulates hematopoietic stem cell quiescence and interaction with the osteoblastic niche. Cell Stem Cell 2007;1(6):685–97.
63. Alexander WS, Roberts AW, Nicola NA, et al. Deficiencies in progenitor cells of multiple hematopoietic lineages and defective megakaryocytopoiesis in mice lacking the thrombopoietic receptor c-Mpl. Blood 1996;87(6):2162–70.
64. Qian H, Buza-Vidas N, Hyland CD, et al. Critical role of thrombopoietin in maintaining adult quiescent hematopoietic stem cells. Cell Stem Cell 2007;1(6): 671–84.
65. Ballmaier M, Germeshausen M, Krukemeier S, et al. Thrombopoietin is essential for the maintenance of normal hematopoiesis in humans: development of aplastic anemia in patients with congenital amegakaryocytic thrombocytopenia. Ann N Y Acad Sci 2003;996:17–25.
66. Kosugi S, Kurata Y, Tomiyama Y, et al. Circulating thrombopoietin level in chronic immune thrombocytopenic purpura. Br J Haematol 1996;93(3):704–6.
67. Feng X, Scheinberg P, Wu CO, et al. Cytokine signature profiles in acquired aplastic anemia and myelodysplastic syndromes. Haematologica 2011;96(4): 602–6.
68. Olnes MJ, Scheinberg P, Calvo KR, et al. Eltrombopag and improved hematopoiesis in refractory aplastic anemia. N Engl J Med 2012;367(1):11–9.
69. Desmond R, Townsley DM, Dumitriu B, et al. Eltrombopag restores trilineage hematopoiesis in refractory severe aplastic anemia that can be sustained on discontinuation of drug. Blood 2014;123(12):1818–25.
70. Townsley DM, Scheinberg P, Winkler T, et al. Eltrombopag added to standard immunosuppression for aplastic anemia. N Engl J Med 2017;376(16):1540–50.
71. Scheinberg P, Rios O, Scheinberg P, et al. Prolonged cyclosporine administration after antithymocyte globulin delays but does not prevent relapse in severe aplastic anemia. Am J Hematol 2014;89(6):571–4.
72. Tichelli A, Schrezenmeier H, Socie G, et al. A randomized controlled study in patients with newly diagnosed severe aplastic anemia receiving antithymocyte globulin (ATG), cyclosporine, with or without G-CSF: a study of the SAA Working Party of the European Group for Blood and Marrow Transplantation. Blood 2011; 117(17):4434–41.
73. Winkler T, Cooper JN, Townsley DM, et al. Eltrombopag for refractory severe aplastic anemia: dosing regimens, long-term follow-up, clonal evolution and somatic mutation profiling. Blood 2017;130(suppl 1):777.

Upfront Matched Unrelated Donor Transplantation in Aplastic Anemia

Katherine Clesham, MD[1], Robin Dowse, MD[1],
Sujith Samarasinghe, MD, PhD*

KEYWORDS

- Aplastic anemia • Hemopoietic stem cell transplantation (HSCT)
- Matched sibling donor • Matched unrelated donor

KEY POINTS

- Idiopathic severe aplastic anemia (SAA) is a rare condition, and hemopoietic stem cell transplantation (HSCT) remains the only curative therapy.
- HSCT is considered first-line treatment in patients less than 35 years old with SAA with a matched sibling donor (MSD).
- Current best practice is less clear in those without an MSD. Immunosuppressive therapy (IST) has traditionally been thought of as first-line treatment in those without an MSD; however, there remains a significant risk of relapse and clonal evolution.
- Outcomes following matched unrelated donor (MUD) HSCT in SAA have improved because of advances in the development of high-resolution HLA typing, developments in supportive care, and implementation of novel conditioning regimens.
- After careful discussion with the patient and parents, MUD HSCT could be considered first-line treatment in selected patients.

INTRODUCTION

Aplastic anemia (AA), defined by pancytopenia and a hypocellular marrow in the absence of reticulin fibrosis or abnormal infiltration, is a rare disorder with an incidence of approximately 2 per million in Europe.[1] Most cases are idiopathic, with T-cell–mediated destruction of hematopoietic stem cells thought to be the underlying pathophysiology. Without treatment, patients are likely to succumb to infection or hemorrhage. In this review, the authors discuss how to approach one of the outstanding questions in the management of patients with severe aplastic anemia (SAA): "What is the role of

Disclosure Statement: None.
Department of Pediatric Hematology, Camelia Botnar Laboratories, UCL Great Ormond Street Hospital, P2.008, Great Ormond Street, London, WC1N 3JH, UK
[1] The authors contributed equally.
* Corresponding author.
E-mail address: Sujith.Samarasinghe@gosh.nhs.uk

upfront matched unrelated donor hematopoietic stem cell transplant in aplastic anemia?"

TREATMENT OF APLASTIC ANEMIA

Allogeneic hematopoietic stem cell transplant (HSCT) from an HLA matched sibling donor (MSD) is the preferred frontline treatment of pediatric and young adult patients with AA.[1,2] In those lacking such a donor, immunosuppressive therapy (IST) has historically been primary treatment, but with improved outcomes after transplants from matched unrelated donors (MUD), many centers now consider upfront MUD HSCT. Although historically MSD HSCT was associated with a higher overall survival (OS) than IST, this is no longer the case in children because of better salvage of IST failures. Recent studies from Japan and the European Blood and Marrow Transplantation (EBMT) indicate that frontline MSD HSCT leads to a better failure-free survival (FFS) than IST but not OS.[2–4] Therefore, because of the excellent OS seen in pediatric SAA, comparisons between IST and HSCT should focus on event-free survival (EFS) rather than OS.

The use of IST as treatment of AA originates from the observation of autologous marrow reconstitution in patients with graft failure who had undergone HCST with antithymocyte globulin (ATG) conditioning.[5] Current guidelines recommend horse antithymocyte globulin (h-ATG) with cyclosporine (CSA), because combination therapy is superior to ATG alone.[6] Pediatric studies using this combination have reported overall response rates of between 59.9% and 77%.[7–10] Factors influencing response rates are shown in **Box 1**.

The use of the more immunosuppressive rabbit ATG is not recommended outside of relapse/refractory cases because it has been associated with inferior outcomes compared with h-ATG.[8,11–13] Response to IST is evaluated between 3 and 4 months after treatment. If there has been a response, CSA can be weaned slowly from 6 months with frequent monitoring of blood for signs of relapse. Between 15% and 25% of children remain CSA dependent.[9] The monitoring required and ensuing subnormal blood counts may have a detrimental effect on children and their families' quality of life. Relapse rates have been reported in 11.9% to 33% of patients undergoing IST. Current practice is to use MUD HSCT for those failing one course of IST, due to superior EFS compared with a second course of IST.[14] In patients who have had a prior response to IST, in those without a suitable donor, a repeat IST has a response rate of 60% to 70%.[13,15] Between 10% and 15% of patients who have undergone IST

Box 1
Good prognostic factors for response to immunosuppressive therapy

Severity (very severe aplastic anemia better than severe aplastic anemia)

Younger age

Higher reticulocyte and lymphocyte count at diagnosis

Male gender

Leukocyte count $<2 \times 10^9/L$

Early treatment

Minor paroxysmal nocturnal hemoglobinuria clone

Longer telomere length

for AA will go on to develop clonal evolution[8,9] with the development of a significant paroxysmal nocturnal hemoglobinuria (PNH) clone, myelodysplastic syndrome, and/or acute myeloid leukemia (AML). This risk does not plateau, making it of particular concern to the pediatric population. Advantages and disadvantages associated with IST and MUD HSCT are shown in **Tables 1** and **2**.

WHY MATCHED UNRELATED DONOR HEMOPOIETIC STEM CELL TRANSPLANTATION HAS IMPROVED

Outcome after MUD HSCT for SAA has significantly improved over time because of several factors.[16] The availability of "high-resolution" (allelic) HLA molecular typing means that donors who appear equally well matched on serologic testing can be distinguished, thereby reducing rejection and graft-versus-host disease (GVHD) rates, and thus improving OS. Development of less toxic conditioning regimens such as Fludarabine, cyclophosphamide, and Campath (alemtuzumab) (FCC) has also significantly reduced rates of GVHD, while not increasing graft rejection, leading to improvements in OS.[17–19] A large EBMT study recently highlighted that OS for MUD HSCT is now approaching that of MSD HSCT, confirming that these developments were leading to tangible improvements.[20] The authors also recently published a report of 44 successive children who received 10-antigen (HLA-A, -B, -C, -DRB1, -DQB1) MUD HSCTs, 40 of whom had previous IST. HSCT conditioning was an FCC regimen and did not include radiotherapy. There was an excellent estimated 5-year FFS of 95% with low rates of acute and chronic GVHD.[21]

EVIDENCE OF UPFRONT MATCHED UNRELATED DONOR HEMOPOIETIC STEM CELL TRANSPLANTATION IN SEVERE APLASTIC ANEMIA

Following on from the excellent results that were seen in MUD HSCT after IST failure, the authors then determined the outcomes of frontline MUD HSCT. Dufour and colleagues[2] explored the feasibility and safety of upfront MUD transplantation in 29 children (aged between 0.5 and 18.6 years) from a UK cohort who received MUD HSCT (5 patients received mismatched unrelated donor [MMUD] HSCT). These patients lacked an MSD and did not receive prior IST. Outcomes measures were OS and EFS, which were derived from standard definitions used in previous AA publications.[22] Outcomes were compared with matched historical controls who had received:

i. Frontline MSD HSCT
ii. Frontline IST with h-ATG and CSA
iii. MUD HSCT after IST failure as second-line therapy

Time to neutrophil recovery in the MUD cohort was on average 18 days (range 9–29), translating to a median time from diagnosis to neutrophil recovery of 0.39 years.

Table 1	
Factors in favor and against immunosuppressive therapy	
Advantages	**Disadvantages**
Low treatment-related mortality	Treatment failure
Excellent long-term survival	High relapse risk
Salvageable with HSCT	3–4 mo until cellular response
	Partial responses
	Clonal evolution

Table 2
Factors in favor and against front-line matched unrelated donor hemopoietic stem cell transplantation

Advantages	Disadvantages
Only curative option	Graft-versus-host disease
Rapid neutrophil recovery	Difficulty finding donor
Low rates of clonal evolution	Treatment-related mortality
High complete remission rates	Longer initial hospitalization
Improvement in quality of life	

Rates of GVHD were low with FCC. The 1-year cumulative incidence of grade II-IV acute GVHD was 10% ± 6%, and 19% ± 8% chronic GVHD (all cases were limited). One patient experienced graft failure after a 1-antigen mismatched transplant (this patient also had preexisting HLA-A antibodies) and subsequently received a second successful HSCT. There was one death following MUD HSCT, due to idiopathic pneumonia syndrome after engraftment. The remaining 27 patients all achieved a complete remission.

There was no significant difference in OS and EFS between the upfront MUD/MMUD versus MSD controls (96% vs 91%, $P = .3$ and 92% vs 87%, $P = .37$, respectively) (**Fig. 1**). Furthermore, the median interval from diagnosis to neutrophil recovery was similar in the upfront MUD cohort compared to MSD controls ($P = 0.93$). Compared with IST controls, there was no significant difference between the OS seen in frontline MUD HSCT cohort (94% vs 96%, $P = .68$). There was, however, significantly higher EFS in the MUD group versus IST control (92% vs 40%, $P = .0001$) (**Fig. 2**). Last, comparison with MUD HSCT after IST failure controls revealed significantly higher OS and EFS (95% vs 74% for both OS and EFS, $P = .02$) in the upfront MUD group (**Fig. 3**). In the MUD after IST failure controls the median interval between diagnosis and HSCT was 1 year. An interval from diagnosis to HSCT greater than 6 months has been shown to adversely affect survival, and this most likely explains the difference in OS seen between the 2 groups.[20] A short interval between diagnosis and HSCT is desirable

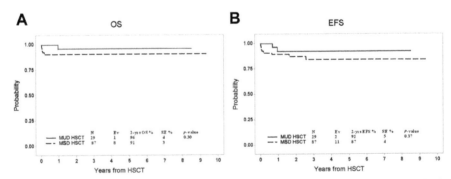

Fig. 1. Outcomes following upfront unrelated donor HSCT are similar to MSD HSCT in childhood idiopathic SAA: (*A*) Kaplan-Meier curve of OS and (*B*) EFS after upfront MUD/MMUD and MSD HSCT controls. (*From* Dufour C, Veys P, Carraro E, et al. Similar outcome of upfront-unrelated and matched sibling stem cell transplantation in idiopathic paediatric aplastic anaemia. A study on behalf of the UK Paediatric BMT Working Party, Paediatric Diseases Working Party and Severe Aplastic Anaemia Working Party of EBMT. Br J Haematol 2015;171(4):589; with permission.)

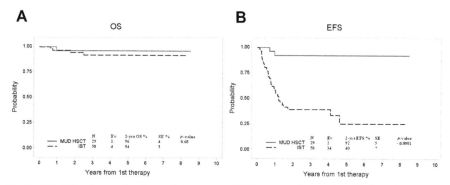

Fig. 2. EFS following upfront unrelated donor HSCT is superior to IST with lymphoglobulin and cyclosporine in childhood idiopathic SAA: (*A*) Kaplan-Meier curve of OS and (*B*) EFS after upfront matched unrelated HSCT and IST controls. (*From* Dufour C, Veys P, Carraro E, et al. Similar outcome of upfront-unrelated and matched sibling stem cell transplantation in idiopathic paediatric aplastic anaemia. A study on behalf of the UK Paediatric BMT Working Party, Paediatric Diseases Working Party and Severe Aplastic Anaemia Working Party of EBMT. Br J Haematol 2015;171(4):590; with permission.)

because it reduces time to acquire infection or development of HLA antibodies from transfusions.

This study and others[17] demonstrate that many of the factors that the previously made frontline MUD HSCT undesirable, that is, severe GVHD, graft failure, treatment-related mortality, are no longer major concerns. Furthermore, the very high complete remission rates seen with MUD HSCT are particularly important in children to enable them to pursue a normal quality of life.

Both the UK studies are limited by being retrospective with the potential for selection bias. To counter this, a US prospective trial (TransIT; trial number NCT02845596) is currently recruiting patients younger than 25 with SAA who lack an MSD to compare IST with h-ATG versus 10/10 or 9/10 MUD HSCT. It is hoped that this study will

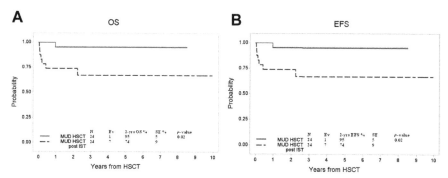

Fig. 3. Superior outcome following upfront unrelated donor HSCT compared with unrelated donor HSCT after IST failure in childhood idiopathic SAA: (*A*) Kaplan-Meier curve of OS and (*B*) EFS after upfront MUD HSCT and after IST failure MUD controls. (*From* Dufour C, Veys P, Carraro E, et al. Similar outcome of upfront-unrelated and matched sibling stem cell transplantation in idiopathic paediatric aplastic anaemia. A study on behalf of the UK Paediatric BMT Working Party, Paediatric Diseases Working Party and Severe Aplastic Anaemia Working Party of EBMT. Br J Haematol 2015;171(4):590; with permission.)

determine the safety and feasibility of frontline MUD HSCT and lead to a comparison of EFS between IST and HSCT.

FACTORS AFFECTING WHETHER TO UNDERTAKE UPFRONT MATCHED UNRELATED DONOR HEMOPOIETIC STEM CELL TRANSPLANTATION

The decision to proceed with MUD or IST should be determined based on patient and donor factors (**Table 3**). Ethnic origin is a major determinant of a patient's likelihood of finding an MUD. In one North American study, donors with a 7 to 8/8 HLA match were found in 90% of white/non-Hispanic patients, 76% of Hispanics, 62% of Black/African Americans, and 33% of Asians.[23] Thus, for some patients from non-Caucasian backgrounds, frontline MUD HSCT may not be a suitable option. Timing is highly relevant in whether to proceed with MUD. Patients should be tissue-typed in the diagnostic workup for SAA to minimize delays in a MUD search if required. If a suitable unrelated donor cannot be found, or delays are anticipated with arranging the donation, then it is preferable to proceed directly to IST, because delays in proceeding with IST could adversely affect response rates.

COUNSELING THE PATIENT AND FAMILY

The study by Dufour and colleagues[2] led the EBMT SAA Working Party and the UK Children's Cancer and Leukemia Group to recommend that if an MUD can be found quickly, then HSCT may be considered an upfront treatment in children who lack an MSD. The UK pediatric idiopathic SAA algorithm is detailed in **Fig. 4**. In the absence of prospective trials, it is crucial to weigh the factors for and against MUD HSCT in each case. It is recommended that all patients with SAA are cared for in centers with specialized experience in the management of children and adolescents with AA. A careful discussion with the patient and family to weigh pros and cons of IST versus frontline MUD HSCT is required. Such counselling can only be done in specialized hematology centers.

ALTERNATIVE STEM CELL SOURCES

Haploidentical transplants are an attractive option because of rapid availability of a potential donor for most children. Retrospective multicenter data comparing haploidentical HSCT with MSD transplants showed similar OS (86.1% vs 91.3%) and FFS (85% vs 89.8%).[24] The haploidentical group did experience significantly higher rates of GVHD; nevertheless, these data points suggest that in experienced centers, frontline haploidentical HSCT is an emerging option especially when h-ATG or an MUD is not readily available.[25,26] A US prospective study (trial number NCT02833805) is currently

Table 3 Factors influencing decision to proceed directly with matched unrelated donor hemopoietic stem cell transplantation	
Patient Factors Favoring MUD over IST	Donors Factors Favoring MUD over IST
Life-threatening infections where rapid and definitive cellular recovery favor HSCT over IST	Donor availability within 3 mo
Presence of cytogenetically abnormal clone suggestive of myelodysplastic syndrome, for example, monosomy 7	Bone marrow as stem cell source
Recurrent fevers/infections	Age of donor <45 y and preferably <30
	Donor not a multiparous woman

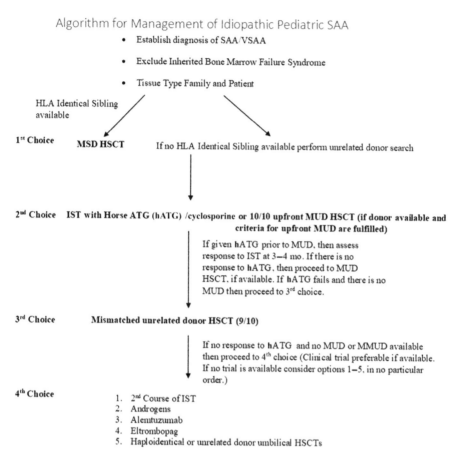

Fig. 4. UK algorithm for children with idiopathic SAA. VSAA, very severe aplastic anemia. (*Adapted from* Samarasinghe S, Veys P, Vora A, et al. Paediatric amendment to adult BSH guidelines for aplastic anaemia. Br J Haematol 2018;180(2):202; with permission.)

recruiting to determine the feasibility and safety of conducting frontline MUD, partially matched and haploidentical HSCT in SAA.

FUTURE DIRECTIONS OF STUDY

Predicting which patients will respond to IST and who might develop clonal evolution may help to refine which patients may benefit from frontline HSCT or IST. A study of 64 children with AA found that short telomere length (STL), as measured by flow cytometry, was a predictor of poor response to IST.[27] A follow-up paper from the same group showed that the presence of a minor PNH clone was a predictor of good response to IST, and this was used to define good-risk (PNH positive and/or longer telomere lengths) and poor-risk (STL and no PNH clone) patients. The good-risk group showed a significantly better response to IST compared with poor risk (70% vs 19%, $P<.001$).[28] A Japanese study is planned to explore frontline transplantation in children who have poor prognostic markers to IST, that is, STL and absence of PNH clone. Other biomarkers of IST response have been investigated. Very high levels of thrombopoietin at diagnosis is an independent predictor of poor response,[29] and the presence of intracellular interferon-gamma in patient lymphocytes may predict a good response to IST.[30]

With the advent of next-generation sequencing, small populations of clonal hematopoiesis have been found in many patients with AA. Specific mutations may be predictive of poor response to IST and/or evolution to MDS/AML via immune escape and increased proliferation.[31] Analysis suggests that BCOR and BCORL1 mutations are associated with a good response to IST, whereas ASXL1, DNMT3A, and RUNX1 mutations are linked with poor progression free survival and OS.[32] Those patients found to harbor these deleterious mutations may benefit most from transplant rather than IST, although this would need to be determined in future studies.

Improving outcomes in those undergoing IST appears to be possible with the addition of eltrombopag, a thrombopoietin mimetic that has induced trilineage hemopoietic recovery in patients with IST-refractory AA.[33] Recent studies have shown that the addition of eltrombopag to IST leads to improved response rates in treatment-naïve patients.[34] Further studies aim to recruit pediatric patients (NCT01623167) to assess efficacy and safety in this group. This development may lead to IST outperforming upfront MUD once again, although clonal evolution remains a potential concern, with some patients in these studies developing monosomy 7 and complex cytogenetic abnormalities.[35]

SUMMARY

Upfront MUD HSCT is a safe and feasible treatment option for children and young adults with AA when a suitable donor is readily available. Thus, all patients who lack an MSD should have a donor search initiated at diagnosis. The decision to proceed with transplant requires careful discussion with the patient and their family and should only be performed in a specialist center experienced in the management of AA.

REFERENCES

1. Killick SB, Bown N, Cavenagh J, et al. Guidelines for the diagnosis and management of adult aplastic anaemia. Br J Haematol 2016;172(2):187–207.
2. Dufour C, Veys P, Carraro E, et al. Similar outcome of upfront-unrelated and matched sibling stem cell transplantation in idiopathic paediatric aplastic anaemia. A study on behalf of the UK Paediatric BMT Working Party, Paediatric Diseases Working Party and Severe Aplastic Anaemia Working Party of EBMT. Br J Haematol 2015;171(4):585–94.
3. Doney K, Leisenring W, Storb R, et al. Primary treatment of acquired aplastic anemia: outcomes with bone marrow transplantation and immunosuppressive therapy. Ann Intern Med 1997;126(2):107–15.
4. Yoshida N, Kobayashi R, Yabe H, et al. First-line treatment for severe aplastic anemia in children: bone marrow transplantation from a matched family donor versus immunosuppressive therapy. Haematologica 2014;99(12):1784–91.
5. Speck B, Gratwohl A, Nissen C, et al. Treatment of severe aplastic anaemia with antilymphocyte globulin or bone-marrow transplantation. Br Med J (Clin Res Ed) 1981;282(6267):860–3.
6. Frickhofen N, Heimpel H, Kaltwasser JP, et al. Antithymocyte globulin with or without cyclosporin A: 11-year follow-up of a randomized trial comparing treatments of aplastic anemia. Blood 2003;101(4):1236–42.

7. Fuhrer M, Rampf U, Baumann I, et al. Immunosuppressive therapy for aplastic anemia in children: a more severe disease predicts better survival. Blood 2005; 106(6):2102-4.
8. Scheinberg P, Nunez O, Wu C, et al. Treatment of severe aplastic anaemia with combined immunosuppression: anti-thymocyte globulin, ciclosporin and mycophenolate mofetil. Br J Haematol 2006;133(6):606-11.
9. Saracco P, Quarello P, Iori AP, et al. Cyclosporin A response and dependence in children with acquired aplastic anaemia: a multicentre retrospective study with long-term observation follow-up. Br J Haematol 2008;140(2):197-205.
10. Kamio T, Ito E, Ohara A, et al. Relapse of aplastic anemia in children after immunosuppressive therapy: a report from the Japan Childhood Aplastic Anemia Study Group. Haematologica 2011;96(6):814-9.
11. Yoshimi A, van den Heuvel-Eibrink MM, Baumann I, et al. Comparison of horse and rabbit antithymocyte globulin in immunosuppressive therapy for refractory cytopenia of childhood. Haematologica 2014;99(4):656-63.
12. Takahashi Y, Muramatsu H, Sakata N, et al. Rabbit antithymocyte globulin and cyclosporine as first-line therapy for children with acquired aplastic anemia. Blood 2013;121(5):862-3.
13. Scheinberg P, Nunez O, Young NS. Retreatment with rabbit anti-thymocyte globulin and ciclosporin for patients with relapsed or refractory severe aplastic anaemia. Br J Haematol 2006;133(6):622-7.
14. Kosaka Y, Yagasaki H, Sano K, et al. Prospective multicenter trial comparing repeated immunosuppressive therapy with stem-cell transplantation from an alternative donor as second-line treatment for children with severe and very severe aplastic anemia. Blood 2008;111(3):1054-9.
15. Tichelli A, Passweg J, Nissen C, et al. Repeated treatment with horse antilymphocyte globulin for severe aplastic anaemia. Br J Haematol 1998;100(2):393-400.
16. Locasciulli A, Oneto R, Bacigalupo A, et al. Outcome of patients with acquired aplastic anemia given first line bone marrow transplantation or immunosuppressive treatment in the last decade: a report from the European Group for Blood and Marrow Transplantation (EBMT). Haematologica 2007;92(1):11-8.
17. Marsh JC, Gupta V, Lim Z, et al. Alemtuzumab with fludarabine and cyclophosphamide reduces chronic graft-versus-host disease after allogeneic stem cell transplantation for acquired aplastic anemia. Blood 2011;118(8):2351-7.
18. Marsh JC, Pearce RM, Koh MB, et al. Retrospective study of alemtuzumab vs ATG-based conditioning without irradiation for unrelated and matched sibling donor transplants in acquired severe aplastic anemia: a study from the British society for blood and marrow transplantation. Bone Marrow Transplant 2014;49(1): 42-8.
19. Samarasinghe S, Iacobelli S, Knol C, et al. Impact of different in vivo T cell depletion strategies on outcomes following hematopoietic stem cell transplantation for idiopathic aplastic anaemia: a study on behalf of the EBMT SAA working party. Blood 2015;126(23):1210.
20. Bacigalupo A, Socie G, Hamladji RM, et al. Current outcome of HLA identical sibling versus unrelated donor transplants in severe aplastic anemia: an EBMT analysis. Haematologica 2015;100(5):696-702.
21. Samarasinghe S, Steward C, Hiwarkar P, et al. Excellent outcome of matched unrelated donor transplantation in paediatric aplastic anaemia following failure with immunosuppressive therapy: a United Kingdom multicentre retrospective experience. Br J Haematol 2012;157(3):339-46.

22. Dufour C, Pillon M, Passweg J, et al. Outcome of aplastic anemia in adolescence: a survey of the severe aplastic anemia working party of the European Group for Blood and Marrow Transplantation. Haematologica 2014;99(10):1574–81.
23. Pidala J, Kim J, Schell M, et al. Race/ethnicity affects the probability of finding an HLA-A, -B, -C and -DRB1 allele-matched unrelated donor and likelihood of subsequent transplant utilization. Bone Marrow Transplant 2013;48(3):346–50.
24. Xu L-P, Jin S, Wang S-Q, et al. Upfront haploidentical transplant for acquired severe aplastic anemia: registry-based comparison with matched related transplant. J Hematol Oncol 2017;10(1):25.
25. Clay J, Kulasekararaj AG, Potter V, et al. Nonmyeloablative peripheral blood haploidentical stem cell transplantation for refractory severe aplastic anemia. Biol Blood Marrow Transplant 2014;20(11):1711–6.
26. Esteves I, Bonfim C, Pasquini R, et al. Haploidentical BMT and post-transplant Cy for severe aplastic anemia: a multicenter retrospective study. Bone Marrow Transplant 2015;50(5):685–9.
27. Sakaguchi H, Nishio N, Hama A, et al. Peripheral blood lymphocyte telomere length as a predictor of response to immunosuppressive therapy in childhood aplastic anemia. Haematologica 2014;99(8):1312–6.
28. Narita A, Muramatsu H, Sekiya Y, et al. Paroxysmal nocturnal hemoglobinuria and telomere length predicts response to immunosuppressive therapy in pediatric aplastic anemia. Haematologica 2015;100(12):1546–52.
29. Elmahdi S, Muramatsu H, Narita A, et al. Markedly high plasma thrombopoietin (TPO) level is a predictor of poor response to immunosuppressive therapy in children with acquired severe aplastic anemia. Pediatr Blood Cancer 2016;63(4): 659–64.
30. Sloand E, Kim S, Maciejewski JP, et al. Intracellular interferon-γ in circulating and marrow T cells detected by flow cytometry and the response to immunosuppressive therapy in patients with aplastic anemia. Blood 2002;100(4):1185–91.
31. Babushok DV, Perdigones N, Perin JC, et al. Emergence of clonal hematopoiesis in the majority of patients with acquired aplastic anemia. Cancer Genet 2015; 208(4):115–28.
32. Yoshizato T, Dumitriu B, Hosokawa K, et al. Somatic mutations and clonal hematopoiesis in aplastic anemia. N Engl J Med 2015;373(1):35–47.
33. Olnes MJ, Scheinberg P, Calvo KR, et al. Eltrombopag and improved hematopoiesis in refractory aplastic anemia. N Engl J Med 2012;367(1):11–9.
34. Townsley DM, Scheinberg P, Winkler T, et al. Eltrombopag added to standard immunosuppression for aplastic anemia. N Engl J Med 2017;376(16):1540–50.
35. Desmond R, Townsley DM, Dumitriu B, et al. Eltrombopag restores trilineage hematopoiesis in refractory severe aplastic anemia that can be sustained on discontinuation of drug. Blood 2014;123(12):1818–25.

Haploidentical Donor Bone Marrow Transplantation for Severe Aplastic Anemia

Amy E. DeZern, MD, MHS[a],*, Robert A. Brodsky, MD[b]

KEYWORDS

- Severe aplastic anemia • Cyclophosphamide • Haploidentical transplant
- Graft versus host disease

KEY POINTS

- Relapsed and refractory SAA carries a grave prognosis if efforts to renew hematopoiesis and avoid clonal evolution are not pursued.
- Allogeneic bone marrow transplantation addresses the acute and chronic complications of SAA, by virtually eliminating the risk of relapse and secondary clonal disease but introduces the risk of acute and chronic GVHD.
- High-dose cyclophosphamide (50 mg/kg/d × 4 days) has a unique history in the context of AA for transplant and nontransplant therapies.
- Use of post-transplantation cyclophosphamide on Days 3 and 4 post-transplant has allowed for expansion of the donor pool to include haploidentical transplants for patient with relapsed and refractory SAA.
- Rates of GVHD and other transplant-related mortality are low with use of post-transplantation cyclophosphamide.

INTRODUCTION

Acquired severe aplastic anemia (SAA) is an immune-mediated hematopoietic stem cell disorder that presents with a hypocellular marrow and pancytopenia.[1,2] The incidence is roughly 1 in 250,000 individuals per year.[3,4] Most newly diagnosed patients are managed with immunosuppressive therapy (IST) unless they are young and have a suitable human leukocyte antigen (HLA)-matched sibling donor for bone marrow

Disclosure Statement: Dr A.E. DeZern has no financial conflicts of interest to disclose. Dr R.A. Brodsky has no financial conflicts of interest to disclose.
[a] Division of Hematologic Malignancies, The Johns Hopkins University School of Medicine, 1650 Orleans Street, CRBI Room 3M87, Baltimore, MD 21287-0013, USA; [b] Division of Hematology, The Johns Hopkins University School of Medicine, 720 Rutland Avenue, Ross 1025, Baltimore, MD 21205, USA
* Corresponding author.
E-mail address: Adezern1@jhmi.edu

transplantation (BMT). IST improves hematopoiesis and decreases the early mortality of the disease. SAA is not considered overtly malignant, but clonal hematopoiesis is present in more than 60% of patients at diagnosis; commonly mutated genes include *PIGA, BCOR/BCORL1, DNMT3A,* and *ASXL1* among others.[5–7] This explains the high rate of paroxysmal nocturnal hemoglobinuria (PNH) and myelodysplastic syndromes (MDS) that frequently arise from SAA 5 years or more after treatment with IST.[8–11] Infection (usually fungal) is the most common cause of early death in patients with SAA; however, hemorrhage, clonal disease (MDS,[12] leukemia, PNH), and transfusional iron overload are other causes of severe morbidity and mortality.[13] Improved supportive care has led to significant progress in controlling the acute aspects of the disease (bleeding and infection), but little progress has been made controlling the late complications of SAA, especially the risk for relapse and secondary clonal disorders following IST. Indeed, SAA that is refractory or relapses after antithymocyte globulin (ATG)/cyclosporine is associated with a high degree of morbidity and mortality. Curative strategies are desperately needed for these patients.

Allogeneic BMT addresses the acute and chronic complications of SAA by virtually eliminating the risk of relapse and secondary clonal disease, but introduces the risk of acute and chronic graft-versus-host disease (GVHD). Thus, allogeneic BMT from an HLA-matched sibling donor is the standard of care for young, newly diagnosed patients with SAA,[2,14] with long-term survival rates approaching 90% in patients younger than 20 years[15,16] and 76% for patients older than 20 years.[16] The less favorable transplant outcomes in older (>30–40 years) patients is attributed to reduced engraftment, and higher rates of GVHD.[17]

When to apply alternative donor BMT has remained an active research question for many years. More recently, there has been an increase in HLA haploidentical BMT (haplo-BMT) from family members globally[18–20] for all diseases. For SAA in particular, a European survey showed that haploidentical donors constituted 6.7%, whereas cord blood is used in 3.2% of transplants in AA.[18] This is only likely to increase as outcomes improve with haploidentical transplant for SAA. Here, we review the outcomes in relapsed and refractory disease and upfront use of haplo-BMT for patients suffering with SAA.

HAPLOIDENTICAL TRANSPLANT STRATEGIES

The ideal BMT regimen in AA is one that results in sustained engraftment, minimal toxicity from the regimen, lack of acute or chronic GVHD, and allows most patients (old and young) to proceed efficiently to this potentially curative option. In a nonmalignant disease, such as AA, it is advantageous to use strategies to minimize GVHD.[21] Multiple approaches are used toward this goal. **Table 1** reviews results of these studies. As in all of BMT, multiple factors require evaluation before alternative donor BMT in AA.

THE ROLE OF HIGH-DOSE CYCLOPHOSPHAMIDE IN THERAPY FOR APLASTIC ANEMIA

High-dose cyclophosphamide (HiCY) (50 mg/kg/d × 4 days) has as unique history in the context of AA for transplant and nontransplant therapies. **Fig. 1** shows the role of cyclophosphamide over the past six decades for AA. The first successful allogeneic BMT in a human was performed for SAA following conditioning with HiCY.[22] Shortly afterward, reports of complete hematopoietic recovery with host hematopoiesis following allogeneic BMT for SAA began to trickle into the literature.[23,24] This suggested that HiCY, with its stem cell–sparing yet highly lymphocytotoxic properties, could achieve durable complete responses in SAA. This hypothesis was confirmed

Table 1

Results of haploidentical bone marrow transplant for severe aplastic anemia

Location	Date	N	Pre-BMT Therapy	Median Age (Range)	Conditioning Regimen	Graft Source	GVHD Prophylaxis	Engraftment	Overall Survival (%)	Median Follow-up	Acute GVHD	Chronic GVHD
Studies using post-transplant cyclophosphamide as GVHD prophylaxis												
Brazil[36]	2010–2014	16	All R/R to IST; no IBMFS included	17 (5–39)	RIC: Flu, CY, TBI (200–600 cGy)	BM 13 PB 3	PTCy +3,4; MMF to D35 CSA/Tacro	15/16; secondary graft loss 2/16	67.1	355 d	13% grade II-IV	20% limited
United Kingdom[37]	Before 2014	8	4 R/R to IST; 4 failed to engraft after previous BMT	32 (19–57)	RIC: Flu, CY, TBI (200 cGy)	PB (G-CSF mobilized)	PTCy +3,4 MMF to D35 CSA/Tacro	6/8	75	14.8 mo (7.2–44.4)	1 grade 2 aGVHD	0
[a]Baltimore[34]	2011–2016	16 (13 haplo)	All R/R to IST; IBMFS included	30 (11–69)	RIC: rATG, Flu, CY, TBI (200 cGy)	BM	PTCy +3,4 MMF to D35 Tacro	100%	100	21 mo (3–64)	2 grade 1–2 aGVHD	2 limited
Studies not using post-transplant cyclophosphamide as GVHD prophylaxis												
China[45]	2007–2010	26	All R/R to IST; no IBMFS included	25.4 (18–41)	RIC: rATG, Flu, CY	BM + PB	CSA to D180 MMF to D90 MTX D+1,3,6,11	92.4%	84.6	1313.2 d (738–2005)	12% grade II-IV	4% extensive
China[48]	2012–2015	89	None	22 (4–51)	RIC: Bu; CY; rATG	BM + PB	CSA to 1 y MMF to D60 MTX D+1,3,6,11	98.9%	86.1	22.6 (7.1–47.6)	30.3% grade II-IV	3.4% extensive
[a]China[38]	2012–2015	101	All R/R to IST; no IBMFS included	19 (2–45)	RIC: Bu; CY; rATG	BM + PB	CSA to 1 y; MMF to D60; MTX D+1,3,6,11	100% of 97 who survived to Day 28	89	18.3 mo (3–43.6)	33.7% grade II-IV	10% extensive

(continued on next page)

Table 1
(continued)

Location	Date	N	Pre-BMT Therapy	Median Age (Range)	Conditioning Regimen	Graft Source	GVHD Prophylaxis	Engraftment	Overall Survival (%)	Median Follow-up	Acute GVHD	Chronic GVHD
Studies in pediatric patients												
China[39]	2002–2013	36	All R/R to first line tx (only 33% had ATG)	5 (0.5–14)	RIC (3 regimens)	PBSCs in 34; 1 BM; 1 UC (matching 3–5/6)	MTX + CSA or tacro or MMF	34/36	86.1 at 5 y	42 mo (20–157)	11 with grade II; 2 with grade III	7 limited; 1 extensive
China[42]	2010–2013	17	All R/R to first line tx (only 5 had ATG)	10 (4–19)	RIC: Bu; Flu; or CY; ATG or ALG	BM + PB	CSA + MTX + basiliximab	17/17 myeloid; 16/17 platelet (1 secondary)	71.6	362 (36–1321) d	12 with grade I–II; 1 with grade III–IV	4 limited
[a]China[46]	2007–2015	52	29 pts R/R (only 15 had ATG); 23 pts upfront	9 (2–17)	RIC: Bu; CY; rATG	BM + PB	CSA to 1 y; MMF to D60; MTX D+1,3,6,11	96.2%	84.5	744.5 (100–3294) d	39.2% grade I–II; 13.7 grade III–IV	34.2% (1 extensive)
Peripheral blood stem cell source												
India[44]	2012–2014	10	50% failed IST	35 (6–46)	Flu; CY; rATG; melphalan	PB	Sirolimus (in 5/10), PTCy, MMF to D35, CSA	90%	60	2 y	1 patient	2 patients
India[43]	2015–2016	10	50% failed IST	12 (4–21)	Flu; CY; rATG; melphalan	PB	Sirolimus, abatacept, PTCy	90%	88.9	NR but >1 y for 8 pts	1 patient grade 2–4	1 patient off IST by 1 y

Abbreviations: BM, bone marrow; BU, busulfan; CSA, cyclosporine; CY, cyclophosphamide; Flu, fludarabine; G-CSF, granulocyte colony stimulating factor; IBMFS, inherited bone marrow failure syndrome; MMF, mycophenolate mofetil; MTX, methotrexate; PB, peripheral blood; PTCy, post-transplant cyclophosphamide at 50 mg/kg per dose; R/R, relapsed or refractory; rATG, rabbit antithymocyte globulin; RIC, reduced-intensity conditioning; Tacro, tacrolimus.
[a] Prospective study.

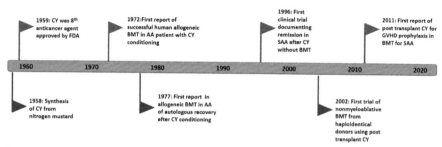

Fig. 1. History of cyclophosphamide in aplastic anemia. CY, cyclophosphamide; FDA, Food and Drug Administration.

in the 1990s. A Johns Hopkins report of complete hematologic remission in 7 of 10 SAA patients treated with HiCY without BMT proved the potential efficacy of this approach.[25] Subsequent reports in larger numbers of patients with SAA confirmed these results[26] but the prolonged aplasia and morbidity of this approach has limited the enthusiasm for HiCY as therapy for SAA.

More recently, the efficacy of HiCY for alloimmunity has been realized. HiCY after BMT was shown to inhibit graft rejection and GVHD in animal models.[27] Based on these data, and the clinical experience demonstrating the efficacy of HiCY in SAA and other severe autoimmune diseases,[28] the use of HiCY or specifically post-transplant cyclophosphamide (PTCy) (50 mg/kg/d on Days +3 and + 4) was found to be highly effective for GVHD prophylaxis. In phase II clinical trials, HiCY after non-myeloablative haplo-BMT is associated with rates of acute or chronic GVHD similar to those seen with matched allogeneic BMT in hematologic malignancies.[29–31] This platform to decrease GVHD has been especially effective in nonmalignant diseases, such as PNH and sickle cell disease,[32,33] where a graft-versus-tumor effect is not necessary. More recently, it has been used for AA.[34–37]

RESULTS OF HAPLO–BONE MARROW TRANSPLANTATION FOR SEVERE APLASTIC ANEMIA

Approaches Using Post-transplant Cyclophosphamide

The first reported use PTCy for treating SAA was by Dezern and colleagues[35] with myeloablative conditioning. In a pilot study, Clay and colleagues[37] reported the use of haplo-BMT in refractory SAA, using a reduced intensity conditioning with PTCy and mobilized peripheral blood stem cells (PBSC) in eight patients, with successful engraftment in six patients with low acute GVHD and no chronic GVHD. Follow-up was 14.8 (7.2–44.4) months. Esteves and colleagues[36] also described haplo-BMT using the Hopkins regimen (described later) in another small cohort with 16 patients, after failure of IST or graft failure following unrelated-donor or cord blood transplant. Their protocol was similar to Clay and colleagues.[37] Graft source was bone marrow in 13 and PBSC in three. The 1-year overall survival (OS) was 67.1% (95% confidence interval, 36.5%–86.4%).

Previous reports with haplo-BMT without PTCy in SAA have produced heterogeneous results depending on the patient population and are limited by small sample sizes (see **Table 1**).[36–44] In these series, rejection has been between 6% and 25%, acute GVHD between 12% and 30%, chronic GVHD between 20% and 40%, and OS between 60% and 100%.[36–45] Limited comparisons can be made across these studies but some differences between studies may be related to infectious complications, donor-specific antibodies, and amount of patients' previous therapies.

Nonetheless, in the relapsed and refractory setting, all patients had previously received IST at the time of diagnosis for their SAA and thus this may have impacted more favorably on engraftment with any of the conditioning regimens. Furthermore, the previous use of multiple lines of therapy could have also contributed to the improved engraftment rates over historical reports.[21] Upfront haploidentical transplant studies are still early with limited reports in the literature. Most studies have short follow-up.

More recently, DeZern and colleagues[34] reported on a prospective phase 2 trial of PTCy for refractory SAA in which 16 patients (median age, 30 years; range, 11–69) underwent transplant from 13 haploidentical and three unrelated donors. The conditioning consisted of rabbit ATG 4.5 mg/kg over 3 days, fludarabine (Flu) 30 mg/m^2 for 5 days, Cy 14.5 mg/kg^2 for 2 days, and total body irradiation (TBI) 200 cGy (**Fig. 2**). Graft source was bone marrow with target yield of 4×10^8 nucleated cells/kg recipient ideal weight. For GVHD prophylaxis, PTCy 50 mg/kg/d intravenous on Days +3 and + 4 was administered along with mycophenolate mofetil (MMF) on Days +5 through 35 and tacrolimus from Day +5 through 1 year. Granulocyte colony–stimulating factor (G-CSF) was given from Day +5 until absolute neutrophil count was more than 1.5×10^9/L for 3 days. There was no graft failure and mild GVHD occurred in two patients. There was evidence for clonality in 37% of the patients pre-BMT and this was eliminated post-BMT. Furthermore, excellent performance status was noted in all patients after recovery. This study is limited by the small sample size and short follow-up. This is similar to what was seen in Brazil using the same regimen, although they did have two patients with secondary graft loss and one primary graft failure.[36] Currently haplo-BMT with PTCy is being studied on a national level in the United States by the Bone Marrow Transplant Clinical Trials Network (NCT02918292).

Other Strategies Including Upfront Haploidentical Transplant

In a prospective, multicenter study of haplo-BMT for SAA refractory to IST, Xu and colleagues[38] analyzed the outcomes of 101 patients. Conditioning was with intravenous busulfan (BU) 6.4 mg/kg, Cy 200 mg/kg, and rabbit ATG 10 mg/kg. Graft source was combined bone marrow and G-CSF-stimulated PBSC. GVHD prophylaxis was with CSA, MMF, and short-term methotrexate. These were compared with 48 patients who had matched-related donor (MRD) BMTs. Haplo-BMT compared with MRD

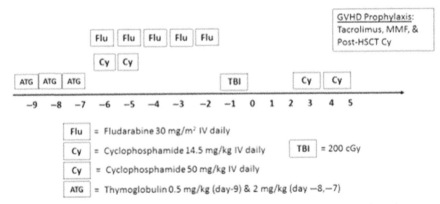

Fig. 2. Schema for nonmyeloablative haploidentical bone marrow transplant for severe aplastic anemia using post-transplantation cyclophosphamide. HSCT, hematopoietic stem cell transplantation; MMF, mycophenolate mofetil.

showed more grade II–IV acute GVHD (33.7 vs 4.2%; P<.001), more chronic GVHD (22.4 vs 6.6%; P = .014) at 1 year, but similar 3-year OS (89.0 vs 91.0%; P = .555) and failure free survival (FFS) (86.8 vs 80.3%; P = .659).[38]

Jaiswal and colleagues[44] looked at a TBI-sparing regimen in 10 patients (median, 35 years; 6–46 years) including horse ATG, at 15 mg/kg from Day −8 to day −6, Flu 30 mg/m^2/day for 5 days, and Cy 15 mg/kg/d for 2 days with melphalan 120 mg/m^2 followed by PBSCs and PTCy. This protocol was modified with the introduction of siro-limus on Day −7.[44] Six of the 10 patients were alive; five of the six received the Day −7 sirolimus. The authors hypothesized that early recovery of regulatory T cells in this small cohort might indicate a tolerance induction mechanism that could have resulted from synergism between PTCY and sirolimus.[44] Additionally, this group used this same platform and added in T-cell costimulation blockade with abatacept, suggesting a further role of transplant tolerance with this approach.[43]

Xu and colleagues[46] reported on 52 children who received haplo-BMT, with 29 receiving it as salvage and the remaining 23 received it as their upfront therapy, using the BU/Cy/rATG protocol described previously.[38] Primary engraftment was achieved in 51 subject. The cumulative incidence of acute GVHD (aGVHD) grade II–IV was 39.2% and of chronic GVHD (cGVHD) was 34.2%, respectively. The 3-year OS and FFS rates were 84.5% and 82.7% for the whole cohort.[46] The upfront and salvage haplo patients did similarly here with nonsignificant benefit for the upfront group. There were 3-year OS and FFS rates of 87% and 82.6% for the upfront group and 82.6% (P = .698) and 82.8% (P = .899) for the salvage cohort. The longer-term FFS of more than 80% of the upfront cohort compares favorably with previous reports of upfront IST FFS rates.[47]

Upfront haplo-BMT in 158 patients with SAA was reported by Xu and colleagues[48] based on the Chinese transplant registry. Here, haplo-BMTs were performed in 89 pa-tients based on the BU/Cy/rATG treatment protocol described previously,[38] and then compared with 69 MRD transplants, conditioned with either Cy + rATG or Cy + Flu + rATG.[48] Haplo-BMT recipients had increased grades II–IV aGVHD (30.3 vs 1.5%; P<.001) and cGVHD (30.6 vs 4.4%; P<.001) at 1 year but similar extensive cGVHD (3.4 vs 0%; P = .426) compared with related transplants. The 3-year OS rates were 86.1% and 91.3% (P = .358), whereas the 3-year FFS rates were 85.0% and 89.8% (P = .413) in the haplo-BMT and MRD cohorts, respectively.[48]

CONDITIONING FOR HAPLOIDENTICAL TRANSPLANT FOR APLASTIC ANEMIA

Reduced intensity or nonmyeloablative conditioning is likely sufficient to balance engraftment and toxicities in this setting. It has previously been shown that TBI- based conditioning regimens reduced the risk of graft rejection but increased GVHD and other late effects.[49] Standard ATG-based conditioning regimens are used to aid in engraftment but have also been associated with up to a 30% incidence of cGVHD.[50,51] Flu has been used in conditioning for patients with both acquired and constitutional aplastic anemia with good results.[52–55] We favor the use of a conditioning regimen including rATG, Flu, and TBI with T-cell replete allografts for patients with SAA (see **Fig. 2**).

In addition, T-cell depleted and T-cell replete[34,44,56] haploidentical strategies have been reported for multiply relapsed SAA patients lacking a matched donor. Im and col-leagues[57] describe 21 patients who underwent Fly, Cy, 400 cGy TBI, and ATG condi-tioning followed by either CD3/19 or CD3alfa beta/CD19 depleted grafts. OS was reported as 94% at 3 years, without cases of chronic GVHD. T-replete haploidentical approaches have been taken by Wang and coworkers[42] (17 children, full intensity conditioning and 4 agent GVHD prophylaxis: OS 71% at 1 year, 20% chronic GVHD) and Gao and coworkers[45] (26 adults, reduced intensity conditioning with three-agent GVHD prophylaxis: OS 82% at 2 years, GVHD 40%).

Increasing data are available for a reduced-intensity approach followed by T-replete haploidentical transplant and PTCy described previously as optimal GVHD prophylaxis with OS approaching 90% and low-GVHD rates.[34,36,37] Thus, although follow-up is short and numbers do remain small, we conclude from these aggregate data that reduced-intensity conditioning regimens followed by haploidentical allografts for patients with SAA are an increasingly viable therapeutic option. The multicenter study through the Bone Marrow Transplant Clinical Trials Network (NCT02918292) of haploidentical transplant in relapsed or refractory SAA modeled after the Hopkins approach[34] will provide additional experience and clinical outcomes in the arena in the United States.

DONOR SELECTION
Stem Cell Choice

Most patients have more than one potential haploidentical donor. The process of choosing among these for the best possibly donor is important but remains a controversial topic. The European Society for Blood and Marrow Transplantation reviewed outcomes in nearly 700 patients with SAA receiving transplants from HLA-matched siblings. In patients younger than 20 years of age, rates of chronic GVHD (relative risk, 2.82; $P = .002$) and overall mortality (relative risk, 2.04; $P = .024$) were higher after transplantation of peripheral blood progenitor cell grafts than after transplantation of bone marrow. In younger patients, the 5-year survival was 85% after marrow transplants but only 73% after PBSC. These data suggest that bone marrow grafts are preferable in this age group[58,59] but this has not been studied systematically in haploidentical donors. Most centers in the United States favor a bone marrow graft to avoid excessive GHVD in a nonmalignant disease; however, in the United Kingdom, PBSC were successfully used without increased rates of GVHD.[37] In China many transplants of this nature follow another procedure to optimize cell counts. Haploidentical donors are treated with subcutaneous G-CSF. Marrow grafts are then collected on Day 1 with a target mononuclear cell count of 2 to 4×10^8/kg of recipient body weight. PBSC are also collected by apheresis. The target mononuclear cell count from BM and PB was 6 to 8×10^8/kg of recipient bodyweight. If the mononuclear cell count is not sufficient, additional PBSC are collected on the following day.[38]

Choice of Best Haploidentical Donor

There are often multiple potential haploidentical donor options. These are first-degree relatives of the patient including biologic parents; siblings or half-siblings; or children with two, three, or four mismatches using DNA-based typing. A unidirectional mismatch in either the graft-versus-host or host-versus-graft direction is considered a mismatch. The donor and recipient are recommended to be identical at a minimum of one allele (at high-resolution DNA-based typing) at the following genetic loci: HLA-A, -B, -C, and DRB1 for haploidentical matching. There is nothing in AA that is unique compared with hematologic malignancies that suggests a nonstandard approach to the choice of donor to an AA patient. When more than one donor is available, the donor with the lowest number of HLA allele mismatches is chosen unless there is HLA crossmatch incompatibility or a medical reason to select otherwise. In cases where there is more than one donor with the least degree of mismatch, donors are selected based on the most favorable combination of HLA compatibility in crossmatch testing and ABO compatibility. Prioritization is given to the lowest number of mismatches in the host-versus-graft direction to minimize the risk of graft rejection. If there is more than one donor with the least amount of host-versus-graft allele mismatches, the suggested prioritization in order of importance includes ABO compatibility, cytomegalovirus status (use a seronegative donor for a seronegative recipient or use a seropositive donor for a seropositive recipient), younger age, lighter weight (this rule applies to donors 18 years or older; however, children may also be used as donors if appropriate), and sex of the donor (if all else is equal, males are preferred over nulliparous females over multiparous females).[60] Youth (age <40 years) is increasingly valued when it comes to choice of any donor and this may begin to take greater priority in the haploidentical donor selection algorithm.[61]

The Challenge of Anti-human Leukocyte Antigen Antibodies

Donor-specific anti-HLA antibodies (DSA) have been implicated in graft rejection in solid organ transplantation for many years. More recently their role in BMT has been better defined.[62] Results in multiple retrospective reviews have suggested that DSA are associated with a higher rate of graft rejection in patients undergoing BMT[63] including those from a haploidentical donor.[64] Thus, donors with high levels DSA should be excluded. Anti-HLA desensitization is used for low-titer DSA in BMT for AA with haploidentical donors but only if there is no haploidentical donor without DSA.[65,66]

GRAFT-VERSUS-HOST DISEASE PROPHYLAXIS

PTCy is becoming standard backbone of GVHD prophylaxis in haplo-BMT. Additionally, oral IST is administered through Day 180 or even 1 year in SAA.[67] This often includes MMF and a calcineurin inhibitor. Most of the more favorable results (seen in **Table 1**) use this approach. Methotrexate remains commonly used.

SUMMARY AND FUTURE OF HAPLOIDENTICAL TRANSPLANTS IN APLASTIC ANEMIA

Haplo-BMT is now a safe and potentially curative option for treating patients with SAA who are refractory to IST, have relapsed after IST, or who have acquired a secondary clonal disorder (MDS/PNH) after IST (**Fig. 3**). Current strategies (including PTCy as

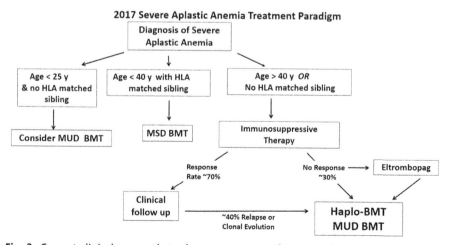

Fig. 3. Current clinical approach to the management of severe aplastic anemia including haploidentical bone marrow transplant. MSD, matched sibling donor.

GVHD prophylaxis) have increased the availability of haplo-BMT to patients previously considered transplant ineligible because they lack a suitable donor or were too high risk for BMT because of the risk GVHD. Ongoing investigations seek to increase this option for these patients through development of further novel therapeutic strategies to optimize haplo-BMT, both in the treatment refractory setting and the upfront setting. Furthermore, haploidentical transplants are attractive because of low cost and early availability of a donor, although issues of DSA may be potentially problematic.[60,68] The current results suggest that haplo-BMT should become standard therapy for refractory SAA patients. Upfront haplo-BMT remains investigational but may be useful for patients with SAA lacking a matched sibling donor or Matched Unrelated Donor who want to consider minimizing risk of clonal evolution post-IST.

REFERENCES

1. Brodsky RA, Jones RJ. Aplastic anaemia. Lancet 2005;365(9471):1647–56.
2. Scheinberg P, Young NS. How I treat acquired aplastic anemia. Blood 2012; 120(6):1185–96.
3. Young NS, Kaufman DW. The epidemiology of acquired aplastic anemia. Haematologica 2008;93(4):489–92.
4. Alter BP. Bone marrow failure syndromes in children. Pediatr Clin North Am 2002; 49(5):973–88.
5. Yoshizato T, Dumitriu B, Hosokawa K, et al. Somatic mutations and clonal hematopoiesis in aplastic anemia. N Engl J Med 2015;373(1):35–47.
6. Marsh JC, Mufti GJ. Clinical significance of acquired somatic mutations in aplastic anaemia. Int J Hematol 2016;104:159–67.
7. Kulasekararaj AG, Jiang J, Smith AE, et al. Somatic mutations identify a subgroup of aplastic anemia patients who progress to myelodysplastic syndrome. Blood 2014;124(17):2698–704.
8. Young NS. Acquired bone marrow failure. Philadelphia: JB Lippincott; 1995.
9. Alter BP. Diagnosis, genetics, and management of inherited bone marrow failure syndromes. Hematology Am Soc Hematol Educ Program 2007;29–39.
10. Tefferi A, Vardiman JW. Myelodysplastic syndromes. N Engl J Med 2009;361(19): 1872–85.
11. Whitman SP, Archer KJ, Feng L, et al. Absence of the wild-type allele predicts poor prognosis in adult de novo acute myeloid leukemia with normal cytogenetics and the internal tandem duplication of FLT3: a cancer and leukemia group B study. Cancer Res 2001;61(19):7233–9.
12. Kim SY, Le Rademacher J, Antin JH, et al. Myelodysplastic syndrome evolving from aplastic anemia treated with immunosuppressive therapy: efficacy of hematopoietic stem cell transplantation. Haematologica 2014;99(12):1868–75.
13. Scheinberg P. Aplastic anemia: therapeutic updates in immunosuppression and transplantation. Hematology Am Soc Hematol Educ Program 2012;2012: 292–300.
14. Eapen M, Horowitz MM. Alternative donor transplantation for aplastic anemia. Hematology Am Soc Hematol Educ Program 2010;2010:43–6.
15. Storb R, Blume KG, O'Donnell MR, et al. Cyclophosphamide and antithymocyte globulin to condition patients with aplastic anemia for allogeneic marrow transplantations: the experience in four centers. Biol Blood Marrow Transplant 2001; 7(1):39–44.

16. Current use and outcomes of hematopoietic stem cell transplantation: CIBMTR Summary Slides 2013. Available in: https://www.cibmtr.org/ReferenceCenter/SlidesReports/SummarySlides/pages/index.aspx. Accessed May 6, 2018.
17. Bacigalupo A. Matched and mismatched unrelated donor transplantation: is the outcome the same as for matched sibling donor transplantation? Hematology Am Soc Hematol Educ Program 2012;2012:223–9.
18. Passweg JR, Baldomero H, Bader P, et al. Use of haploidentical stem cell transplantation continues to increase: the 2015 European Society for Blood and Marrow Transplant activity survey report. Bone Marrow Transplant 2017;52(6): 811–7.
19. Niederwieser D, Baldomero H, Szer J, et al. Hematopoietic stem cell transplantation activity worldwide in 2012 and a SWOT analysis of the Worldwide Network for Blood and Marrow Transplantation Group including the global survey. Bone Marrow Transplant 2016;51(6):778–85.
20. Xu LP, Wu DP, Han MZ, et al. A review of hematopoietic cell transplantation in China: data and trends during 2008-2016. Bone Marrow Transplant 2017; 52(11):1512–8.
21. Ciceri F, Lupo-Stanghellini MT, Korthof ET. Haploidentical transplantation in patients with acquired aplastic anemia. Bone Marrow Transplant 2013;48(2):183–5.
22. Thomas ED, Storb R, Fefer A, et al. Aplastic anaemia treated by marrow transplantation. Lancet 1972;1(7745):284–9.
23. Gmur J, Vonfelten A, Rhyner K, et al. Autologous hematologic recovery from aplastic-anemia following high-dose cyclophosphamide and HLA-matched allogeneic bone-marrow transplantation. Acta Haematol 1979;62(1):20–4.
24. Sensenbrenner LL, Steele AA, Santos GW. Recovery of hematologic competence without engraftment following attempted bone-marrow transplantation for aplastic-anemia: report of a case with diffusion chamber studies. Exp Hematol 1977;5(1):51–8.
25. Brodsky RA, Sensenbrenner LL, Smith BD, et al. Durable treatment-free remission following high-dose cyclophosphamide for previously untreated severe aplastic anemia. Ann Intern Med 2001;135:477–83.
26. Brodsky RA, Chen AR, Dorr D, et al. High-dose cyclophosphamide for severe aplastic anemia: long-term follow-up. Blood 2010;115(11):2136–41.
27. Luznik L, Engstrom LW, Iannone R, et al. Posttransplantation cyclophosphamide facilitates engraftment of major histocompatibility complex-identical allogeneic marrow in mice conditioned with low-dose total body irradiation. Biol Blood Marrow Transplant 2002;8(3):131–8.
28. DeZern AE, Petri M, Drachman DB, et al. High-dose cyclophosphamide without stem cell rescue in 207 patients with aplastic anemia and other autoimmune diseases. Medicine (Baltimore) 2011;90(2):89–98.
29. Kasamon YL, Bolanos-Meade J, Prince GT, et al. Outcomes of nonmyeloablative HLA-haploidentical blood or marrow transplantation with high-dose post-transplantation cyclophosphamide in older adults. J Clin Oncol 2015;33(28):3152–61.
30. Luznik L, Jones RJ, Fuchs EJ. High-dose cyclophosphamide for graft-versus-host disease prevention. Curr Opin Hematol 2010;17(6):493–9.
31. Luznik L, O'Donnell PV, Symons HJ, et al. HLA-haploidentical bone marrow transplantation for hematologic malignancies using nonmyeloablative conditioning and high-dose, posttransplantation cyclophosphamide. Biol Blood Marrow Transplant 2008;14(6):641–50.
32. Tisdale JF, Eapen M, Saccardi R. HCT for nonmalignant disorders. Biol Blood Marrow Transplant 2013;19(1 Suppl):S6–9.

33. Bolanos-Meade J, Fuchs EJ, Luznik L, et al. HLA-haploidentical bone marrow transplantation with posttransplant cyclophosphamide expands the donor pool for patients with sickle cell disease. Blood 2012;120(22):4285–91.

34. DeZern AE, Zahurak M, Symons H, et al. Alternative donor transplantation with high-dose post-transplantation cyclophosphamide for refractory severe aplastic anemia. Biol Blood Marrow Transplant 2017;23(3):498–504.

35. Dezern AE, Luznik L, Fuchs EJ, et al. Post-transplantation cyclophosphamide for GVHD prophylaxis in severe aplastic anemia. Bone Marrow Transplant 2011; 46(7):1012–3.

36. Esteves I, Bonfim C, Pasquini R, et al. Haploidentical BMT and post-transplant Cy for severe aplastic anemia: a multicenter retrospective study. Bone Marrow Transplant 2015;50(5):685–9.

37. Clay J, Kulasekararaj AG, Potter V, et al. Nonmyeloablative peripheral blood haploidentical stem cell transplantation for refractory severe aplastic anemia. Biol Blood Marrow Transplant 2014;20(11):1711–6.

38. Xu LP, Wang SQ, Wu DP, et al. Haplo-identical transplantation for acquired severe aplastic anaemia in a multicentre prospective study. Br J Haematol 2016;175(2): 265–74.

39. Zhu H, Luo RM, Luan Z, et al. Unmanipulated haploidentical haematopoietic stem cell transplantation for children with severe aplastic anaemia. Br J Haematol 2016;174(5):799–805.

40. Zhang Y, Guo Z, Liu XD, et al. Comparison of haploidentical hematopoietic stem cell transplantation and immunosuppressive therapy for the treatment of acquired severe aplastic anemia in pediatric patients. Am J Ther 2017;24(2):e196–201.

41. Sarmiento M, Ramirez PA. Unmanipulated haploidentical hematopoietic cell transplantation with post-transplant cyclophosphamide in a patient with paroxysmal nocturnal hemoglobinuria and secondary aplastic anemia. Bone Marrow Transplant 2016;51(2):316–8.

42. Wang Z, Zheng X, Yan H, et al. Good outcome of haploidentical hematopoietic SCT as a salvage therapy in children and adolescents with acquired severe aplastic anemia. Bone Marrow Transplant 2014;49(12):1481–5.

43. Jaiswal SR, Bhakuni P, Zaman S, et al. T cell costimulation blockade promotes transplantation tolerance in combination with sirolimus and post-transplantation cyclophosphamide for haploidentical transplantation in children with severe aplastic anemia. Transpl Immunol 2017;43-44:54–9.

44. Jaiswal SR, Chatterjee S, Mukherjee S, et al. Pre-transplant sirolimus might improve the outcome of haploidentical peripheral blood stem cell transplantation with post-transplant cyclophosphamide for patients with severe aplastic anemia. Bone Marrow Transplant 2015;50(6):873–5.

45. Gao L, Li Y, Zhang Y, et al. Long-term outcome of HLA-haploidentical hematopoietic SCT without in vitro T-cell depletion for adult severe aplastic anemia after modified conditioning and supportive therapy. Bone Marrow Transplant 2014; 49(4):519–24.

46. Xu LP, Zhang XH, Wang FR, et al. Haploidentical transplantation for pediatric patients with acquired severe aplastic anemia. Bone Marrow Transplant 2017;52(3): 381–7.

47. Yoshida N, Kobayashi R, Yabe H, et al. First-line treatment for severe aplastic anemia in children: bone marrow transplantation from a matched family donor versus immunosuppressive therapy. Haematologica 2014;99(12):1784–91.

48. Xu LP, Jin S, Wang SQ, et al. Upfront haploidentical transplant for acquired severe aplastic anemia: registry-based comparison with matched related transplant. J Hematol Oncol 2017;10(1):25.

49. Sanders JE, Woolfrey AE, Carpenter PA, et al. Late effects among pediatric patients followed for nearly 4 decades after transplantation for severe aplastic anemia. Blood 2011;118(5):1421–8.

50. Konopacki J, Porcher R, Robin M, et al. Long-term follow up after allogeneic stem cell transplantation in patients with severe aplastic anemia after cyclophosphamide plus antithymocyte globulin conditioning. Haematologica 2012;97(5):710–6.

51. Champlin RE, Perez WS, Passweg JR, et al. Bone marrow transplantation for severe aplastic anemia: a randomized controlled study of conditioning regimens. Blood 2007;109(10):4582–5.

52. Kharfan-Dabaja MA, Otrock ZK, Bacigalupo A, et al. A reduced intensity conditioning regimen of fludarabine, cyclophosphamide, antithymocyte globulin, plus 2 Gy TBI facilitates successful hematopoietic cell engraftment in an adult with dyskeratosis congenita. Bone Marrow Transplant 2012;47(9):1254–5.

53. Dietz AC, Orchard PJ, Baker KS, et al. Disease-specific hematopoietic cell transplantation: nonmyeloablative conditioning regimen for dyskeratosis congenita. Bone Marrow Transplant 2011;46(1):98–104.

54. Marsh JC, Gupta V, Lim Z, et al. Alemtuzumab with fludarabine and cyclophosphamide reduces chronic graft-versus-host disease after allogeneic stem cell transplantation for acquired aplastic anemia. Blood 2011;118(8):2351–7.

55. Wang SB, Li L, Pan XH, et al. Engraftment of heavily transfused patients with severe aplastic anemia with a fludarabine-based regimen. Clin Transplant 2013; 27(2):E109–15.

56. Gupta N, Choudhary D, Sharma SK, et al. Haploidentical hematopoietic SCT for acquired severe aplastic anemia using post-transplant high-dose CY. Bone Marrow Transplant 2015;50(1):155–6.

57. Im HJ, Koh KN, Seo JJ. Haploidentical hematopoietic stem cell transplantation in children and adolescents with acquired severe aplastic anemia. Korean J Pediatr 2015;58(6):199–205.

58. Schrezenmeier H, Passweg JR, Marsh JC, et al. Worse outcome and more chronic GVHD with peripheral blood progenitor cells than bone marrow in HLA-matched sibling donor transplants for young patients with severe acquired aplastic anemia. Blood 2007;110(4):1397–400.

59. Bacigalupo A, Socie G, Schrezenmeier H, et al. Bone marrow versus peripheral blood as the stem cell source for sibling transplants in acquired aplastic anemia: survival advantage for bone marrow in all age groups. Haematologica 2012; 97(8):1142–8.

60. McCurdy SR, Fuchs EJ. Selecting the best haploidentical donor. Semin Hematol 2016;53(4):246–51.

61. Kollman C, Spellman SR, Zhang MJ, et al. The effect of donor characteristics on survival after unrelated donor transplantation for hematologic malignancy. Blood 2016;127(2):260–7.

62. Morin-Zorman S, Loiseau P, Taupin JL, et al. Donor-specific anti-HLA antibodies in allogeneic hematopoietic stem cell transplantation. Front Immunol 2016;7:307.

63. Ciurea SO, Thall PF, Wang X, et al. Donor-specific anti-HLA Abs and graft failure in matched unrelated donor hematopoietic stem cell transplantation. Blood 2011; 118(22):5957–64.

64. Ciurea SO, Thall PF, Milton DR, et al. Complement-binding donor-specific anti-HLA antibodies and risk of primary graft failure in hematopoietic stem cell transplantation. Biol Blood Marrow Transplant 2015;21(8):1392–8.

65. Gladstone DE, Zachary AA, Fuchs EJ, et al. Partially mismatched transplantation and human leukocyte antigen donor-specific antibodies. Biol Blood Marrow Transplant 2013;19(4):647–52.

66. Leffell MS, Jones RJ, Gladstone DE. Donor HLA-specific Abs: to BMT or not to BMT? Bone Marrow Transplant 2015;50(6):751–8.

67. Bacigalupo A, Brand R, Oneto R, et al. Treatment of acquired severe aplastic anemia: bone marrow transplantation compared with immunosuppressive therapy: the European Group for Blood and Marrow Transplantation experience. Semin Hematol 2000;37(1):69–80.

68. Ciurea SO, Champlin RE. Donor selection in T cell-replete haploidentical hematopoietic stem cell transplantation: knowns, unknowns, and controversies. Biol Blood Marrow Transplant 2013;19(2):180–4.

Significance of Clonal Mutations in Bone Marrow Failure and Inherited Myelodysplastic Syndrome/Acute Myeloid Leukemia Predisposition Syndromes

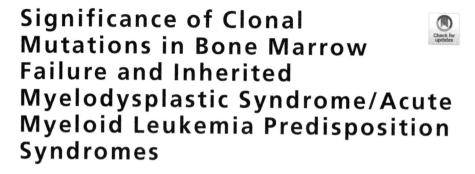

Eva J. Schaefer, MD, R. Coleman Lindsley, MD, PhD*

KEYWORDS

- Myelodysplastic syndrome • Bone marrow failure syndromes
- Genetic predisposition • Clonal hematopoiesis

KEY POINTS

- Clonal evolution in myelodysplastic syndromes can be driven by specific extrinsic and intrinsic selective pressures.
- Acquired somatic mutations in inherited bone marrow failure syndromes can partially complement underlying cellular defects leading to a selective clonal advantage that might be distinct from myeloid transformation.
- Long-term mutational studies with systematic analysis of serial samples in a larger number of patients are required to define prognostic and therapeutic implications of clonal hematopoiesis in patients with bone marrow failure syndromes.

INTRODUCTION
Myelodysplastic Syndrome Pathogenesis

Myelodysplastic syndrome (MDS) is a heterogeneous group of clonal hematopoietic disorders characterized by dysfunctional hematopoiesis, bone marrow dysplasia, and an increased risk of development of acute myeloid leukemia (AML).[1] Although MDS is most common in older patients (>70 years), it can occur in all age

Disclosure Statement: The authors have no relationship with a commercial company that has a direct financial interest in subject matter or materials discussed.
Department of Medical Oncology, Dana-Farber Cancer Institute, 450 Brookline Avenue, Boston, MA 02215, USA
* Corresponding author. Dana-Farber Cancer Institute, 450 Brookline Avenue, DA-530C, Boston, MA 02115.
E-mail address: coleman_lindsley@dfci.harvard.edu

Hematol Oncol Clin N Am 32 (2018) 643–655
https://doi.org/10.1016/j.hoc.2018.03.005
0889-8588/18/© 2018 Elsevier Inc. All rights reserved.

groups, including children and young adults. Primary MDS emerges without known predisposing cause and is associated with advanced age, whereas secondary and therapy-related MDS (t-MDS) are proportionally more common in younger MDS patients and develop in the context of inherited or acquired bone marrow failure or after exposure to chemotherapy, respectively.

Genetic studies have demonstrated that MDS molecular alterations are closely associated with clinical outcomes and disease characteristics.[2,3] Indeed, the spectrum of genetic alterations in young MDS patients is different than that of older MDS patients, consistent with the distinct age-associated mechanisms of MDS pathogenesis.[2] Whereas older patients more frequently harbor somatic mutations in genes encoding epigenetic modifiers (*TET2* and *DNMT3A*) or RNA splicing (*SRSF2* and *SF3B1*), younger patients have much higher frequency of genes associated with germline conditions (*GATA2* and *SBDS*) and acquired predispositions (*PIGA*). Mutations in other genes, such as *TP53*, *RUNX1*, or *RAS*, are common across all age groups.[2]

Clonal Hematopoiesis and Aging

Advancing age is the most established risk factor for developing clonally restricted hematopoiesis. During normal aging, individual hematopoietic stem cells (HSCs) steadily accumulate somatic mutations. By age 60, it is estimated that each HSC harbors 8 mutations affecting its coding genome.[4] Although most of these mutations do not measurably alter stem cell function, some confer a competitive advantage over normal HSCs and cause preferential contribution to mature hematopoietic cells. This phenomenon, when occurring in otherwise healthy individuals, is termed Clonal Hematopoiesis of Indeterminate Potential (CHIP), which has several key properties:

1. A strong association with advancing age,
2. An increased risk of developing frank hematologic malignancy (overall risk = 1% per year),
3. An increase in all-cause mortality related to an elevated risk of cardiovascular events.[5]

The age-dependent accumulation of somatic mutations may underlie the increasing prevalence of MDS among older individuals; the median age at MDS diagnosis is 71 to 76 years.[6] The close genetic and epidemiologic concordance between CHIP and primary MDS has engendered a model whereby clinically unapparent clonal HSC expansion is caused by an initiating mutation affecting particular genes, such as *DNMT3A*, *TET2*, and *ASXL1*, whereas transformation to frank myeloid malignancy is mediated by subsequent stepwise acquisition of additional myeloid driver mutations.[3,5] The factors that influence the frequency, genetic spectrum, and clinical implications of CHIP remain incompletely understood.

Extrinsic Selection and Clonal Hematopoiesis: Clonal Hematopoiesis of Indeterminate Potential and Therapy-Related Myelodysplastic Syndrome

Changes in cell extrinsic selection pressures due to specific therapeutic exposures or disease characteristics may influence the development and clinical implications of clonal hematopoiesis. For example, CHIP is present in about 30% of patients with non-Hodgkin lymphoma who undergo autologous stem cell transplantation, reflecting a rate more than 5 times higher than healthy adults of similar age spectrum.[7] Similarly, clonal hematopoiesis is common among patients with nonhematologic cancers.[8] The genetic spectrum of CHIP that arises in the context of therapeutic exposure is distinct, showing an enrichment of mutations affecting *TP53* and *PPM1D*, genes that are important for the cellular stress response. Mutations in *TP53* and *PPM1D* are also highly associated with t-MDS, compared with primary MDS, suggesting a mechanistic link between CHIP arising in the context of exposure and the subsequent development of t-MDS.[2]

Clonal Hematopoiesis in Inherited Bone Marrow Failure and Familial Myelodysplastic Syndrome/Acute Myeloid Leukemia Predisposition Syndromes

The ability of a cell to persist within a specific selective environment defines its "fitness" and reflects aggregate characteristics of cell survival, differentiation, and proliferation. Importantly, cellular fitness is functionally defined only relative to surrounding cells. In healthy individuals, clonal hematopoiesis and MDS arise in the competitive backdrop of normal hematopoiesis. In this context, clonal expansion is based on a gain of fitness relative to otherwise fit cells. By contrast, bone marrow failure syndromes can display subtle or profound alterations of HSC function and microenvironment. Therefore, even mutations that cause modest enhancement of fitness may manifest as clonal hematopoiesis or drive myeloid transformation. Moreover, disease-specific cellular defects (**Fig. 1**) may create context-dependent selective environments that result in distinct opportunities for somatic genetic cooperation (**Fig. 2**).

In later discussion, the authors discuss how inherited bone marrow failure syndromes and MDS/AML predisposition syndromes may exert an influence on the incidence and genetic spectrum of clonal hematopoiesis and myeloid transformation. Furthermore, the authors consider how disease-specific selective pressures, driven by diverse underlying pathogenetic mechanisms, may define distinct selective pressures that are intrinsic and extrinsic to the HSC.

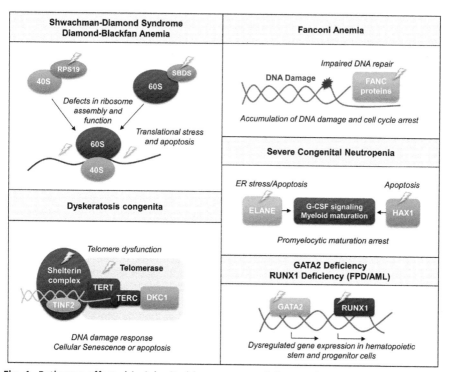

Fig. 1. Pathways affected in inherited bone marrow failure and MDS/AML predisposition syndromes. ER, endoplasmic reticulum.

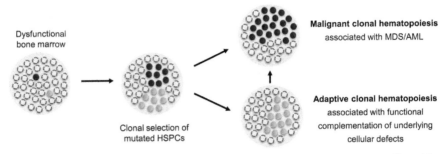

Fig. 2. Clonal hematopoiesis in inherited bone marrow failure and MDS/AML predisposition syndromes. Bone marrow failure syndromes are associated with dysfunctional hematopoiesis that may drive a strong selective pressure that favors mutated hematopoietic stem and progenitor cells with enhanced fitness. Although some mutations cause leukemic transformation (*red circles*), others may enable clonal expansion due to functional complementation of disease-specific cellular defects (*green circles*). The latter may involve biological pathways that are distinct from leukemic transformation and not associated with elevated risk of progression to MDS or AML. HSPCs, hematopoietic stem and progenitor cell.

SHWACHMAN-DIAMOND SYNDROME

Shwachman-Diamond syndrome (SDS) is an autosomal recessive bone marrow failure syndrome that is caused by biallelic inactivating mutations in the *SBDS* gene on chromosome 7 (q11.21) and is associated with short stature, exocrine pancreatic dysfunction, and a strong predisposition to MDS/AML transformation.[9] In a cohort of 55 SDS patients, 36% of patients developed MDS or AML by the age of 30 years.[10] Cellular deficiency of the SBDS protein results in ribosomal dysfunction and translational inefficiency, which is linked to Fas ligand–induced apoptosis and induction of TP53-mediated cellular senescence pathways.[11,12]

Recurrent clonal cytogenetic alterations are commonly identified in the bone marrow of SDS patients, including isochromosome 7 (i7(q10)), monosomy 7, and del(20q). Although monosomy 7 is associated with rapid clonal progression, del(20q) and i7(q10) correlate with a benign clinical course,[13,14] suggesting that development of clonal hematopoiesis with somatic genetic alterations may not be deterministic of leukemic transformation.

In SDS patients with compound heterozygosity for the 2 most common SBDS mutations, the presence of i(7)(q10) favored the allele with c.258+2T>C (a splice site mutation causing decreased SBDS levels) over the c.183_184TA>CT allele (a nonsense mutation causing complete SBDS loss). As such, i(7)(q10) may cause a relative increase of SBDS protein, thereby improving the underlying cellular dysfunction and driving a selective clonal advantage.[14] Similarly, the minimally deleted region of del(20q) involves the *EIF6* gene locus. It has been hypothesized that EIF6 haploinsufficiency promotes partial rescue of impaired ribosome biogenesis in SDS cells by favoring ejection of EIF6 from the nascent 60S ribosome.[13,15] In each of these scenarios, the selective fitness of somatically mutated clones may be driven by functional complementation of underlying cellular defects, rather than by alteration of pathways directly involved in biological transformation.[13,15] Consistent with this model, neither i(7)(q10) nor del(20q) alterations are associated with an increased risk of leukemic transformation.

In the authors' genetic analysis of samples obtained before transplantation from 1514 patients with MDS, they identified 7 patients with canonical biallelic *SBDS* mutations.[2] These SDS patients were significantly younger than other MDS patients (median age 25.1 years) and had poor clinical outcomes (median survival of 1.2 years) compared with other young patients (median survival not reached). Consistent with their poor survival, all patients with biallelic *SBDS* mutations had at least one somatic *TP53* mutation. Moreover, *TP53* mutations were significantly more frequent in patients with biallelic *SBDS* mutations than in patients without *SBDS* mutations. The high frequency of *TP53* mutations in this cohort suggests that there may be a specific cooperative effect between SBDS deficiency and *TP53* alterations that mediates clinical progression to MDS.

A subsequent study of 27 patients used a barcoded sequencing approach to confirm that somatic *TP53* mutations are highly recurrent in SDS, affecting 48% of patients.[16] The incidence of *TP53* mutations in this SDS cohort correlated with increased age, and several patients harbored multiple *TP53* mutations. Importantly, the investigators identified *TP53* mutations even among patients without clinical or morphologic evidence of transformation, and the presence of *TP53* mutations was not associated with worse hematologic function. *TP53* mutations were not detected in severe congenital neutropenia (SCN) and cyclic neutropenia patients,[16] suggesting that *TP53* mutations are not broadly associated with neutropenic conditions, but rather may be specifically linked to SDS biology.

TP53 is a central effector of the cellular response to ribosomal dysfunction.[17] Indeed, TP53 overexpression is observed in bone marrow biopsies from SDS patients[12] and Sbds deficiency in mice was shown to induce Tp53-dependent apoptosis in myeloid cells,[18] suggesting that ribosomal dysfunction and translational inefficiency in SDS patients induce TP53-dependent cellular senescence. Consistent with the role of TP53 in mediating the SDS phenotype, genetic ablation of Trp53 in mice attenuates the atrophy seen in Sbds-deficient pancreatic acinar cells.[11] It is possible that somatic acquisition of *TP53* mutations in SBDS-deficient hematopoietic cells similarly rescues inefficient hematopoiesis, resulting in selection and clonal expansion of mutated cells.

DIAMOND-BLACKFAN ANEMIA

Diamond-Blackfan Anemia (DBA) is characterized by red blood cell aplasia and is associated with infantile onset of isolated, severe, macrocytic anemia, as well as short stature and congenital anomalies.[9] DBA is inherited in an autosomal dominant pattern and is most frequently caused by mutations affecting genes that encode ribosomal proteins, which are important for 18S or 28S rRNA maturation and small or large ribosomal subunit synthesis, respectively.[9] Approximately 25% of DBA patients have a mutation in *RPS19*, although more than 10 causative genes have been identified.[9] The Diamond-Blackfan Anemia Registry reports that DBA patients have a cumulative incidence for AML of 5% by the age of 46 years.[19]

In the authors' MDS transplant cohort, only one patient had DBA (defined by the presence of a heterozygous frameshift mutation in the *RPS17* gene).[2] In this case, the authors identified 6 distinct somatic mutations involving *TP53* and *PPM1D*, which encodes a serine-threonine protein phosphatase that regulates TP53 and the cellular stress response. This observation is consistent with a mechanistic link between ribosomal dysfunction and *TP53*-dependent transformation that has been observed in SDS patients that develop MDS.

In bone marrow specimens from DBA patients without transformation, TP53 has been shown to accumulate in erythroid progenitor cells, and *TP53* was induced selectively in primary human erythroid progenitor cells after *RPS19* knockdown.[20]

Moreover, the erythroid phenotype in mouse models of DBA is rescued by concomitant inactivation of *Tp53*.[21] Mutations in the TP53 pathway may thus drive clonal expansion by attenuating DBA-related erythroid apoptosis.[20,22] However, specific characteristics of clonal evolution in DBA patients and mechanistic links between DBA-related ribosomal dysfunction and TP53-dependent myeloid transformation remain to be elucidated.

SEVERE CONGENITAL NEUTROPENIA

SCN is most commonly caused by germline mutations in *ELANE* or *HAX1* and leads to promyelocytic maturation arrest, dysfunctional production of neutrophils in the bone marrow, and a heighted risk of life-threatening infections.[9] Supportive therapy involves administration of granulocyte colony-stimulating factor (G-CSF), which results in most cases in significant improvement of neutrophil counts.[23] The risk of myeloid transformation is high, with a cumulative incidence of 22% after 15 years of G-CSF treatment, and correlates with a poor response to G-CSF therapy.[23]

In a study of 148 SCN patients, 13 out of 23 patients (78%) who developed MDS or AML carried somatic activating *CSF3R* receptor mutations.[24] However, disease latency was highly variable, and several patients harbored *CSF3R* mutations for many years without evidence of transformation. Similarly, serial analysis of one patient showed that 5 different *CSF3R* mutations were present 15 years before transformation, and that eventual development of leukemia was associated with outgrowth of a single clone that had gained additional myeloid driver mutations.[25] Together, these data suggest that *CSF3R* mutations may require cooperating genetic events to cause leukemia.

Most *CSF3R* mutations cause a truncation of the cytoplasmic domain mediating enhanced cell proliferation and survival.[26] By potentiating G-CSF signaling, *CSF3R* mutations may thus result in functional compensation for ELANE- and HAX1-related defects in neutrophil production, providing a potential explanation for the high prevalence of *CSF3R* mutations in SCN patients.[20,27] A definite role for *CSF3R* mutations in initiating SCN-related leukemogenesis, independent of enabling adaptive hematopoiesis, and the link to G-CSF therapy, remains to be determined.

Somatic *RUNX1* mutations were recently identified in 64.5% of SCN patients with MDS or AML, often occurring in clones that had already acquired *CSF3R* mutations.[28] In contrast, no *RUNX1* mutations were seen in a cohort of 40 SCN patients without leukemic transformation.[16] These data strongly support a role for *RUNX1* mutations as a late step in leukemic transformation in the context of SCN. The variable latency between acquisition of somatic *CSF3R* mutations and the development of *RUNX1* mutations suggests that additional cooperating clinical or genetic variables may not yet be identified.[25,28]

FANCONI ANEMIA

Fanconi anemia (FA) is a disorder of chromosomal instability caused by germline mutations in DNA repair genes of the FA/BRCA pathway.[9] Clinical features can vary widely, with some individuals manifesting bone marrow failure, short statue, skin and upper limb abnormalities, and others (25%–40%) having no abnormal physical findings.[29] Patients with FA have elevated cumulative incidence of various cancers by the age of 50 years, including MDS (40%), AML (10%), and solid tumors (20%–30%).[30]

Somatic reversion of germline FANC gene mutations in hematopoietic cells has been reported in 15% of FA patients.[31] Cells with one functionally corrected allele may have a selective clonal advantage over cells with 2 pathogenic alleles, thus causing functional rescue with enhanced contribution to the HSC pool and to hematopoiesis, resulting in stabilization of blood counts.[31] Importantly, reversion events were not detected in FA-related MDS or AML, suggesting that restoration of Fanconi pathway function may drive relative clonal advantage in the context of impaired hematopoiesis, but is biologically distinct from malignant transformation.[32]

The frequency of somatic chromosomal gains and losses in 57 FA patients was evaluated using high-density genome-wide CGH/SNP arrays.[32] In this study, alterations were identified in 61% of patients with diverse clinical phenotypes, demonstrating that clonal hematopoiesis is common in FA patients, irrespective of hematologic status. Highly recurrent alterations in this cohort included gains of 1q (45%) and 3q (41%), monosomy 7/del(7q) (17%), 11q- (13.8%), and abnormalities involving *RUNX1* (21%), although the distribution of alterations across hematologic phenotypes was distinct. Whereas clonal hematopoiesis involving somatic genetic reversions of mutated FANC genes or 1q+ was associated with an indolent clinical course, the presence of *RUNX1* lesions, 3q+, or −7/del(7q) were more common in MDS and AML.[32–34] Moreover, the presence of molecular genetic alterations associated with non-FA AML, such as oncogenic *NRAS* mutations, FLT3 internal tandem duplication, or MLL partial tandem duplication, was restricted to patients with frank AML.[32]

Gains of 1q and 3q are specifically enriched in FA patients, suggesting that they may confer a distinct clonal advantage in the context of impaired FA/BRCA pathways.[32] Moreover, 1q+ can be observed in FA patients with clonal hematopoiesis with and without myeloid transformation and could reflect an uncharacterized mechanism of functional complementation of Fanconi abnormalities in HSCs. Conversely, gain of 3q is highly associated with malignant transformation, possibly because of the amplification of the leukemogenic oncogene EVI1.[32,35]

DYSKERATOSIS CONGENITA

Dyskeratosis congenita (DC) is caused by germline mutations in a set of genes involved in telomere maintenance, including *TINF2* (12%), *TERT* (5%), *TERC* (5%), *RTEL1* (2%), and *DKC1* (25%).[9] Characteristic clinical features include abnormal skin pigmentation, oral leukoplakia and nail dystrophy, hypoplastic bone marrow, pulmonary fibrosis, and liver disease.[9] DC patients have a high risk of developing hematologic complications, such as aplastic anemia (AA), MDS, and AML, as well as solid tumors.[9]

The role of acquired somatic genetic alterations in myeloid transformation in DC patients has not been systematically characterized. In 16 DC patients analyzed using a combination of X-inactivation analyses, comparative whole exome sequencing (WES) and single nucleotide polymorphism arrays, 8 out of 9 female patients showed skewed X-inactivation, suggesting that clonal hematopoiesis is common.[36] Among 6 patients evaluated by whole exome sequencing, no somatic mutations affecting recurrently mutated genes associated with hematologic cancers were identified. Importantly, one patient showed somatic reversion in *DKC1*, suggesting that restoration of normal telomere length maintenance affords a selective advantage in hematopoietic cells.[36] None of the patients in this study had clinical or morphologic evidence of myeloid transformation.

In the authors' analysis of MDS patients receiving allogeneic transplantation, 1% of adults harbored pathogenic germline mutations affecting genes involved in telomere maintenance, including *TERT*, *TERC*, or *DKC1*, whereas at least another 2% of cases had rare variants of uncertain biological significance.[2] Among 11 adult patients with germline *TERT* or *TERC* mutations, 8 (73%) had somatic mutations in established myeloid driver genes, including 7 with mutations affecting *TP53* or *PPM1D*. TP53 plays a critical role in enforcing senescence and apoptotic responses to telomere dysfunction, whereas PPM1D is a serine-threonine protein phosphatase that negatively regulates the DNA damage response via dephosphorylation of specific residues on ATM, CHK1, and TP53.[37] Mutations in *PPM1D* are localized to exon 6 and cause C-terminal truncations that may cause an increase in phosphatase activity that aberrantly inhibits checkpoint and DNA damage response pathways.[38] Similar to SDS and DBA, where the mechanism of bone marrow failure drives activation of TP53 activity, data suggest that severe telomere attrition may select for somatic clones with genetic inactivation of *TP53*.

GATA2 DEFICIENCY

Germline mutations of *GATA2* cause a spectrum of clinical phenotypes defined by GATA2 haploinsufficiency with autosomal dominant inheritance. GATA2 regulates HSC function in a dose-dependent manner, and mutations lead to inactivation via truncation or impairment of functional DNA binding.[39] Patients with GATA2 haploinsufficiency have a 70% risk of progression to early-onset myeloid malignancies along with immune deficiencies and variable systemic features.[40]

Myeloid transformation in GATA2 deficiency syndromes is associated with somatic mutations in typical myeloid driver genes, including chromosomal abnormalities, such as monosomy 7 and trisomy 8.[41] Among young MDS patients, the association between monosomy 7 and germline *GATA2* mutations is particularly striking: 70% of adolescent patients with monosomy 7 have an underlying GATA2 deficiency.[42] *ASXL1* mutations are most common, identified in 14 out of 48 patients (29%) in one study, and associated with monosomy 7 and trisomy 8, young age, female gender, and poor survival.[41] Other smaller studies have seen similar association with *ASXL1* mutations as well as recurrent mutations affecting other hematologic driver genes, including *SETBP1*, *RUNX1*, *NRAS*, and *STAG2*.[43–45]

FAMILIAL PLATELET DISORDER WITH PREDISPOSITION TO ACUTE MYELOID LEUKEMIA

The Familial Platelet Disorder with Predisposition to Acute Myeloid Leukemia (FPD/AML) is an autosomal dominant disease caused by inactivating germline alterations affecting the hematopoietic transcription factor RUNX1. Typical clinical manifestations include thrombocytopenia with defects of platelet function leading to a mild to moderate bleeding tendency and a propensity to develop MDS or AML.[46] In a study of 10 families with 5 pedigrees harboring *RUNX1* germline mutations, the median incidence of MDS/AML was 35%.[47]

In the context of germline *RUNX1* mutations, acquisition of somatic mutations is a common, if not ubiquitous characteristic of MDS/AML transformation. In focused genetic analyses, acquired mutations in FPD/AML patients have been identified in a typical spectrum of myeloid driver genes, but the most frequent progression mutation affects the second *RUNX1* allele.[48–50] In a study of 9 asymptomatic individuals with germline *RUNX1* mutations, 6 (67%) had evidence of clonal hematopoiesis, reflected by detectable somatic mutations in the blood or bone marrow.[51] However, only one patient harbored a mutation in a canonical myeloid driver gene, suggesting existence of novel cooperating drivers of clonal hematopoiesis or other factors that favor development of clonally restricted hematopoiesis in RUNX1-deficient HSCs. Although these data suggest a high cumulative risk of developing clonal hematopoiesis,[51] a direct link between clonal hematopoiesis and development of subsequent myeloid malignancies with recurrent drivers has not been established.

ACQUIRED APLASTIC ANEMIA

Acquired AA is caused by HLA restricted destruction of HSCs by autoreactive T cells.[52] Immunosuppression therapy (IST), supportive therapies, and allogeneic hematopoietic stem cell transplantation have improved the outcome of the disease. However, even after successful IST, patients remain at high risk of developing clonal disorders such as MDS/AML and paroxysmal nocturnal hemoglobinuria, with a 10-year cumulative incidence of 10% to 15% and 50%, respectively.[53,54]

Clonal hematopoiesis in AA patients most frequently involves mutations in *BCOR*, *BCORL1*, *PIGA*, *DNMT3A*, *ASXL1*, *RUNX1*, and HLA genes and is often detectable at diagnosis and dynamic over time.[54–56] *ASXL1*, *RUNX1*, and *DNMT3A* mutations are associated with advanced age, progression to MDS, and an inferior overall survival, whereas mutations in *PIGA* and *BCOR/BCORL1* correlate with a better response to immunosuppressive therapy and a better overall outcome.[54,55] Although clonal dynamics detected in serial samples of 35 AA patients were highly variable, clones harboring PIGA or *BCOR/BCORL1* mutations tended to remain stable or to decrease over time, suggesting a specific clonal advantage in the setting of autoimmune destruction, which is lost during effective IST.[54]

Frequent uniparental disomy involving the HLA locus and recurrent loss-of-function HLA mutations support a model whereby escape from T-cell–mediated destruction can drive selective clonal advantage in some AA patients.[54,56–58] However, expansion of HLA-mutated clones has not been linked to myeloid transformation, suggesting that immune evasion might drive a biologically distinct pathway of clonal dominance (**Fig. 3**). Clonal hematopoiesis in AA may thus be driven by a range of selection contexts, including immune evasion, aberrant survival in an altered microenvironment, or stem cell attrition.

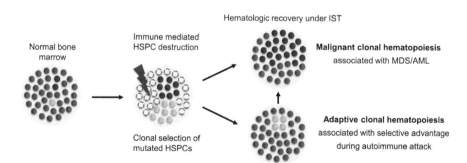

Fig. 3. Clonal hematopoiesis in acquired AA. Immune-mediated selection pressure drives expansion of HSPCs with context-specific growth advantage. Some clones may expand during the initial phase of disease due to a capacity for immune evasion, but may recede after successful immunosuppressive therapy (IST) and hematologic recovery (*green circles*). Other clones with typical myeloid driver mutations may display more context-independent expansion (*red circles*).

SUMMARY

Development of clonal hematopoiesis represents the hallmark initiation of myeloid transformation. However, the timing, genetic spectrum, and clinical implications of clonal hematopoiesis can be influenced by a range of cell-intrinsic and cell-extrinsic factors. Importantly, context-specific variables, such as germline mutations in inherited bone marrow failure or immune-mediated cell destruction in AA, can exert a strong selection pressure on the development and progression of clonal hematopoiesis. Global hematopoietic dysfunction or bone marrow microenvironmental abnormalities may enable expansion of clones that are better adapted to specific extrinsic or intrinsic selection (see **Figs. 2** and **3**).

Clinical Implications

Based on the genetic data outlined earlier, several outstanding questions remain to be answered. What clinical or genetic factors mediate myeloid transformation in patients with inherited bone marrow diseases? How can adaptive clonal hematopoiesis best be distinguished from incipient malignant degeneration? Can identification of specific somatic genetic characteristics be integrated prospectively into clinical care of individual patients? Unbiased genetic analysis of patient samples using whole exome or whole genome sequencing approaches, paired with systematic longitudinal analysis of samples obtained from patients at multiple times during the course of life, may provide answers to these questions. An improved understanding of the role of acquired somatic mutations in clonal progression of bone marrow failure syndromes has the potential to improve outcomes in this high-risk patient group by identifying novel therapeutic vulnerabilities or enabling improved clinical decision making based on objectively measurable molecular characteristics.

REFERENCES

1. Arber DA, Orazi A, Hasserjian R, et al. The 2016 revision to the World Health Organization classification of myeloid neoplasms and acute leukemia. Blood 2016; 127(20):2391–406.
2. Lindsley RC, Saber W, Mar BG, et al. Prognostic mutations in myelodysplastic syndrome after stem-cell transplantation. N Engl J Med 2017;376(6):536–47.
3. Makishima H, Yoshizato T, Yoshida K, et al. Dynamics of clonal evolution in myelodysplastic syndromes. Nat Genet 2016;49(2):204–12.
4. Welch J, Ley T, Link D, et al. The origin and evolution of mutations in acute myeloid leukemia. Cell 2012;150(2):264–78.
5. Jaiswal S, Fontanillas P, Flannick J, et al. Age-related clonal hematopoiesis associated with adverse outcomes. N Engl J Med 2014;371(26):2488–98.
6. Sekeres MA. The epidemiology of myelodysplastic syndromes. Hematol Oncol Clin North Am 2010;24(2):287–94.
7. Gibson CJ, Lindsley RC, Tchekmedyian V, et al. Clonal hematopoiesis associated with adverse outcomes after autologous stem-cell transplantation for lymphoma. J Clin Oncol 2017;35(14):1598–605.
8. Coombs CC, Zehir A, Devlin SM, et al. Therapy-related clonal hematopoiesis in patients with non-hematologic cancers is common and associated with adverse clinical outcomes. Cell Stem Cell 2017;21(3):374–82.
9. Wegman-Ostrosky T, Savage SA. The genomics of inherited bone marrow failure: from mechanism to the clinic. Br J Haematol 2017;177(4):526–42.
10. Donadieu J, Leblanc T, Meunier BB, et al. Analysis of risk factors for myelodysplasias, leukemias and death from infection among patients with congenital

neutropenia. Experience of the French Severe Chronic Neutropenia Study Group. Haematologica 2005;90(1):45–53.

11. Tourlakis ME, Zhang S, Ball HL, et al. In vivo senescence in the Sbds-deficient murine pancreas: cell-type specific consequences of translation insufficiency. PLoS Genet 2015;11(6):e1005288.

12. Elghetany MT, Alter BP. p53 protein overexpression in bone marrow biopsies of patients with Shwachman-Diamond syndrome has a prevalence similar to that of patients with refractory anemia. Arch Pathol Lab Med 2002;126(4):452–5.

13. Pressato B, Valli R, Marletta C, et al. Deletion of chromosome 20 in bone marrow of patients with Shwachman-Diamond syndrome, loss of the EIF6 gene and benign prognosis Shwachman-Diamond. Br J Haematol 2012;157(4):501–3.

14. Minelli A, Maserati E, Nicolis E, et al. The isochromosome i(7)(q10) carrying c.258+2t>c mutation of the SBDS gene does not promote development of myeloid malignancies in patients with Shwachman syndrome. Leukemia 2009; 23(4):708–11.

15. Valli R, Pressato B, Marletta C, et al. Different loss of material in recurrent chromosome 20 interstitial deletions in Shwachman-Diamond syndrome and in myeloid neoplasms. Mol Cytogenet 2013;6:56.

16. Xia J, Miller CA, Baty J, et al. Somatic mutations and clonal hematopoiesis in congenital neutropenia. Blood 2018;131(4):408–16.

17. McGowan KA, Pang WW, Bhardwaj R, et al. Reduced ribosomal protein gene dosage and p53 activation in low-risk myelodysplastic syndrome. Blood 2011; 118(13):3622–33.

18. Zambetti NA, Bindels EMJ, Van Strien PMH, et al. Deficiency of the ribosome biogenesis gene Sbds in hematopoietic stem and progenitor cells causes neutropenia in mice by attenuating lineage progression in myelocytes. Haematologica 2015;100(10):1285–93.

19. Vlachos A, Rosenberg PS, Atsidaftos E, et al. Incidence of neoplasia in Diamond Blackfan anemia: a report from the Diamond Blackfan Anemia Registry. Blood 2012;119(16):3815–9.

20. Dutt S, Narla A, Lin K, et al. Haploinsufficiency for ribosomal protein genes causes selective activation of p53 in human erythroid progenitor cells. Blood 2011;117(9):2567–76.

21. McGowan KA, Li JZ, Park CY, et al. Ribosomal mutations cause p53-mediated dark skin and pleiotropic effects. Nat Genet 2008;40(8):963–70.

22. Danilova N, Sakamoto KM, Lin S. Ribosomal protein S19 deficiency in zebrafish leads to developmental abnormalities and defective erythropoiesis through activation of p53 protein family. Blood 2008;112(13):5228–37.

23. Rosenberg PS, Alter BP, Bolyard AA, et al. The incidence of leukemia and mortality from sepsis in patients with severe congenital neutropenia receiving long-term G-CSF therapy. Blood 2006;107(12):4628–35.

24. Germeshausen M, Ballmaier M, Welte K. Incidence of CSF3R mutations in severe congenital neutropenia and relevance for leukemogenesis: results of a long-term survey. Blood 2007;109:93–9.

25. Beekman RE, Valkhof MG, Sanders MA, et al. Sequential gain of mutations in severe congenital neutropenia progressing to acute myeloid leukemia. Blood 2012; 119(22):5071–7.

26. Germeshausen M, Ballmaier M, Welte K. Implications of mutations in hematopoietic growth factor receptor genes in congenital cytopenias. Ann N Y Acad Sci 2001;938:305–20 [discussion: 320–1].

27. Qiu Y, Zhang Y, Hu N, et al. A truncated granulocyte colony-stimulating factor receptor (G-CSFR) inhibits apoptosis induced by neutrophil elastase G185R mutant. J Biol Chem 2017;292(8):3496–505.

28. Skokowa J, Steinemann D, Katsman-Kuipers JE, et al. Cooperativity of RUNX1 and CSF3R mutations in severe congenital neutropenia: a unique pathway in myeloid leukemogenesis. Blood 2014;123(14):2229–38.

29. Shimamura A, Alter BP. Pathophysiology and management of inherited bone marrow failure syndromes. Blood Rev 2010;24(3):101–22.

30. Alter BP, Giri N, Savage SA, et al. Malignancies and survival patterns in the National Cancer Institute inherited bone marrow failure syndromes cohort study. Br J Haematol 2010;150(2):179–88.

31. Soulier J, Leblanc T, Jubert C, et al. Detection of somatic mosaicism and classification of Fanconi anemia patients by analysis of the FA/BRCA pathway. Blood 2005;105(3):1329–37.

32. Quentin S, Cuccuini W, Ceccaldi R, et al. Myelodysplasia and leukemia of Fanconi anemia are associated with a specific pattern of genomic abnormalities that includes cryptic RUNX1/AML1 lesions. Blood 2011;117(15):e161–70.

33. Cioc AM, Wagner JE, MacMillan ML, et al. Diagnosis of myelodysplastic syndrome among a cohort of 119 patients with Fanconi anemia: morphologic and cytogenetic characteristics. Am J Clin Pathol 2010;133(1):92–100.

34. Tönnies H, Huber S, Kühl JS, et al. Clonal chromosomal aberrations in bone marrow cells of Fanconi anemia patients: gains of the chromosomal segment 3q26q29 as an adverse risk factor. Blood 2003;101(10):3872–4.

35. Meyer S, Bristow CWM, Pepper S, et al. Fanconi anemia (FA)–associated 3q gains in leukemic transformation consistently target EVI1, but do not affect low TERC expression in FA. Blood 2011;117(22):6047–50.

36. Perdigones N, Perin JC, Schiano I, et al. Clonal hematopoiesis in patients with dyskeratosis congenita. Am J Hematol 2016;91(12):1227–33.

37. Lu X, Nannenga B, Donehower LA. PPM1D dephosphorylates Chk1 and p53 and abrogates cell cycle checkpoints. Genes Dev 2005;19(10):1162–74.

38. Kleiblova P, Shaltiel IA, Benada J, et al. Gain-of-function mutations of PPM1D/Wip1 impair the p53-dependent G1 checkpoint. J Cell Biol 2013;201(4):511–21.

39. Rodrigues NP, Janzen V, Forkert R, et al. Haploinsufficiency of GATA-2 perturbs adult hematopoietic stem-cell homeostasis. Blood 2005;106(2):477–84.

40. Micol JB, Abdel-Wahab O. Collaborating constitutive and somatic genetic events in myeloid malignancies: ASXL1 mutations in patients with germline GATA2 mutations. Haematologica 2014;99(2):201–3.

41. West RR, Hsu AP, Holland SM, et al. Acquired ASXL1 mutations are common in patients with inherited GATA2 mutations and correlate with myeloid transformation. Haematologica 2014;99(2):276–81.

42. Wlodarski MW, Hirabayashi S, Pastor V, et al. Prevalence, clinical characteristics and prognosis of GATA2-related myelodysplastic syndromes (MDS) in children and adolescents. Blood 2016;127(11):1387–98.

43. Wang X, Muramatsu H, Okuno Y, et al. GATA2 and secondary mutations in familial myelodysplastic syndromes and pediatric myeloid malignancies. Haematologica 2015;100(10):e398–401.

44. Ding L, Ikezoe T, Tan K, et al. Mutational profiling of a MonoMAC syndrome family with GATA2 deficiency. Leukemia 2017;31(1):244–5.

45. Fisher KE, Hsu AP, Williams CL, et al. Somatic mutations in children with GATA2-associated myelodysplastic syndrome who lack other features of GATA2 deficiency. Blood Adv 2017;1(7):10–2.

46. Porter CC, Druley TE, Erez A, et al. Recommendations for surveillance for children with leukemia-predisposing conditions. Clin Cancer Res 2017;23(11): e14–22.

47. Owen CJ, Toze CL, Koochin A, et al. Five new pedigrees with inherited RUNX1 mutations causing familial platelet disorder with propensity to myeloid malignancy. Blood 2008;112(12):4639–45.

48. Preudhomme C, Renneville A, Bourdon V, et al. High frequency of RUNX1 biallelic alteration in acute myeloid leukemia secondary to familial platelet disorder. Blood 2009;113(22):5583–7.

49. Knudson AG. Mutation and cancer: statistical study of retinoblastoma. Proc Natl Acad Sci U S A 1971;68(4):820–3.

50. Antony-Debré I, Duployez N, Bucci M, et al. Somatic mutations associated with leukemic progression of familial platelet disorder with predisposition to acute myeloid leukemia. Leukemia 2015;30(August 2015):999–1002.

51. Churpek JE, Pyrtel K, Kanchi KL, et al. Genomic analysis of germline and somatic variants in familial myelodysplasia/acute myeloid leukemia. Blood 2015;126(22): 2484–91.

52. Risitano AM, Maciejewski JP, Green S, et al. In-vivo dominant immune responses in aplastic anaemia: molecular tracking of putatively pathogenetic T-cell clones by TCR beta-CDR3 sequencing. Lancet 2004;364(9431):355–64.

53. Li Y, Li X, Ge M, et al. Long-term follow-up of clonal evolutions in 802 aplastic anemia patients: a single-center experience. Ann Hematol Oncol 2011;90(5):529–37.

54. Yoshizato T, Dumitriu B, Hosokawa K, et al. Somatic mutations and clonal hematopoiesis in aplastic anemia. N Engl J Med 2015;373(1):35–47.

55. Negoro E, Nagata Y, Clemente MJ, et al. Origins of myelodysplastic syndromes after aplastic anemia. Blood 2011;118(9):2492–501.

56. Babushok DV, Duke JL, Xie HM, et al. Somatic HLA mutations expose the role of class I-mediated autoimmunity in aplastic anemia and its clonal complications. Blood Adv 2017;1(22):1900–10.

57. Katagiri T, Sato-Otsubo A, Kashiwase K, et al. Frequent loss of HLA alleles associated with copy number-neutral 6pLOH in acquired aplastic anemia. Blood 2011;118(25):6601–9.

58. Stanley N, Olson TS, Babushok DV. Recent advances in understanding clonal haematopoiesis in aplastic anaemia. Br J Haematol 2017;177(4):509–25.

Myelodysplastic Syndrome, Acute Myeloid Leukemia, and Cancer Surveillance in Fanconi Anemia

Sharon A. Savage, MD[a], Michael F. Walsh, MD[b,c,d],*

KEYWORDS

- Bone marrow failure • Myelodysplastic syndrome • Leukemia
- Exquisite therapeutic sensitivity • DNA repair • BRCA1/2 • Fanconi complex
- Fanconi anemia

KEY POINTS

- Fanconi anemia is a DNA damage repair syndrome caused by pathogenic variants in key components of the Fanconi DNA repair complex.
- Patients with Fanconi anemia are at very high risk of bone marrow failure, myelodysplastic syndrome, leukemia, head and neck squamous cell carcinoma, and other malignancies.
- Treatment of patients with Fanconi anemia and cancer must be carefully tailored because of exquisite sensitivity to ionizing radiation and alkylating drugs.

INTRODUCTION TO FANCONI ANEMIA

Fanconi anemia (FA; MIM 607139) is a rare, cancer-prone inherited bone marrow failure syndrome with a wide range of clinical presentations, including radial ray anomalies, short stature, microcephaly, café au lait spots, and other medical problems. The condition is eponymous for Dr Guido Fanconi, who originally described the syndrome in 1927. At present, there are more than 2000 patients reported in the literature.[1] Advances in supportive care, including hematopoietic cell transplantation (HCT), have improved the lifespan for patients with FA, but cancer, HCT-related complications,

---

[a] Clinical Genetics Branch, Division of Cancer Epidemiology and Genetics, National Cancer Institute, 9609 Medical Center Drive, Room 6E456, MSC 9772, Bethesda, MD 20892-9772, USA; [b] Department of Medicine, Division of Solid Tumor, Memorial Sloan Kettering Cancer Center, 222 70th Street Room 412, New York, NY 10021, USA; [c] Department of Medicine, Division of Clinical Cancer Genetics, Memorial Sloan Kettering Cancer Center, 222 70th Street Room 412, New York, NY 10021, USA; [d] Department of Pediatrics, Memorial Sloan Kettering Cancer Center, 222 70th Street Room 412, New York, NY 10021, USA
* Corresponding authors. 222 70th Street Room 412, New York, NY 10021.
E-mail address: walshm2@mskcc.org

Hematol Oncol Clin N Am 32 (2018) 657–668
https://doi.org/10.1016/j.hoc.2018.04.002
0889-8588/18/Published by Elsevier Inc.
hemonc.theclinics.com

and other complex medical problems remain significant causes of mortality. Herein, the authors review the underlying biology and clinical manifestations of FA as well as the current recommendations for cancer surveillance and management.

The Biology of Fanconi Anemia

FA is a chromosomal instability disorder caused predominantly by autosomal recessive inheritance of pathogenic variants in key components of the DNA damage response.[2,3] There is one gene, *FANCB*, associated with X-linked recessive inheritance.[4] Germline mutations (ie, pathogenic variants) in at least 22 genes are associated with FA. There is consensus in the field regarding 18 genes (*FANCA, B, C, D1, D2, E, F, G, I, J, L, N, P, Q, T, U, V,* and *W*)[4–26] (**Table 1**).[27] An additional 4 genes (*FANCM, FANCO, FANCR,* and *FANCS*) are considered FA-like, because they have not been described in patients with bone marrow failure (BMF).[25,28,29] *FANCM* is not considered a bonafide FA gene, because it only has only occurred in a patient also reported to harbor biallelic *FANCA* mutations. Biallelic pathogenic variants in *FANCA* are the most common cause of FA, with 65% of patients harboring mutations in this gene. *FANCC* (14%) and *FANCG* (9%) follow *FANCA* for genes most frequently mutated in Fanconi Anemia patients with all other only reported rarely[30] (see **Table 1**).

The proteins of the FA pathway create a biochemical circuit that function in DNA repair, DNA damage response, and other cellular processes. As DNA is replicated, nucleotide incorporation and processing of the replication fork are prone to errors including wrong nucleotides, damaged bases within the DNA, abnormal DNA-protein complexes, creation of DNA-RNA hybrids (R-loops), and aberrant DNA structures, such as G quadraplexes.[31] The specific role of proteins in the Fanconi pathway is removal of DNA interstrand cross-links. Interstrand cross-links may arise from endogenous and exogenous compounds, such as aldehydes and platinum drugs, respectively. Interstrand cross-links prevent DNA strand separation and can act to block the DNA replication process and/or transcription. These aberrant DNA strands, if left intact, promote cell death.[32]

Clinical Manifestations

Clinical characteristics of FA may vary significantly from patient to patient. Typical FA findings include radial ray abnormalities with missing or unusual thumbs, café au lait macules, and typical "Fanconi" facies. Abnormal thumbs are an important differentiating feature of FA and differentiate this syndrome from thrombocytopenia absent radius syndrome in which thumbs are present.[33] Other significant FA-associated anomalies include kidney and urinary tract malformations, vertebral anomalies, esophageal atresia, hydrocephalus, short stature, and small eyes. Almost all organ systems may be involved with the highest number of congenital malformations associated with the *FANCD1/BRCA2* genotype.[34] Clinical features of FA may significantly overlap with those of the VACTERL-H association: VACTERL-H is the acronym for vertebral anomalies, anal atresia, cardiac anomalies, trachea-esophageal fistula, esophageal or duodenal atresia, renal structural anomalies, limb deformities, and hydrocephalus.[35] Additional manifestations of FA may include metabolic abnormalities, endocrinopathies, and hearing impairments. Although patients with FA may exhibit the VACTERL-H phenotype, it is not specific to FA. Alter and Giri[36] distinguished PHENOS (Pigmentation, small Head, small Eyes, central Nervous system [not hydrocephalus], Otology, and Short stature) as an acronym that includes the major dysmorphic features of FA as an aid to identify FA patients within the VACTERL-H phenotype.

Patients with FA are at very high risk of BMF, myelodysplastic syndrome (MDS), acute myeloid leukemia (AML), head and neck squamous cell carcinoma (HNSCC),

Table 1
The biology of Fanconi anemia

Fanconi Genes	Inheritance Patterns	Classic Features (BMF, Chromosomal Fragility, Malformations)	Number of Patients with Specific Mutation and Cancer Reported by NCI (Without History of Transplant) (n = 163 Patients)	Adult Onset Cancers for Carriers	Key References
FANCA	AR	Yes	11/70	—	Apostolu et al, 1996[5]
FANCB	X-Linked Recessive	Yes	1	—	Meetei et al, 2004[4]
FANCC	AR	Yes	3/19	—	Strathdee et al,[7] 1992
FANCD1/BRCA2	AR/AD	Yes	2/3	Breast, ovarian, prostate, pancreatic, skin	Timmers et al,[6] 2001; Kauff et al,[69] 2002; Pritchard et al,[70] 2016
FANCD2	AR	Yes	7	—	Timmers et al,[6] 2001
FANCE	AR	Yes	—	—	de Winter et al,[8] 2000; de Winter et al,[9] 2000
FANCF	AR	Yes	2	—	de Winter et al,[8] 2000; de Winter et al,[9] 2000
FANCG	AR	Yes	1/7	—	Garcia-Higuera et al,[10] 1999
FANCI	AR	Yes	2/3	—	Dorsman et al,[11] 2007; Sims et al,[12] 2007; Smogorzewska et al,[13] 2007
FANCJ/BRIP1	AR/AD	Yes	—	Ovarian	Cantor et al,[14] 2001; Tung et al,[71] 2016

(continued on next page)

Table 1
(continued)

Fanconi Genes	Inheritance Patterns	Classic Features (BMF, Chromosomal Fragility, Malformations)	Number of Patients with Specific Mutation and Cancer Reported by NCI (Without History of Transplant) (n = 163 Patients)	Adult Onset Cancers for Carriers	Key References
FANCL	AR	Yes	—	—	Meetei et al,[15] 2003
FANCN/PALB2	AR/AD	Yes	—	Breast, pancreatic, metastatic prostate	Xia et al,[16] 2006; Tung et al,[71] 2016
FANCP/SLX4	AR	Yes	—	—	Svendsen et al,[17] 2009
FANCQ/ERCC4	AR	Yes	—	—	Bogliolo et al,[18] 2013
FANCT/UBE2T	AR	Yes	—	—	Zhang et al,[19] 2000; Hira et al,[20] 2015
FANCU/XRCC2	AR	Yes	—	—	Jones et al,[21] 1995; Shamseldin et al,[22] 2012
FANCV/REV7	AR	Yes	—	—	Li & Benezra,[23] 1996; Bluteau et al,[24] 2016
FANCW/RFWD3	AR	Yes	—	—	Knies et al,[26] 2017
FANCM	AR	No	—	—	Meetei et al,[25] 2005
FACNO/RAD51 C	AR/AD	No	—	Ovarian/metastatic prostate	Vaz et al,[28] 2010; Tung et al,[71] 2016
FANCR/RAD51	AR/AD	No	1	Ovarian/metastatic prostate	Ameziane et al,[29] 2015; Tung et al,[71] 2016

Abbreviations: AR, autosomal recessive; AD, autosomal dominant.

and other malignancies. In some patients, BMF or cancer may be the first presenting sign of FA. It should be suspected in patients who have higher than expected toxicities related to cancer treatment.

Diagnosing Fanconi Anemia

FA is diagnosed by chromosome breakage studies on patient-derived cells. In this assay, the patient's peripheral blood T lymphocytes are exposed to diepoxybutane or mitomycin C, and the number of resultant abnormal chromosomes is counted. False negatives may occur in samples obtained from individuals with hematopoietic somatic mosaicism, and in such instances, testing of skin fibroblasts is required to diagnose FA.[37]

Genetic testing for FA now includes multiplex (ie, gene panel) testing as well as whole exome or whole genome sequencing. Identification of the causative pathogenic variants is helpful in confirming the diagnosis of FA and essential for genetic counseling of the patient and their family members. The availability of multiplex genetic testing has led to widespread testing of patients in whom FA may not have been considered. In such instances, chromosomal breakage studies have been particularly important in confirming whether the genetic variants are contributory to disease.

CONSEQUENCES AND MANAGEMENT OF HEMATOPOIETIC STEM CELL ATTRITION
Bone Marrow Failure and Leukemia

BMF in FA is attributed to attrition of the hematopoietic stem and progenitor cell compartment due to elevated DNA damage response and apoptosis.[38] The bone marrow of patients with FA has been shown to be proinflammatory; specifically, tumor necrosis factor-α (TNF-α) may contribute to apoptosis of FA hematopoietic stem cells (HSCs) through activation of the extrinsic apoptotic pathway.[38] Moreover, functional studies have illustrated that aberrantly activated oligoclonal T-cell populations suppress hematopoiesis by releasing cytokines (including interferon-γ [INF-γ] and TNF-α).[39,40] This cascade of events is cytotoxic to HSCs and subsequently to lymphoid populations.[41] The toxic environment likely leads to a stem cell compartment favoring the evolution of somatically mutated cells with the capacity to resist the attack of T cells and the evolution of covert leukemic clones (**Fig. 1**).[42–45]

In addition to adverse effects of INF-γ, TNF-α, and other cytokines in FA patients, there is evidence that BMF may be exacerbated by endogenous aldehyde-induced toxicity and/or DNA damage-induced p53 activation, both of which result in HSC attrition.[46,47] One report found that FA patients with *ALDH2* mutations have accelerated

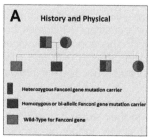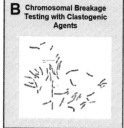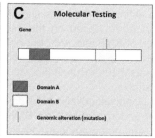

Fig. 1. Fanconi triple assessment: patients being evaluated for FA require a triple assessment, including (A) history/physical examination, (B) clastogenic testing or chromosomal breakage testing with diepoxybutane ± mitomycin C, and (C) genetic testing.

progression of BMF, and murine models harboring *ALDH2* mutations independent of FA genetics have exhibited BMF.[48]

In the absence of typical congenital anomalies, cytopenias may be a presenting sign of FA. In addition, a clue to inherited bone marrow failure syndromes may also be elevated hemoglobin F and high mean corpuscular volume for age without another cause. Most patients with FA manifest clinically significant cytopenias during their lifetimes. The cumulative incidence of severe BMF is 70% by age 50, and a peak hazard rate of 4% at 12 to 15 years of age.[49] The age of BMF onset varies among patients with FA, even among siblings.[50]

Patients with FA and BMF should be monitored for the development of MDS and progression to AML by following both cytogenetic and morphologic abnormalities. Long-term studies of FA have shown that the risk of developing MDS or AML within 3 years of observing an abnormal clone was roughly 1 in 3 (35%) compared with 1 in 30 (3.3%) for those without an identifiable clone.[49,51] Cytogenetic findings in the bone marrow samples of FA patients may reveal recurring chromosomal changes of 1, 3, and 7, and these findings need to be followed closely given the risk of AML in FA. A notable finding in bone marrow of FA patients is the presence of aberrations of chromosome 3.[52,53] In these patients with identifiable chromosome 3 abnormalities, the 3-year risk of MDS/AML was 90% and 17%, respectively.

In general, the classification scheme for AML is evolving and becoming more molecularly centric.[54] How applicable this evolving schema will be to FA patients is still to be determined and needs to be further analyzed in larger numbers of FA patients.

MDS and AML occur in a significant percentage of patients with FA.[51] In a recent report from Alter and colleagues,[49] interrogating the National Cancer Institute's registry between 1945 and 2014, 130 families have been reported to date with FA, with approximately 160 individuals who are presently living. Leukemia had a cumulative incidence of 5% in FA by the age of 30. The cumulative incidence of MDS in FA patients by the age of 50 was 50% (confidence interval 35%–65%).

Of note, AML is significantly more common in FA than acute lymphoblastic leukemia and lymphomas. The latter hematopoietic malignancies have been reported in patients with FA harboring *FANCD1/BRCA2* gene mutations.[51,52,55–57]

Clinical Management

In general, patients with BMF require treatment for the time when BMF becomes severe, which is generally defined as hemoglobin less than 8 g/dL, platelets less than 30,000/mm^3, and absolute neutrophil count less than 500/mm^3.[2] The decision to undergo HCT is a serious one, which requires a multidisciplinary approach and assessment. The complexities of decision making in the context of FA-associated comorbidities led to the development of an interesting mathematical decision model to estimate event free-survival conditional on age and per-year cause-specific hazard rates, based on the assumption that bone marrow transplant eliminates the risk of BMF and AML but not the risk of solid tumors.[2,49,58] This approach provides perspective in deciding when or if a patient with FA should undergo HCT and suggests that transplantation at a younger age offers a benefit that is not as clear in older patients.

Nonmyeloablative HCT conditioning regimens are recommended for patients with FA undergoing HCT for BMF without MDS or AML due to their exquisite sensitivity to chemotherapy and ionizing radiation.[56,59–64] Matched sibling donors are recommended, when available, and mutation identification and testing are essential in this context. It is important for patients and their families to understand that HCT can cure BMF, but it does not cure nonhematopoietic complications of FA.[49]

All patients with FA in whom HCT is considered should be evaluated and treated at a center specializing in FA.[2] Given the rarity of FA, optimal supportive care and clinical expertise in the management of the complex FA co-morbidities are best managed at centers specializing in FA. Patients with FA who evolved to MDS or AML require a highly specialized approach because of their sensitivity to standard cancer therapeutics.[2,65]

Androgens are an option for BMF in patients with FA who cannot undergo HCT.[66,67] There are multiple well-recognized side effects of androgens, including but not limited to virilization, premature closure of growth plates, behavioral changes, elevated liver enzymes, hepatic adenomas, hepatocellular carcinoma, peliosis hepatis, acne, and hypertension. One-half to three-quarters of patients respond to androgens within 3 months. Androgens do not prevent progression to AML, which once developed, may increase the risks associated with transplant, and when patients are older, additional viral infections may have been acquired that may impact transplant outcome.[68]

SOLID MALIGNANCIES

FA patients are at very high risk of solid tumors. In the prospective longitudinal cohort study by the National Cancer Institute (NCI) at the National Institutes of Health (NIH) of 130 families including 163 patients, 21/163 (12%) patients were diagnosed with solid tumors: HNSCC (n = 10), vulva (n = 3), esophagus (n = 2), brain (n = 2), anus (n = 1), lung (n = 1), cervix (n = 1), and breast (n = 1), and an additional 35/163 (21%) were diagnosed including squamous cell cancer (SCC) (n = 23) and basal cell cancer (BCC) (n = 12).[49] The observed to expected ratio, for any malignancy in nontransplanted patients for FA, was 19. In FA patients having undergone HSC transplant (n = 63/163), the frequency of solid tumors was higher at 33 (51%): HNSCC (n = 5), larynx (n = 1), vulva (n = 2), brain (n = 1), thyroid (n = 2), BCC (n = 9), and SCC (n = 12). The effect of HSCT on increased cancer rates is reflected in the higher observed to expected ratios for transplanted versus the nontransplanted FA patients 55 versus 19.[49] According to Alter and colleagues, the cumulative incidence of solid tumors reported in FA patients is roughly 20% by the age of 65. Because FA patients exhibit extreme sensitivity to alkylating and radiation therapies, there continue to be significant challenges in treating patients and avoiding second malignancies.

CANCER SCREENING AND RISK REDUCTION

The guidelines for diagnosis management of FA are described in detail at http://fanconi.org/index.php/publications/guidelines. FA patients require multidisciplinary care and self-directed screening. Proper health maintenance includes coordination of care with ear, nose, and throat physicians, hematologists, oncologists, gastroenterologists, orthopedic surgeons, gynecologists (for female patients), endocrinologists, dermatologists, dentists, and pediatric developmental physicians.

HNSCC is the most common solid tumor in FA patients. Approximately 1 in 7 (14%) patients with FA who survive to the age 40 will be diagnosed with HNSCC during their lifetime.[49,51] Surveillance should begin at age 10 years, which is based on literature reports of the earliest age of diagnosis with head and neck cancer. The sites at risk for the development of HNSCC include all areas of the upper aerodigestive tract. Therefore, all mucosal surfaces of the head and neck should be examined. This examination should also include the proximal and distal oropharynx and appropriate equipment such as a transoral mirror and flexible fiber-optic laryngoscope. This examination should occur every 6 months, and suspicious lesions should be biopsied. In instances whereby a premalignant or malignant lesion is identified, it should be appropriately treated, and screening should increase to every 2 to 3 months. Patients need to be

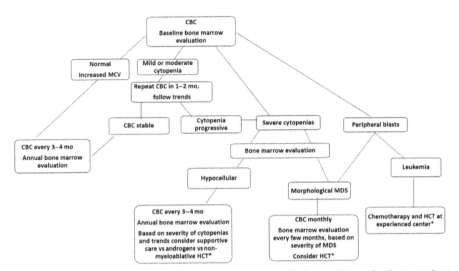

Fig. 2. Suggested hematologic evaluation for patients with Fanconi Anemia. Every patient will have specific needs that require adaptation by an experienced physician. There should be a low threshold for referral to a center with expertise in Fanconi anemia. Bone marrow evaluation includes an aspirate and a biopsy for cellularity and assessment of chromosomal abnormalities. The presence of bone marrow chromosomal clonal abnormalities should be monitored closely. *Potential related HCT donors should be evaluated with chromosomal breakage studies and Fanconi anemia gene testing based on patient's gene. CBC, complete blood count; HCT, hematopoietic cell transplantation; MCV, mean corpuscular volume; MDS, myelodysplastic syndrome.

diligent and perform self-examination, bringing any suspicious findings to their physicians' attention (http://fanconi.org/index.php/publications/guidelines_for_diagnosis_and_management).

Fanconi patients are at increased risk of skin cancers; thus, individuals should perform routine skin checks for suspicious lesions following the ABCD acronym for nevus inspection (asymmetry, bleeding/border changes, color changes, and difference in diameter). Patients should also protect their skin with hats, clothing, and sunscreen. FA patients require application of sunscreen with an SPF of at least 30. Individuals should see their dermatologist once a year and strive to maintain adequate vitamin D levels through supplements if necessary.

In regard to hematologic monitoring, most physicians agree that a complete blood count (CBC) and bone marrow aspirate and biopsy are recommended at diagnosis. The bone marrow evaluation should be repeated annually. The CBC should be monitored more frequently for proactive management of cytopenias and MDS (**Fig. 2**).[65]

SUMMARY

FA is a DNA damage syndrome. FA in inherited in an autosomal recessive inheritance disease except for patients with *FANCB* mutations, in which case the disease is X linked. Multidisciplinary care for FA patients is required.[65] The field's understanding of FA continues to evolve with greater than 20 genes described to play a role in Fanconi biology, a description of the environmental milieu of FA patient's bone marrow, tailored nonmyeloablative bone marrow transplant regimens, and candidate therapeutics.

At present, HCT continues to be the only curative treatment of hematopoietic disease in FA patients.

Chromosomal breakage studies are the gold standard testing assay, and there is a continued need for genotypic/phenotypic description and studies. Triple assessment, including clinical characteristics, chromosomal breakage studies, and molecular testing, provides the greatest context for advancing the understanding of FA and better understanding atypical findings. Studies need to be powered well in order to make valid conclusions from integrated genotype/phenotype analyses. Moreover, uniform annotation of variant calling following rigorous classification guidelines will allow for meaningful clinical translation. At present, identification of FANC complex carriers has broad clinical relevance depending on the specific gene and variant detected. In some instances, such as *FANCD1, PALB2, RAD51C, RAD51*, and *BRIP1*, heterozygous carriers are at risk for adult onset cancers, but the extent to which heterozygous carriers of pathogenic variants in other FA genes are at risk is not known and is an area of active study. Carriers should be counseled for reproductive risks as well.[69–71] The continued international effort focused on comprehensive care for FA patients is crucial given the rarity of this disease and for further advancements in caring for patients to be made.

ACKNOWLEDGMENTS

We would like to acknowledge Dr. Neelam Giri, National Cancer Institute, for assistance with creating Figure 2. The work of S.A.S. is supported by the intramural research program of the Division of Cancer Epidemiology and Genetics, National Cancer Institute.

REFERENCES

1. Alter BP. Fanconi anemia and the development of leukemia. Best Pract Res Clin Haematol 2014;27(3–4):214–21.
2. Fanconi anemia reserach fund. Guidelines for diagnosis and management, 2008. Eugene (OR): Fanconi Anemia Reserach Fund, Inc; 2008. Fanconi Anemia.
3. Perona G, Cetto GL, Bernardi F, et al. Fanconi's anaemia in adults: study of three families. Haematologica 1977;62(6):615–28.
4. Meetei AR, Levitus M, Xue Y, et al. X-linked inheritance of Fanconi anemia complementation group B. Nat Genet 2004;36(11):1219–24.
5. Fanconi anaemia/Breast cancer consortium. Positional cloning of the Fanconi anaemia group A gene. Nat Genet 1996;14(3):324–8.
6. Timmers C, Taniguchi T, Hejna J, et al. Positional cloning of a novel Fanconi anemia gene, FANCD2. Mol Cell 2001;7(2):241–8.
7. Strathdee CA, Gavish H, Shannon WR, et al. Cloning of cDNAs for Fanconi's anaemia by functional complementation. Nature 1992;358(6385):434.
8. de Winter JP, Leveille F, van Berkel CG, et al. Isolation of a cDNA representing the Fanconi anemia complementation group E gene. Am J Hum Genet 2000;67(5):1306–8.
9. de Winter JP, Rooimans MA, van Der Weel L, et al. The Fanconi anaemia gene FANCF encodes a novel protein with homology to ROM. Nat Genet 2000;24(1):15–6.
10. Garcia-Higuera I, Kuang Y, Naf D, et al. Fanconi anemia proteins FANCA, FANCC, and FANCG/XRCC9 interact in a functional nuclear complex. Mol Cell Biol 1999;19(7):4866–73.
11. Dorsman JC, Levitus M, Rockx D, et al. Identification of the Fanconi anemia complementation group I gene, FANCI. Cell Oncol 2007;29(3):211–8.

12. Sims AE, Spiteri E, Sims RJ 3rd, et al. FANCI is a second monoubiquitinated member of the Fanconi anemia pathway. Nat Struct Mol Biol 2007;14(6):564–7.
13. Smogorzewska A, Matsuoka S, Vinciguerra P, et al. Identification of the FANCI protein, a monoubiquitinated FANCD2 paralog required for DNA repair. Cell 2007;129(2):289–301.
14. Cantor SB, Bell DW, Ganesan S, et al. BACH1, a novel helicase-like protein, interacts directly with BRCA1 and contributes to its DNA repair function. Cell 2001; 105(1):149–60.
15. Meetei AR, de Winter JP, Medhurst AL, et al. A novel ubiquitin ligase is deficient in Fanconi anemia. Nat Genet 2003;35(2):165–70.
16. Xia B, Sheng Q, Nakanishi K, et al. Control of BRCA2 cellular and clinical functions by a nuclear partner, PALB2. Mol Cell 2006;22(6):719–29.
17. Svendsen JM, Smogorzewska A, Sowa ME, et al. Mammalian BTBD12/SLX4 assembles a Holliday junction resolvase and is required for DNA repair. Cell 2009; 138(1):63–77.
18. Bogliolo M, Schuster B, Stoepker C, et al. Mutations in ERCC4, encoding the DNA-repair endonuclease XPF, cause Fanconi anemia. Am J Hum Genet 2013; 92(5):800–6.
19. Zhang QH, Ye M, Wu XY, et al. Cloning and functional analysis of cDNAs with open reading frames for 300 previously undefined genes expressed in CD34+ hematopoietic stem/progenitor cells. Genome Res 2000;10(10):1546–60.
20. Hira A, Yoshida K, Sato K, et al. Mutations in the gene encoding the E2 conjugating enzyme UBE2T cause Fanconi anemia. Am J Hum Genet 2015;96(6):1001–7.
21. Jones NJ, Zhao Y, Siciliano MJ, et al. Assignment of the XRCC2 human DNA repair gene to chromosome 7q36 by complementation analysis. Genomics 1995;26(3):619–22.
22. Shamseldin HE, Elfaki M, Alkuraya FS. Exome sequencing reveals a novel Fanconi group defined by XRCC2 mutation. J Med Genet 2012;49(3):184–6.
23. Li Y, Benezra R. Identification of a human mitotic checkpoint gene: hsMAD2. Science 1996;274(5285):246–8.
24. Bluteau D, Masliah-Planchon J, Clairmont C, et al. Biallelic inactivation of REV7 is associated with Fanconi anemia. J Clin Invest 2016;126(9):3580–4.
25. Meetei AR, Medhurst AL, Ling C, et al. A human ortholog of archaeal DNA repair protein Hef is defective in Fanconi anemia complementation group M. Nat Genet 2005;37(9):958–63.
26. Knies K, Inano S, Ramirez MJ, et al. Biallelic mutations in the ubiquitin ligase RFWD3 cause Fanconi anemia. J Clin Invest 2017;127(8):3013–27.
27. Bogliolo M, Surralles J. Fanconi anemia: a model disease for studies on human genetics and advanced therapeutics. Curr Opin Genet Dev 2015;33:32–40.
28. Vaz F, Hanenberg H, Schuster B, et al. Mutation of the RAD51C gene in a Fanconi anemia-like disorder. Nat Genet 2010;42(5):406–9.
29. Ameziane N, May P, Haitjema A, et al. A novel Fanconi anaemia subtype associated with a dominant-negative mutation in RAD51. Nat Commun 2015;6:8829.
30. Dong H, Nebert DW, Bruford EA, et al. Update of the human and mouse Fanconi anemia genes. Hum Genomics 2015;9:32.
31. Rodriguez A, D'Andrea A. Fanconi anemia pathway. Curr Biol 2017;27(18): R986–8.
32. Noll DM, Mason TM, Miller PS. Formation and repair of interstrand cross-links in DNA. Chem Rev 2006;106(2):277–301.
33. Shaw S, Oliver RA. Primary heamorrhagic thrombocythaemia. Proc R Soc Med 1958;51(9):768–72.

34. Savage SA, Dufour C. Classical inherited bone marrow failure syndromes with high risk for myelodysplastic syndrome and acute myelogenous leukemia. Semin Hematol 2017;54(2):105–14.
35. Bluteau D, Masliah-Planchon J, Clairmont C, et al. Biallelic inactivation of REV7 is associated with Fanconi anemia. J Clin Invest 2017;127(3):1117.
36. Alter BP, Giri N. Thinking of VACTERL-H? Rule out Fanconi anemia according to PHENOS. Am J Med Genet A 2016;170(6):1520–4.
37. Alter BP, Joenje H, Oostra AB, et al. Fanconi anemia: adult head and neck cancer and hematopoietic mosaicism. Arch Otolaryngol Head Neck Surg 2005;131(7): 635–9.
38. Ceccaldi R, Sarangi P, D'Andrea AD. The Fanconi anaemia pathway: new players and new functions. Nat Rev Mol Cell Biol 2016;17(6):337–49.
39. Young NS, Calado RT, Scheinberg P. Current concepts in the pathophysiology and treatment of aplastic anemia. Blood 2006;108(8):2509–19.
40. Risitano AM, Maciejewski JP, Green S, et al. In-vivo dominant immune responses in aplastic anaemia: molecular tracking of putatively pathogenetic T-cell clones by TCR beta-CDR3 sequencing. Lancet 2004;364(9431):355–64.
41. Sloand E, Kim S, Maciejewski JP, et al. Intracellular interferon-gamma in circulating and marrow T cells detected by flow cytometry and the response to immunosuppressive therapy in patients with aplastic anemia. Blood 2002;100(4):1185–91.
42. Dufour C, Corcione A, Svahn J, et al. Interferon gamma and tumour necrosis factor alpha are overexpressed in bone marrow T lymphocytes from paediatric patients with aplastic anaemia. Br J Haematol 2001;115(4):1023–31.
43. Dufour C, Corcione A, Svahn J, et al. TNF-alpha and IFN-gamma are overexpressed in the bone marrow of Fanconi anemia patients and TNF-alpha suppresses erythropoiesis in vitro. Blood 2003;102(6):2053–9.
44. Mori H, Colman SM, Xiao Z, et al. Chromosome translocations and covert leukemic clones are generated during normal fetal development. Proc Natl Acad Sci U S A 2002;99(12):8242–7.
45. Whitney MA, Royle G, Low MJ, et al. Germ cell defects and hematopoietic hypersensitivity to gamma-interferon in mice with a targeted disruption of the Fanconi anemia C gene. Blood 1996;88(1):49–58.
46. Ceccaldi R, Parmar K, Mouly E, et al. Bone marrow failure in Fanconi anemia is triggered by an exacerbated p53/p21 DNA damage response that impairs hematopoietic stem and progenitor cells. Cell Stem Cell 2012;11(1):36–49.
47. Langevin F, Crossan GP, Rosado IV, et al. Fancd2 counteracts the toxic effects of naturally produced aldehydes in mice. Nature 2011;475(7354):53–8.
48. Hira A, Yabe H, Yoshida K, et al. Variant ALDH2 is associated with accelerated progression of bone marrow failure in Japanese Fanconi anemia patients. Blood 2013;122(18):3206–9.
49. Alter BP, Giri N, Savage SA, et al. Cancer in the National Cancer Institute inherited bone marrow failure syndrome cohort after 15 years of follow-up. Haematologica 2018;103(1):30–9.
50. Faivre L, Guardiola P, Lewis C, et al. Association of complementation group and mutation type with clinical outcome in Fanconi anemia. European Fanconi Anemia Research Group. Blood 2000;96(13):4064–70.
51. Kutler DI, Singh B, Satagopan J, et al. A 20-year perspective on the International Fanconi Anemia Registry (IFAR). Blood 2003;101(4):1249–56.
52. Tonnies H, Huber S, Kuhl JS, et al. Clonal chromosomal aberrations in bone marrow cells of Fanconi anemia patients: gains of the chromosomal segment 3q26q29 as an adverse risk factor. Blood 2003;101(10):3872–4.

53. Cioc AM, Wagner JE, MacMillan ML, et al. Diagnosis of myelodysplastic syndrome among a cohort of 119 patients with Fanconi anemia: morphologic and cytogenetic characteristics. Am J Clin Pathol 2010;133(1):92–100.

54. Papaemmanuil E, Gerstung M, Bullinger L, et al. Genomic classification and prognosis in acute myeloid leukemia. N Engl J Med 2016;374(23):2209–21.

55. Alter BP, Rosenberg PS, Brody LC. Clinical and molecular features associated with biallelic mutations in FANCD1/BRCA2. J Med Genet 2007;44(1):1–9.

56. Myers K, Davies SM, Harris RE, et al. The clinical phenotype of children with Fanconi anemia caused by biallelic FANCD1/BRCA2 mutations. Pediatr Blood Cancer 2012;58(3):462–5.

57. Wagner JE, Tolar J, Levran O, et al. Germline mutations in BRCA2: shared genetic susceptibility to breast cancer, early onset leukemia, and Fanconi anemia. Blood 2004;103(8):3226–9.

58. Khan NE, Rosenberg PS, Alter BP. Preemptive bone marrow transplantation and event-free survival in Fanconi anemia. Biol Blood Marrow Transplant 2016;22(10):1888–92.

59. Ayas M, Saber W, Davies SM, et al. Allogeneic hematopoietic cell transplantation for Fanconi anemia in patients with pretransplantation cytogenetic abnormalities, myelodysplastic syndrome, or acute leukemia. J Clin Oncol 2013;31(13):1669–76.

60. Chaudhury S, Auerbach AD, Kernan NA, et al. Fludarabine-based cytoreductive regimen and T-cell-depleted grafts from alternative donors for the treatment of high-risk patients with Fanconi anaemia. Br J Haematol 2008;140(6):644–55.

61. MacMillan ML, DeFor TE, Young JA, et al. Alternative donor hematopoietic cell transplantation for Fanconi anemia. Blood 2015;125(24):3798–804.

62. MacMillan ML, Hughes MR, Agarwal S, et al. Cellular therapy for Fanconi anemia: the past, present, and future. Biol Blood Marrow Transplant 2011;17(1 Suppl):S109–14.

63. Stepensky P, Shapira MY, Balashov D, et al. Bone marrow transplantation for Fanconi anemia using fludarabine-based conditioning. Biol Blood Marrow Transplant 2011;17(9):1282–8.

64. Mehta PA, Davies SM, Leemhuis T, et al. Radiation-free, alternative-donor HCT for Fanconi anemia patients: results from a prospective multi-institutional study. Blood 2017;129(16):2308–15.

65. Walsh MF, Chang VY, Kohlmann WK, et al. Recommendations for childhood cancer screening and surveillance in DNA repair disorders. Clin Cancer Res 2017;23(11):e23–31.

66. Diamond LK, Shahidi NT. Treatment of aplastic anemia in children. Semin Hematol 1967;4(3):278–88.

67. Shahidi NT, Diamond LK. Testosterone-induced remission in aplastic anemia of both acquired and congenital types. Further observations in 24 cases. N Engl J Med 1961;264:953–67.

68. Guidelines FA. Chapter 3: hematologic abnormalities in patients with Fanconi anemia. 2014.

69. Kauff ND, Satagopan JM, Robson ME, et al. Risk-reducing salpingo-oophorectomy in women with a BRCA1 or BRCA2 mutation. N Engl J Med 2002;346(21):1609–15.

70. Pritchard CC, Mateo J, Walsh MF, et al. Inherited DNA-repair gene mutations in men with metastatic prostate cancer. N Engl J Med 2016;375(5):443–53.

71. Tung N, Domchek SM, Stadler Z, et al. Counselling framework for moderate-penetrance cancer-susceptibility mutations. Nat Rev Clin Oncol 2016;13(9):581–8.

Evaluation and Management of Hematopoietic Failure in Dyskeratosis Congenita

Suneet Agarwal, MD, PhD

KEYWORDS

- Dyskeratosis congenita • Telomeres • Bone marrow failure
- Bone marrow transplantation • Aplastic anemia

KEY POINTS

- Genetic discovery in the rare inherited bone marrow failure syndrome dyskeratosis congenita (DC) has revealed a spectrum of diseases caused by mutations in genes regulating telomere maintenance.
- Defects in telomere maintenance provide a molecular framework for understanding hematopoietic stem cell failure in DC.
- Timely diagnosis of an underlying telomere biology disorder greatly affects patient management and is facilitated by telomere length testing and genetic testing.
- Prospective trials and coordinated efforts are driving therapeutic advancements for hematopoietic failure in DC.

INTRODUCTION

Dyskeratosis congenita (DC) is a rare, inherited bone marrow failure (BMF) syndrome characterized by variable manifestations and ages of onset, and predisposition to cancer. Genetic discoveries in the past 20 years have revealed DC as one of a spectrum of diseases caused by mutations in genes regulating telomere maintenance, collectively referred to here as telomere biology disorders (TBDs). Hematologic disease is a frequent finding in patients with DC and in children presenting with TBD. Timely diagnosis of an underlying TBD in patients with BMF affects treatment and has been facilitated by increased awareness and availability of diagnostic tests in recent years. This article summarizes the pathophysiology, evaluation, and management of hematopoietic failure in patients with DC/TBD.

Division of Hematology/Oncology, Harvard Medical School, Dana-Farber Boston Children's Cancer and Blood Disorders Center, Boston Children's Hospital, 1 Blackfan Circle, Karp 07214, Boston, MA 02115, USA
E-mail address: suneet.agarwal@childrens.harvard.edu

Hematol Oncol Clin N Am 32 (2018) 669–685
https://doi.org/10.1016/j.hoc.2018.04.003
0889-8588/18/© 2018 Elsevier Inc. All rights reserved.

A SPECTRUM OF TELOMERE DISEASES

DC in its classic form was described more than 100 years ago and is characterized by manifestations regarded as the diagnostic triad of reticular skin pigmentation abnormalities, oral leukoplakia, and dystrophic nails. These symptoms are now recognized as the outward manifestations of a systemic degenerative disease with myriad disorders emerging variably over the lifespan.[1] Hematologic disease is frequent: clinically significant BMF manifested in 50% of patients with DC by age 50 year in one prospective cohort, whereas 90% of patients with DC developed at least a single lineage cytopenia by the fourth decade of life in a registry study.[2,3] Patients with DC have increased risks of myelodysplastic syndrome (MDS) (>500 times) and acute myeloid leukemia (AML) (~73 times) compared with the general population.[4] The elucidation of gene mutations in classic DC led to the discovery of a broad and variable spectrum of disease, affecting individuals of all ages.[5,6] Early-onset, multisystem disorders manifesting as Hoyeraal-Hreidarsson syndrome, Revesz syndrome, or Coats plus disease are caused by mutations in genes also disrupted in patients presenting with classic DC.[7–10] In contrast, some patients without overt syndromic features diagnosed in childhood or adulthood with idiopathic aplastic anemia or familial MDS/AML carry germline mutations in the same telomere biology genes implicated in DC.[11–14] Still other patients with TBDs may remain asymptomatic from a hematologic standpoint throughout life, but present in the fifth to seventh decades of life with progressive and ultimately fatal hepatic or pulmonary fibrosis.[15,16] An increasing awareness of the highly variable presentation of TBD and the availability of clinically validated telomere length and genetic testing have led to refined estimates of the rarity of TBD. Although early-onset phenotypes with multisystem disease such as DC are generally said to affect ~1 in 1 million children, the prevalence of the broader spectrum of TBD that includes adults with late-onset manifestations may be 10 to 100 times higher.[17] In these individuals, recognizing subtle hematologic defects in the absence of overt symptoms can have important clinical consequences, such as anticipating complications of medical therapy for other TBD-associated disorders (eg, organ transplant for lung or liver disease), and assessing their suitability as bone marrow donors for affected family members.[18,19]

TELOMERES IN STEM CELL SELF-RENEWAL

Telomeres are repetitive protein-DNA structures that protect the ends of chromosomes (**Fig. 1**). Hundreds to thousands of copies of the hexanucleotide repeat TTAGGG are complexed with shelterin proteins (TRF1, TRF2, RAP1, TIN2, POT1, TPP1) to prevent the recognition of free DNA ends as double-stranded breaks. The ends of linear DNA cannot be replicated by DNA polymerase, and therefore telomere length decreases with each cell cycle. At a critically short telomere length, senescence is triggered and cells stop dividing.[20,21] Adult self-renewing cells such as hematopoietic stem cells (HSCs) counteract telomere-associated senescence by activating telomerase (encoded by the *TERT* gene), a ribonucleoprotein that replaces hexanucleotide repeats by reverse transcription of an RNA template (encoded by the *TERC* gene). The balance of replication-associated telomere attrition and telomerase-mediated repeat addition is an important determinant of stem cell self-renewal capacity and therefore tissue regenerative capacity throughout the lifespan. Telomere length can be considered an endowment from a tissue-specific stem cell that determines the number of times its telomerase-negative, differentiated progeny can divide.

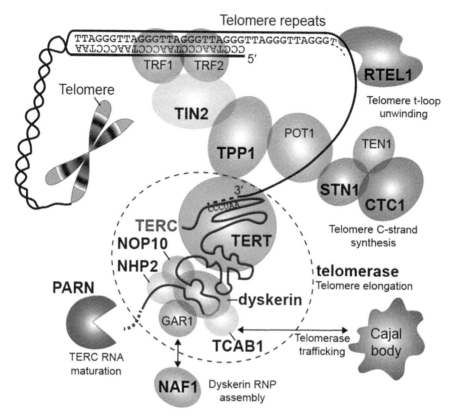

Fig. 1. Components of telomere biology disrupted in DC. Telomeres are composed of thousands of TTAGGG repeats. The telomere repeats are bound by several proteins (TRF1, TRF2, TIN2, RAP1 [not shown], TPP1, and POT1), collectively called shelterin. The telomere ends in a loop (t loop) with a 3′ overhang, which must be unwound by RTEL1 for telomere replication. The figure depicts the unwound telomere end bound by telomerase, a ribonucleoprotein (RNP) complex that elongates telomeres by reverse transcription. Telomerase is composed of the reverse transcriptase TERT and the RNA template TERC, which add telomere repeats to the 3′ end. Several other proteins make up the telomerase RNP (dyskerin, NOP10, NHP2, GAR1, TCAB1), and are responsible for stabilizing and trafficking telomerase to the Cajal body, where telomeres are elongated. NAF1 is responsible for early assembly of the dyskerin RNP but is replaced by GAR1 in the mature RNP. PARN is required for maturation and stabilization of nascent TERC RNA. Components of the CST (CTC1, STN1, TEN1) complex are responsible for filling in the lagging C-strand of the elongating telomere end. Components of the telomere maintenance machinery that have been found to be disrupted in DC are shown in color with bold labels.

GENETICS OF DYSKERATOSIS CONGENITA/TELOMERE BIOLOGY DISORDERS

The pioneering work of Dokal, Vulliamy and colleagues[22,23] in the 1990s established a registry of patients with DC that enabled genetic linkage studies and led to the discovery of *DKC1*, the first DC-associated gene. The protein encoded by *DKC1*, dyskerin, was found to have homology to Cbf5p, a yeast pseudouridine synthase that binds an RNA motif called the H/ACA box. Independently, Mitchell and Collins[24] identified an H/ACA box motif in the long noncoding RNA component of human telomerase, TERC, leading to their insight that disruption of telomere maintenance pathways may underlie DC. This hypothesis was confirmed by their subsequent demonstrations that dyskerin was indeed a novel component of human telomerase, and that TERC RNA levels were decreased in *DKC1*-mutant cells in patients with DC.[25] Subsequently, the discovery of germline *TERC* mutations in autosomal dominant DC pedigrees solidified a role for defective telomere maintenance in DC.[26] In the ensuing 20 years, mutations in 13 genes involved in various aspects of telomere maintenance have been identified to account for ~70% of DC cases[27–30] (**Table 1**), including genes encoding telomerase-associated components (TERC, TERT, DKC1, NOP10, NHP2, TCAB1, NAF1, PARN), shelterin proteins (TIN2, TPP1), and other regulators of telomere length and replication (RTEL1, CTC1, STN1) (see **Fig. 1**).

The inheritance of short telomeres has been shown to contribute to disease manifestations and patient phenotypes. Genetic anticipation is seen in autosomal dominant forms of DC/TBD, with hematopoietic and multisystem disease presenting earlier in life, and with an increasing penetrance in each generation.[31,32] This anticipation is thought to be caused by the combined effect of inheriting shortened telomeres (ie, diminished telomere endowment) in addition to a telomere maintenance defect caused by the underlying genetic mutation. Intriguingly, it has also been observed in animal models and human studies of pedigrees with known autosomal dominant mutations that inheritance of short telomeres without the genetic mutation may result in hematologic or nonhematologic phenotypes of DC.[33–35]

CAUSE OF HEMATOPOIETIC FAILURE IN DYSKERATOSIS CONGENITA

Genetically determined defects in telomere length provide an intuitive pathophysiologic link between premature telomere attrition, compromised HSC self-renewal, and hematopoietic failure. HSC self-renewal and differentiation are required to maintain the homeostatic production of billions of blood cells per day. HSCs express telomerase, and HSC self-renewal is governed in part by telomere length.[36–38] Blood cell telomere length decreases as people age, indicating that telomerase levels are limiting in the HSC compartment.[36] Telomere length of donor hematopoietic cells decreases rapidly on transplant into another host, consistent with accelerated telomere attrition in human HSCs during periods of replicative stress.[39–41] Defects in telomere length inheritance and/or maintenance are therefore consistent with impairments in hematopoietic output over the lifespan. Across the spectrum of TBD, hematopoietic failure as a presenting manifestation tends to correlate with the severity of telomere shortening.[42]

Several correlative studies have linked short telomere length in the hematopoietic compartment to various diseases perhaps reflective of external pressures such as high turnover and immune attack. Shorter than normal telomere length is found in the blood cells of patients with aplastic anemia and MDS, and is associated with evolution of acquired aplastic anemia to MDS.[43–47] Short telomere length also portends poor outcome to therapeutic interventions such as immunosuppressive therapy (IST)[48] and bone marrow transplant,[49] independent of germline mutations in telomere biology genes. These findings indicate a direct role of telomere attrition in hematopoietic failure and transformation.

The observation of clonal dominance in carriers of DC-associated mutations provides strong evidence for a causal role of HSC-intrinsic telomere maintenance defects in BMF. Early studies of maternal carriers of pathogenic X-linked *DKC1* gene mutations showed skewing of X inactivation in the peripheral blood.[50] This finding indicates that hematopoietic progenitors expressing the mutant *DKC1* allele are compromised

Hematopoietic Failure in Dyskeratosis Congenita

Table 1
Genetics of dyskeratosis congenita

#	Gene (Product)	Inheritance	Presenting Manifestations/Syndrome and Genetic Features	Frequency Estimate in DC[a]	Functional Consequence
1	*DKC1* (dyskerin)	X-linked recessive	DC, HHS, AA, PF; female carriers may have subtle findings	More common	Reduced TERC and telomerase activity[b]
2	*TERC* (TERC)	AD	DC, AA, PF, LD, CA; genetic anticipation	Less common	Reduced telomerase activity
3	*TERT* (TERT)	AD	DC, HHS, AA, PF, LD, CA; genetic anticipation	Less common	Reduced telomerase activity or recruitment to telomeres
		AR	DC, HHS	Less common	Reduced telomerase activity or recruitment to telomeres
4	*NOP10* (NOP10)	AR	DC	Very rare	Reduced TERC and telomerase activity[b]
5	*NHP2* (NHP2)	AR	DC	Very rare	Reduced TERC and telomerase activity[b]
6	*TINF2* (TIN2)	AD, often de novo	DC, HHS, RS, PF; mutations clustered in exon 6	More common	Unclear
7	*WRAP53* (TCAB1)	AR	DC	Very rare	Impaired telomerase trafficking to Cajal body[b]
8	*CTC1* (CTC1)	AR	DC, CP	Less common	Impaired telomere replication; telomere fragility

(continued on next page)

Table 1
(continued)

#	Gene (Product)	Inheritance	Presenting Manifestations/Syndrome and Genetic Features	Frequency Estimate in DC[a]	Functional Consequence
9	*RTEL1* (RTEL1)	AD	PF, AA	NA	Impaired telomere replication; telomere fragility
		AR	DC, HHS, AA, PF	Less common	Impaired telomere replication; telomere fragility
10	*ACD* (TPP1)	AD	AA	NA	Impaired telomerase recruitment to telomeres
		AR	DC, HHS	Very rare	Impaired telomerase recruitment to telomeres
11	*PARN* (PARN)	AD	PF, AA	NA	Reduced TERC and telomerase activity[c]
		AR	DC, HHS, AA, PF, LD	Less common	Reduced TERC and telomerase activity[c]
12	*NAF1* (NAF1)	AD	DC, AA, PF, LD, CA; genetic anticipation	Very rare	Reduced TERC and telomerase activity[b]
13	*STN1* (STN1)	AR	DC, CP	Very rare	Impaired telomere replication; telomere fragility

Presenting manifestations. DC: mucocutaneous triad (dystrophic nails, leukoplakia, and skin pigmentation abnormalities); BMF; or other associated features, including increased risk of malignancy, pulmonary fibrosis, vascular abnormalities; includes atypical forms with some features but not full triad.

Abbreviations: AA, plastic anemia; AD, autosomal dominant; AR, autosomal recessive; CA, Myelodysplastic syndrome, acute leukemia, head/neck squamous cell cancers; CP, Coats plus syndrome - cerebroretinal microangiopathy with calcification and cysts; gastrointestinal bleeding; osteopenia; DC, mucocutaneous triad (dystrophic nails, leukoplakia, and skin pigmentation abnormalities); BMF; or other associated features, including increased risk of malignancy, pulmonary fibrosis, vascular abnormalities; includes atypical forms with some features but not full triad; HHS, Hoyeraal-Hreidarsson syndrome - early onset with multiple manifestations with cerebellar hypoplasia, immunodeficiency; LD, liver disease including cirrhosis; NA, not applicable; PF, pulmonary fibrosis and other interstitial lung diseases; RS, Revesz syndrome - early-onset with multiple manifestations including retinal vascular disease.

[a] Frequency estimates. "More common": found mutated in greater than 10% of patients with classic DC. "Less common": found mutated in less than 10% of patients with classic DC. "Very rare": case reports of approximately 1 to 5 patients presenting with classic DC.

[b] Potential dysregulation of other box H/ACA RNAs.

[c] Potential dysregulation of other RNAs.

in survival, self-renewal, and/or differentiation compared with those expressing the normal allele. In autosomal dominant DC, somatic reversion of pathogenic *TERC* mutations has been observed in the peripheral blood.[51] Multiple independent episodes of reversion by somatic recombination were documented to occur at the level of a multipotent hematopoietic progenitor, and the derivatives of individual clones could be shown to comprise most of the peripheral blood cells. Collectively, these striking observations indicate a strong selective pressure for intact telomere maintenance mechanisms in HSCs to ensure adequate hematopoietic output.

DIAGNOSTIC TESTING FOR TELOMERE BIOLOGY DISORDER

Patients presenting with persistent peripheral blood cytopenias and a hypocellular bone marrow undergo extensive testing for infectious, immune, genetic, and other causes of BMF. Because of the implications for management, this evaluation should routinely include testing for constitutional defects in telomere maintenance. The absence of classic mucocutaneous or other signs of DC does not exclude the possibility of an inherited TBD. With the increased availability of appropriate diagnostic testing in the past several years, it has become clear that a substantial number of patients diagnosed with a TBD do not manifest the classic DC triad or other overt findings at the time of presentation with hematopoietic failure.[42]

Telomere length measurement (TLM) provides a functional test for constitutional telomere maintenance, and is an important adjunct to a comprehensive clinical assessment of patients presenting with BMF and/or suspected TBD. Several methods exist to measure telomere length, including Southern blot, quantitative polymerase chain reaction (qPCR), and flow cytometry-fluorescence in situ hybridization (flow-FISH).[52] Flow-FISH of peripheral blood cells is a clinically validated diagnostic test for DC. Flow-FISH entails hybridization of fluorescent probes to telomere ends in blood cells. The overall fluorescent intensity of a cell reflects the telomere length of all of the chromosome ends in the cell. A mean fluorescence intensity is measured for a population of cells (eg, total nucleated blood cells or particular blood cell lineage such as lymphocytes) and compared with age-adjusted normal values. Applying flow-FISH to a registry of patients with known or suspected inherited BMF syndromes, Alter and colleagues[53,54] determined that a mean lymphocyte telomere length less than or equal to 1st percentile (%ile) for age was highly sensitive for identifying patients with a constitutional TBD among patients with various forms of BMF. On this basis, age-adjusted mean lymphocyte telomere length less than or equal to 1%ile has been proposed to be diagnostic of DC/TBD when evaluating children with BMF.[54]

Although clinical flow-FISH has transformed diagnostic testing for DC since it became available approximately 10 years ago, the results must be taken within the clinical context. The diagnostic performance of flow-FISH as defined by the studies described earlier depends largely on the assumption that very low lymphocyte telomere length reflects a constitutional telomere length defect in patients with myeloid failure. However, other acquired or genetic disorders that cause high HSC turnover, or primary immunodeficiency syndromes that affect lymphoid development or homeostasis, may also manifest very low lymphocyte telomere length. In these cases, caution is warranted in interpreting lymphocyte TLM. There remains a need for a constitutional TLM strategy that does not involve hematopoietic cells, which may avoid these confounding situations. A recent study has shown that some children and most older patients with TBD can manifest leukocyte telomere length greater than the 1%ile.[42] In this study, TLM was always less than the 50%ile for age and usually less than 10%ile in patients with TBD. These data argue that, taking all ages and presentations into account, the majority of patients with a genetic disorder of telomere biology will not have telomere length less than 1%ile by flow-FISH. Therefore, the finding of lymphocyte TLM greater than 1%ile should not be used to rule out TBD in adult patients. Other limitations to flow-FISH telomere length testing include the geographic locations of the test centers, need for transport of a fresh specimen within a certain time frame to the testing center, sensitivity of the sample to environmental effects in transit, and lack of insurance coverage for this specialized test.

In terms of other approaches for TLM, qPCR of blood cell telomere length has been shown in several recent studies to be inferior to flow-FISH in diagnostic performance and is therefore not recommended for clinical decision making.[55,56] Southern blot can be considered a gold standard of telomere length measurement but is technically cumbersome and has not been standardized for specific tissues or across age distributions, and therefore its clinical utility is not yet realized.

Genetic testing is an important complement to functional telomere length testing in establishing a diagnosis of TBD. The development of next-generation sequencing panels targeting BMF genes by several investigators and centers has ushered in an era in which genetic testing might be pursued early in the clinical assessment, perhaps before or instead of telomere length testing. However, a major limitation of these exome capture panels is the incomplete genetic characterization of DC/TBD. Other confounders include incomplete coverage of genes of interest, incorrect filtering of potentially pathogenic variants, the interpretation of variants of uncertain significance, and failure to capture noncoding mutations or germline mutations because of somatic reversion. Simultaneous Sanger sequencing or orthogonal methods are useful to address coverage issues. Family studies combined with telomere length testing could be helpful in establishing the pathogenicity of variants of undetermined significance and addressing somatic reversion. Whole-genome sequencing may reveal relevant noncoding variants in patients suspected to have DC/TBD. Given these considerations, our usual practice is to send both the flow-FISH telomere length testing and a BMF genetics panel early in the evaluation of patients with BMF whenever possible.

EVALUATION OF CYTOPENIAS IN PATIENTS WITH DYSKERATOSIS CONGENITA

Peripheral blood cytopenias are common in DC and TBD, more frequently in children and in patients with multisystem disease. Characteristic findings in children presenting with hematopoietic failure caused by DC typically include myeloid defects with a predominance of thrombocytopenia; a high mean corpuscular volume; and more variably anemia, neutropenia, and reticulocytopenia. Lymphocyte numbers may be normal, but in early-onset forms of TBD such as Hoyeraal-Hreidarsson syndrome, a characteristic T cell–positive, B cell–deficient, and natural killer cell–deficient lymphopenia may be present, with or without immune dysregulation or immunodeficiency.

Although hematopoietic failure predominates, other disorders may contribute to low blood counts in patients with DC and TBD, and these are important to evaluate. Pancytopenia may result from transformation to MDS or AML. Hematologic malignancy is a less frequent manifestation of DC than BMF in children, whereas it may be the presenting manifestation of TBD in adults.[2] In patients with liver disease and splenomegaly caused by portal hypertension, hypersplenism may contribute to thrombocytopenia and neutropenia, and may also cause delayed hematopoietic reconstitution after bone marrow transplant. Gastrointestinal bleeding caused by esophageal varices from liver disease or caused by gastric vascular abnormalities, as is seen in Coats plus syndrome,[30,57] may contribute to anemia. Cytopenias from these causes can accompany and be exacerbated by concurrent hematopoietic failure. Bone marrow evaluation on presentation and serially is thus essential to evaluate for morphologic and cytogenetic changes to help distinguish aplasia versus transformation versus consumptive causes of cytopenias in DC.

MANAGEMENT OF HEMATOPOIETIC FAILURE IN DYSKERATOSIS CONGENITA

The optimal management of hematopoietic failure in patients with DC or TBD depends first and foremost on diagnosing the underlying genetic disease. For this reason, all patients presenting with BMF should be assessed for DC/TBD by telomere length and genetic testing in conjunction with a careful clinical assessment. Arguably, the same may hold true for patients with MDS and AML presenting at any age because of the implications for patient management and family counseling. However, the frequency of TBD in these patients, and therefore the diagnostic yield, is unknown. Careful assessment of the family history for pulmonary or liver disease, hematologic defects or malignancy, and other manifestations such as early graying should be undertaken, and may be the primary findings that lead to testing and eventual diagnosis of DC/TBD.

Supportive Care

Transfusion support with red blood cells and platelets may be required for patients with severe cytopenias. Platelet refractoriness following transfusion may reflect hypersplenism caused by liver disease. Exposure to a large number of transfusions increases the risk of allosensitization and graft failure in hematopoietic stem cell transplant (HSCT). Transfusion dependence is therefore considered an indication for intervention with androgens or allogeneic HSCT (discussed later). Erythropoietin and granulocyte colony-stimulating factor are not expected to produce durable improvements in red cell or neutrophil production in patients with DC, and generally are not used.

Immunosuppressive Therapy

IST with cyclosporine and antithymocyte globulin is a standard therapy for patients with severe aplastic anemia (SAA) who do not have a suitable sibling donor for HSCT. Anecdotally some patients with DC who were initially diagnosed with SAA and treated with IST may have had a transient response to IST. However, in general, IST has not been shown to yield a response in patients with DC,[58] and a priority of early diagnosis in DC is to avoid unnecessary exposure to IST and delays to more appropriate therapies.

Eltrombopag

Eltrombopag is a small molecule agonist of the thrombopoietin receptor (c-Mpl), which initially gained approval for the treatment of refractory immune thrombocytopenic purpura. Trials undertaken to determine whether eltrombopag could decrease platelet transfusion requirements in patients with acquired SAA unexpectedly revealed trilineage improvement in a number cases.[59] Based on the fact that the c-Mpl receptor is present on HSCs, it is thought that eltrombopag may directly stimulate HSC self-renewal to improve hematopoietic function in SAA. Recently, based on additional clinical trial experience, eltrombopag has gained US Food and Drug Administration approval as front-line therapy in combination with IST for SAA. With respect to DC, however, anecdotes and case reports suggest there may be no response to eltrombopag in patients with TBD.[60] The use of eltrombopag in patients with DC is therefore not recommended outside of a clinical trial.

Androgens

Based on the observation that males of various species generally have higher hemoglobin levels than females, male sex steroids were trialed in patients with SAA several decades ago.[61] In some patients, improvements in multiple lineages were seen. It is now apparent that androgens can elicit a hematologic response in a substantial proportion of patients with specific inherited BMF syndromes, namely Fanconi anemia (FA) and DC.[62,63] In retrospective reports in DC, various androgens (eg, oxymetholone, fluoxymesterone, nandrolone, and danazol) have been documented to produce hematologic response rates of 60% to 70%, frequently yielding transfusion independence.[64,65] Common and therapy-limiting side effects of androgens such as oxymetholone include dyslipidemia and virilization, which may limit use in female patients and requires careful monitoring.[64,65] In the only prospective trial of androgen therapy for DC/TBD, adult patients were treated with high doses of danazol over a 24-month period, and a hematologic response was achieved in ~80% of patients during the period of evaluation.[66] However, several patients (10 of 24) discontinued therapy before the 24-month time point, and liver enzyme abnormalities were common (41%). Based on its efficacy in this report and apparently decreased side effect profile, danazol can be considered the androgen of choice for treatment of DC/TBD. In general, the timeline to effect of androgens differs between lineages but is on the order of 1 to 3 months.[64-66] The durability of response to androgens is difficult to predict; some patients require dose escalation or lose their response altogether. Although androgens can sustain patients in a transfusion-independent state for months to years, they are not considered curative for hematopoietic defects in DC.

The mechanisms by which androgens improve hematopoietic function in different BMF syndromes are not clear. It has been shown in vitro that androgens that are aromatized into estrogens can upregulate the *TERT* gene via nuclear hormone receptors,[67] which would in theory counteract telomere attrition and restore HSC self-renewal in patients with DC/TBD. In keeping with this, adults with TBD treated with danazol in the prospective trial were found to have telomere elongation in peripheral blood cell DNA over the course of the treatment period, as measured by qPCR.[66] However, several issues have been raised about the proposed mechanism and effect seen in this study:

1. Neither danazol nor its derivatives aromatize to an estrogen.[68]
2. Overexpression of *TERT* alone is insufficient to elongate telomeres in *DKC1* or *TERC* mutant patient cells.[69,70]
3. Telomere length was measured in DNA from total peripheral blood cells, which are likely to differ in composition between pretreatment and convalescent states.
4. Telomere length was measured by qPCR, which may be inferior to methods such as flow-FISH.[55,56]

A prior report on the effects of androgens in patients with DC showed no increase in telomere length when measured longitudinally by flow-FISH, albeit with small numbers of patients.[64] Thus, it remains unknown whether telomere restoration is the mechanism by which androgens exert their hematologic benefits in DC/TBD. Moreover, it is unclear whether androgens affect telomere length or organ function in patients with DC/TBD outside the blood. Therefore, androgens should only be trialed for non-hematopoietic manifestations in patients with DC/TBD in the context of a proper clinical study.

In summary, androgen therapy can be considered a standard transfusion-sparing approach for hematopoietic failure in patients with DC/TBD. The utility of androgens is limited by variability in response; durability of response; side effects, including liver toxicity; and adherence to the medication. There are no clear extra-hematopoietic benefits of androgens in patients with DC. Whether or not androgens should be tried before HSCT in patients with DC is not clear and depends on individual patient characteristics, available HSCT options, and physician and patient choice.

Hematopoietic Stem Cell Transplant

HSCT is the only definitive therapy for the hematopoietic and immunologic defects in DC. Case reports as early as the 1980s and 1990s showed that BMF in DC could be cured with HSCT.[71–81] The observation of long-term hematologic reconstitution after allogeneic HSCT indicates an HSC-intrinsic defect as the major contributor to hematopoietic failure in DC and children with TBD. However, a high morbidity and mortality from conventional HSCT approaches was apparent across the experience. In retrospective analyses, more than 50% of patients died within 4 months of the HSCT procedure, most often because of infections, graft failure, or graft-versus-host disease (GVHD).[82,83] The 5-year overall survival was approximately 45%, with no long-term survivors of unrelated donor HSCT.[82,83] An unusual frequency of fatal lung and vascular complications was noted, attributed to both predisposition to pulmonary and endothelial disease in patients with DC and increased sensitivity to myeloablative conditioning with DNA alkylating agents and radiation.[72,77,78,82] Other factors that likely contributed to poor outcomes in the early experience include the long time interval from onset of BMF to transplant,[76] and inferior unrelated donor matching capabilities and supportive care. DC also sometimes went undiagnosed until after HSCT, because the clinical syndrome was not recognized at the time of hematopoietic failure, and genetic and functional testing were unavailable.[75]

With more awareness of the increased transplant-related mortality in DC, better diagnostics, and application of lessons learned from FA,[84] HSCT outcomes seem to be improving. Reduced-intensity conditioning regimens have been used increasingly in patients with DC since the early 2000s. Progress has been attributed in large part to reduction of DNA alkylating agents (cyclophosphamide, busulfan, melphalan, thiotepa) and ionizing radiation in preparative regimens, and an increasing use of fludarabine and antibody-based immunosuppressive conditioning.[85–92] In a retrospective study of data reported to the Center for International Blood and Marrow Transplantation Research (CIBMTR), the 5-year probability of overall survival for patients with DC undergoing HSCT from 2000 to 2009 was 65%.[83] Similarly, in a review of DC transplants using reduced-intensity conditioning regimens after 2000, approximately two-thirds of patients were alive with a median follow-up of 16 months, and included survivors of unrelated donor and cord blood transplants.[87] A retrospective case series of 7 patients with DC undergoing HSCT with a preparative regimen of fludarabine, alemtuzumab, and lower-dose melphalan showed a 100% engraftment rate and survival of 5 out of 7 patients at a median follow-up of 44 months.[93] However, a retrospective review of 109 patients with DC transplanted since 1976 was unable to show a statistically significant improvement in overall survival using reduced-intensity versus myeloablative conditioning in HSCT for DC, possibly due to short follow-up and small numbers of patients.[94]

In the past decade, prospective HSCT trials tailored for patients with DC with BMF have been developed and executed in the United States. The first (clinicaltrials.gov NCT00455312) was conducted by the University of Minnesota and featured fludarabine and alemtuzumab-based immunosuppression, decreased (50 mg/kg) cyclophosphamide dosing, and a single 200-cGy fraction of total-body irradiation with anatomic lung shielding. GVHD prophylaxis was tailored to avoid cytotoxic agents such as methotrexate and corticosteroids. Early interim results reported by Dietz and colleagues[87] in

2010 described 6 patients treated on this regimen, 5 of whom received unrelated bone marrow or cord blood; 4 patients had successful HSCT, whereas 2 had early mortality from graft rejection and infection. Short-term pulmonary and liver toxicity were not seen, and 3 of the 5 unrelated donor transplants were successful. This trial is completed and results of longer follow-up are expected. A second prospective trial for BMF in DC/TBD originated at Boston Children's Hospital (BCH)/Dana-Farber Cancer Institute in 2012 (clinicaltrials.gov NCT01659606). The study asks whether myeloid engraftment can be achieved in HSCT for BMF in patients with DC without any exposure to radiation or DNA alkylating agents. This approach is based on the theory that, in the context of BMF, defective telomere maintenance and cellular replication results in a competitive disadvantage of HSCs in patients with DC compared with healthy donor HSCs, which could enable engraftment without using nontargeted cytotoxic agents. This regimen, consisting of alemtuzumab and fludarabine conditioning alone, if successful, would represent the first time a series of patients achieved myeloid engraftment in allogeneic HSCT without alkylators or radiation. An early report in 2014 of 4 patients who received unrelated HSCT under this protocol indicated durable engraftment.[95] The protocol has been expanded to the first multicenter, prospective treatment trial for patients with DC, with completion expected in 2018.

Based on the early results of these prospective trials, it can be anticipated that outcomes will continue to improve in HSCT for BMF in DC. Important questions remain. What is the optimal HSCT regimen for patients with TBDs presenting with MDS/AML? Can patients with TBDs with simultaneous hematopoietic failure and comorbidities such as lung and liver disease tolerate and benefit from minimal intensity HSCT? Does a successful minimal intensity HSCT for BMF alter the overall survival and natural history of the disease? Answers to these questions will come from carefully planned prospective trials and coordinated efforts designed to decrease adverse events and increase overall length and quality of life for patients with DC/TBD.

SUMMARY AND FUTURE PROSPECTS

Advances in diagnosing and treating BMF caused by DC have been driven by genetic discovery in the past 2 decades, and the ensuing translation of basic biology to the bedside. Hematopoietic failure caused by an impairment in telomere maintenance "makes sense" and has provided a conceptual framework that has been useful for tailoring therapy and generating hypotheses to be tested in prospective clinical trials. Much remains to learned about the pathophysiology and treatment of other disease manifestations in the TBDs. With a continued focus on understanding DC, new insights into normal human telomere biology can be expected, that will lead to novel therapeutic approaches to restore telomere maintenance in TBD and other disorders.

REFERENCES

1. Kirwan M, Dokal I. Dyskeratosis congenita: a genetic disorder of many faces. Clin Genet 2008;73(2):103–12.
2. Alter BP, Giri N, Savage SA, et al. Malignancies and survival patterns in the National Cancer Institute inherited bone marrow failure syndromes cohort study. Br J Haematol 2010;150(2):179–88.
3. Dokal I. Dyskeratosis congenita in all its forms. Br J Haematol 2000;110(4):768–79.
4. Alter BP, Giri N, Savage SA, et al. Cancer in the National Cancer Institute Inherited Bone Marrow Failure Syndrome Cohort After Fifteen Years of Follow-up. Haematologica 2018;103:30–9.

5. Armanios M, Blackburn EH. The telomere syndromes. Nat Rev Genet 2012; 13(10):693–704.

6. Calado RT, Young NS. Telomere diseases. N Engl J Med 2009;361(24):2353–65.

7. Keller RB, Gagne KE, Usmani GN, et al. CTC1 Mutations in a patient with dyskeratosis congenita. Pediatr Blood Cancer 2012;59(2):311–4.

8. Knight SW, Heiss NS, Vulliamy TJ, et al. Unexplained aplastic anaemia, immunodeficiency, and cerebellar hypoplasia (Hoyeraal-Hreidarsson syndrome) due to mutations in the dyskeratosis congenita gene, DKC1. Br J Haematol 1999; 107(2):335–9.

9. Glousker G, Touzot F, Revy P, et al. Unraveling the pathogenesis of Hoyeraal-Hreidarsson syndrome, a complex telomere biology disorder. Br J Haematol 2015;170(4):457–71.

10. Savage SA, Giri N, Baerlocher GM, et al. TINF2, a component of the shelterin telomere protection complex, is mutated in dyskeratosis congenita. Am J Hum Genet 2008;82(2):501–9.

11. Du HY, Pumbo E, Ivanovich J, et al. TERC and TERT gene mutations in patients with bone marrow failure and the significance of telomere length measurements. Blood 2009;113(2):309–16.

12. Kirwan M, Vulliamy T, Marrone A, et al. Defining the pathogenic role of telomerase mutations in myelodysplastic syndrome and acute myeloid leukemia. Hum Mutat 2009;30(11):1567–73.

13. Yamaguchi H, Baerlocher GM, Lansdorp PM, et al. Mutations of the human telomerase RNA gene (TERC) in aplastic anemia and myelodysplastic syndrome. Blood 2003;102(3):916–8.

14. Yamaguchi H, Calado RT, Ly H, et al. Mutations in TERT, the gene for telomerase reverse transcriptase, in aplastic anemia. N Engl J Med 2005;352(14):1413–24.

15. Armanios MY, Chen JJ, Cogan JD, et al. Telomerase mutations in families with idiopathic pulmonary fibrosis. N Engl J Med 2007;356(13):1317–26.

16. Tsakiri KD, Cronkhite JT, Kuan PJ, et al. Adult-onset pulmonary fibrosis caused by mutations in telomerase. Proc Natl Acad Sci U S A 2007;104(18):7552–7.

17. Armanios M. Telomerase and idiopathic pulmonary fibrosis. Mutat Res 2012; 730(1–2):52–8.

18. Fogarty PF, Yamaguchi H, Wiestner A, et al. Late presentation of dyskeratosis congenita as apparently acquired aplastic anaemia due to mutations in telomerase RNA. Lancet 2003;362(9396):1628–30.

19. Parry EM, Alder JK, Qi X, et al. Syndrome complex of bone marrow failure and pulmonary fibrosis predicts germline defects in telomerase. Blood 2011; 117(21):5607–11.

20. Allsopp RC, Harley CB. Evidence for a critical telomere length in senescent human fibroblasts. Exp Cell Res 1995;219(1):130–6.

21. Harley CB, Futcher AB, Greider CW. Telomeres shorten during ageing of human fibroblasts. Nature 1990;345(6274):458–60.

22. Heiss NS, Knight SW, Vulliamy TJ, et al. X-linked dyskeratosis congenita is caused by mutations in a highly conserved gene with putative nucleolar functions. Nat Genet 1998;19(1):32–8.

23. Knight SW, Vulliamy TJ, Heiss NS, et al. 1.4 Mb candidate gene region for X linked dyskeratosis congenita defined by combined haplotype and X chromosome inactivation analysis. J Med Genet 1998;35(12):993–6.

24. Mitchell JR, Cheng J, Collins K. A box H/ACA small nucleolar RNA-like domain at the human telomerase RNA 3' end. Mol Cell Biol 1999;19(1):567–76.

25. Mitchell JR, Wood E, Collins K. A telomerase component is defective in the human disease dyskeratosis congenita. Nature 1999;402(6761):551–5.

26. Vulliamy T, Marrone A, Goldman F, et al. The RNA component of telomerase is mutated in autosomal dominant dyskeratosis congenita. Nature 2001; 413(6854):432–5.

27. Stanley SE, Gable DL, Wagner CL, et al. Loss-of-function mutations in the RNA biogenesis factor NAF1 predispose to pulmonary fibrosis-emphysema. Sci Transl Med 2016;8(351):351ra107.

28. Townsley DM, Dumitriu B, Young NS. Bone marrow failure and the telomeropathies. Blood 2014;124(18):2775–83.

29. Bertuch AA. The molecular genetics of the telomere biology disorders. RNA Biol 2016;13(8):696–706.

30. Simon AJ, Lev A, Zhang Y, et al. Mutations in STN1 cause coats plus syndrome and are associated with genomic and telomere defects. J Exp Med 2016;213(8): 1429–40.

31. Vulliamy T, Marrone A, Szydlo R, et al. Disease anticipation is associated with progressive telomere shortening in families with dyskeratosis congenita due to mutations in TERC. Nat Genet 2004;36(5):447–9.

32. Diaz de Leon A, Cronkhite JT, Katzenstein AL, et al. Telomere lengths, pulmonary fibrosis and telomerase (TERT) mutations. PLoS One 2010;5(5):e10680.

33. Collopy LC, Walne AJ, Cardoso S, et al. Triallelic and epigenetic-like inheritance in human disorders of telomerase. Blood 2015;126(2):176–84.

34. Armanios M, Alder JK, Parry EM, et al. Short telomeres are sufficient to cause the degenerative defects associated with aging. Am J Hum Genet 2009;85(6): 823–32.

35. Hao LY, Armanios M, Strong MA, et al. Short telomeres, even in the presence of telomerase, limit tissue renewal capacity. Cell 2005;123(6):1121–31.

36. Vaziri H, Dragowska W, Allsopp RC, et al. Evidence for a mitotic clock in human hematopoietic stem cells: loss of telomeric DNA with age. Proc Natl Acad Sci U S A 1994;91(21):9857–60.

37. Broccoli D, Young JW, de Lange T. Telomerase activity in normal and malignant hematopoietic cells. Proc Natl Acad Sci U S A 1995;92(20):9082–6.

38. Chiu CP, Dragowska W, Kim NW, et al. Differential expression of telomerase activity in hematopoietic progenitors from adult human bone marrow. Stem Cells 1996;14(2):239–48.

39. Notaro R, Cimmino A, Tabarini D, et al. In vivo telomere dynamics of human hematopoietic stem cells. Proc Natl Acad Sci U S A 1997;94(25):13782–5.

40. Brummendorf TH, Rufer N, Baerlocher GM, et al. Limited telomere shortening in hematopoietic stem cells after transplantation. Ann N Y Acad Sci 2001;938:1–7 [discussion: 7–8].

41. Akiyama M, Asai O, Kuraishi Y, et al. Shortening of telomeres in recipients of both autologous and allogeneic hematopoietic stem cell transplantation. Bone Marrow Transplant 2000;25(4):441–7.

42. Alder JK, Hanumanthu VS, Strong MA, et al. Diagnostic utility of telomere length testing in a hospital-based setting. Proc Natl Acad Sci U S A 2018;115(10): E2358–65.

43. Calado RT, Cooper JN, Padilla-Nash HM, et al. Short telomeres result in chromosomal instability in hematopoietic cells and precede malignant evolution in human aplastic anemia. Leukemia 2012;26(4):700–7.

44. Scheinberg P, Cooper JN, Sloand EM, et al. Association of telomere length of peripheral blood leukocytes with hematopoietic relapse, malignant transformation, and survival in severe aplastic anemia. JAMA 2010;304(12):1358–64.
45. Lange K, Holm L, Vang Nielsen K, et al. Telomere shortening and chromosomal instability in myelodysplastic syndromes. Genes Chromosomes Cancer 2010; 49(3):260–9.
46. Ohyashiki JH, Ohyashiki K, Fujimura T, et al. Telomere shortening associated with disease evolution patterns in myelodysplastic syndromes. Cancer Res 1994; 54(13):3557–60.
47. Ball SE, Gibson FM, Rizzo S, et al. Progressive telomere shortening in aplastic anemia. Blood 1998;91(10):3582–92.
48. Sakaguchi H, Nishio N, Hama A, et al. Peripheral blood lymphocyte telomere length as a predictor of response to immunosuppressive therapy in childhood aplastic anemia. Haematologica 2014;99(8):1312–6.
49. Peffault de Latour R, Calado RT, Busson M, et al. Age-adjusted recipient pre-transplantation telomere length and treatment-related mortality after hematopoietic stem cell transplantation. Blood 2012;120(16):3353–9.
50. Vulliamy TJ, Knight SW, Dokal I, et al. Skewed X-inactivation in carriers of X-linked dyskeratosis congenita. Blood 1997;90(6):2213–6.
51. Jongmans MC, Verwiel ET, Heijdra Y, et al. Revertant somatic mosaicism by mitotic recombination in dyskeratosis congenita. Am J Hum Genet 2012;90(3): 426–33.
52. Aubert G, Hills M, Lansdorp PM. Telomere length measurement-caveats and a critical assessment of the available technologies and tools. Mutat Res 2012; 730(1–2):59–67.
53. Alter BP, Baerlocher GM, Savage SA, et al. Very short telomere length by flow fluorescence in situ hybridization identifies patients with dyskeratosis congenita. Blood 2007;110(5):1439–47.
54. Alter BP, Rosenberg PS, Giri N, et al. Telomere length is associated with disease severity and declines with age in dyskeratosis congenita. Haematologica 2012; 97(3):353–9.
55. Gadalla SM, Khincha PP, Katki HA, et al. The limitations of qPCR telomere length measurement in diagnosing dyskeratosis congenita. Mol Genet Genomic Med 2016;4(4):475–9.
56. Gutierrez-Rodrigues F, Santana-Lemos BA, Scheucher PS, et al. Direct comparison of flow-FISH and qPCR as diagnostic tests for telomere length measurement in humans. PLoS One 2014;9(11):e113747.
57. Anderson BH, Kasher PR, Mayer J, et al. Mutations in CTC1, encoding conserved telomere maintenance component 1, cause Coats plus. Nat Genet 2012;44(3): 338–42.
58. Al-Rahawan MM, Giri N, Alter BP. Intensive immunosuppression therapy for aplastic anemia associated with dyskeratosis congenita. Int J Hematol 2006; 83(3):275–6.
59. Olnes MJ, Scheinberg P, Calvo KR, et al. Eltrombopag and improved hematopoiesis in refractory aplastic anemia. N Engl J Med 2012;367(1):11–9.
60. Trautmann K, Jakob C, von Grunhagen U, et al. Eltrombopag fails to improve severe thrombocytopenia in late-stage dyskeratosis congenita and diamond-black-fan-anaemia. Thromb Haemost 2012;108(2):397–8.
61. Shahidi NT, Diamond LK. Testosterone-induced remission in aplastic anemia of both acquired and congenital types. Further observations in 24 cases. N Engl J Med 1961;264:953–67.

62. Allen DM, Fine MH, Necheles TF, et al. Oxymetholone therapy in aplastic anemia. Blood 1968;32(1):83–9.
63. Shimamura A, Alter BP. Pathophysiology and management of inherited bone marrow failure syndromes. Blood Rev 2010;24(3):101–22.
64. Khincha PP, Wentzensen IM, Giri N, et al. Response to androgen therapy in patients with dyskeratosis congenita. Br J Haematol 2014;165(3):349–57.
65. Islam A, Rafiq S, Kirwan M, et al. Haematological recovery in dyskeratosis congenita patients treated with danazol. Br J Haematol 2013;162(6):854–6.
66. Townsley DM, Dumitriu B, Liu D, et al. Danazol treatment for telomere diseases. N Engl J Med 2016;374(20):1922–31.
67. Calado RT, Yewdell WT, Wilkerson KL, et al. Sex hormones, acting on the TERT gene, increase telomerase activity in human primary hematopoietic cells. Blood 2009;114(11):2236–43.
68. Grossmann M. Danazol treatment for telomere diseases. N Engl J Med 2016; 375(11):1095.
69. Westin ER, Chavez E, Lee KM, et al. Telomere restoration and extension of proliferative lifespan in dyskeratosis congenita fibroblasts. Aging Cell 2007;6(3): 383–94.
70. Wong JM, Collins K. Telomerase RNA level limits telomere maintenance in X-linked dyskeratosis congenita. Genes Dev 2006;20(20):2848–58.
71. Mahmoud HK, Schaefer UW, Schmidt CG, et al. Marrow transplantation for pancytopenia in dyskeratosis congenita. Blut 1985;51(1):57–60.
72. Berthou C, Devergie A, D'Agay MF, et al. Late vascular complications after bone marrow transplantation for dyskeratosis congenita. Br J Haematol 1991;79(2): 335–6.
73. Chessells JM, Harper J. Bone marrow transplantation for dyskeratosis congenita. Br J Haematol 1992;81(2):314.
74. Dokal I, Bungey J, Williamson P, et al. Dyskeratosis congenita fibroblasts are abnormal and have unbalanced chromosomal rearrangements. Blood 1992; 80(12):3090–6.
75. Phillips RJ, Judge M, Webb D, et al. Dyskeratosis congenita: delay in diagnosis and successful treatment of pancytopenia by bone marrow transplantation. Br J Dermatol 1992;127(3):278–80.
76. Langston AA, Sanders JE, Deeg HJ, et al. Allogeneic marrow transplantation for aplastic anaemia associated with dyskeratosis congenita. Br J Haematol 1996; 92(3):758–65.
77. Yabe M, Yabe H, Hattori K, et al. Fatal interstitial pulmonary disease in a patient with dyskeratosis congenita after allogeneic bone marrow transplantation. Bone Marrow Transplant 1997;19(4):389–92.
78. Rocha V, Devergie A, Socie G, et al. Unusual complications after bone marrow transplantation for dyskeratosis congenita. Br J Haematol 1998;103(1):243–8.
79. Ghavamzadeh A, Alimoghadam K, Nasseri P, et al. Correction of bone marrow failure in dyskeratosis congenita by bone marrow transplantation. Bone Marrow Transplant 1999;23(3):299–301.
80. Lau YL, Ha SY, Chan CF, et al. Bone marrow transplant for dyskeratosis congenita. Br J Haematol 1999;105(2):571.
81. Shaw PH, Haut PR, Olszewski M, et al. Hematopoietic stem-cell transplantation using unrelated cord-blood versus matched sibling marrow in pediatric bone marrow failure syndrome: one center's experience. Pediatr Transplant 1999; 3(4):315–21.

82. de la Fuente J, Dokal I. Dyskeratosis congenita: advances in the understanding of the telomerase defect and the role of stem cell transplantation. Pediatr Transplant 2007;11(6):584–94.
83. Gadalla SM, Sales-Bonfim C, Carreras J, et al. Outcomes of allogeneic hematopoietic cell transplantation in patients with dyskeratosis congenita. Biol Blood Marrow Transplant 2013;19(8):1238–43.
84. Socie G, Devergie A, Girinski T, et al. Transplantation for Fanconi's anaemia: long-term follow-up of fifty patients transplanted from a sibling donor after low-dose cyclophosphamide and thoraco-abdominal irradiation for conditioning. Br J Haematol 1998;103(1):249–55.
85. Ayas M, Nassar A, Hamidieh AA, et al. Reduced intensity conditioning is effective for hematopoietic SCT in dyskeratosis congenita-related BM failure. Bone Marrow Transplant 2013;48(9):1168–72.
86. Cossu F, Vulliamy TJ, Marrone A, et al. A novel DKC1 mutation, severe combined immunodeficiency (T+B-NK- SCID) and bone marrow transplantation in an infant with Hoyeraal-Hreidarsson syndrome. Br J Haematol 2002;119(3):765–8.
87. Dietz AC, Orchard PJ, Baker KS, et al. Disease-specific hematopoietic cell transplantation: nonmyeloablative conditioning regimen for dyskeratosis congenita. Bone Marrow Transplant 2011;46(1):98–104.
88. Dror Y, Freedman MH, Leaker M, et al. Low-intensity hematopoietic stem-cell transplantation across human leucocyte antigen barriers in dyskeratosis congenita. Bone Marrow Transplant 2003;31(10):847–50.
89. Gungor T, Corbacioglu S, Storb R, et al. Nonmyeloablative allogeneic hematopoietic stem cell transplantation for treatment of dyskeratosis congenita. Bone Marrow Transplant 2003;31(5):407–10.
90. Nishio N, Takahashi Y, Ohashi H, et al. Reduced-intensity conditioning for alternative donor hematopoietic stem cell transplantation in patients with dyskeratosis congenita. Pediatr Transplant 2011;15(2):161–6.
91. Nobili B, Rossi G, De Stefano P, et al. Successful umbilical cord blood transplantation in a child with dyskeratosis congenita after a fludarabine-based reduced-intensity conditioning regimen. Br J Haematol 2002;119(2):573–4.
92. Vuong LG, Hemmati PG, Neuburger S, et al. Reduced-intensity conditioning using fludarabine and antithymocyte globulin alone allows stable engraftment in a patient with dyskeratosis congenita. Acta Haematol 2010;124(4):200–3.
93. Nelson AS, Marsh RA, Myers KC, et al. A reduced-intensity conditioning regimen for patients with dyskeratosis congenita undergoing hematopoietic stem cell transplantation. Biol Blood Marrow Transplant 2016;22(5):884–8.
94. Barbaro P, Vedi A. Survival after hematopoietic stem cell transplant in patients with dyskeratosis congenita: systematic review of the literature. Biol Blood Marrow Transplant 2016;22(7):1152–8.
95. Agarwal S, Williams DA, London WB, et al. Full donor myeloid engraftment with minimal toxicity in dyskeratosis congenita patients undergoing allogeneic bone marrow transplantation without radiation or alkylating agents. Blood 2014; 124(21):2941.

Diagnosis, Treatment, and Molecular Pathology of Shwachman-Diamond Syndrome

Adam S. Nelson, MBBS, FRACP, Kasiani C. Myers, MD*

KEYWORDS

- Shwachman-Diamond syndrome • Bone marrow failure • Ribosome
- Pancreatic dysfunction • Neutropenia • Failure to thrive

KEY POINTS

- SDS is a challenging marrow failure disorder with exocrine pancreatic dysfunction and diverse clinical phenotype.
- Ongoing advances in ribosomal biogenesis and cellular function contribute to defining the pathogenesis of the molecular phenotype of SDS, with novel candidate genes recently described.
- Further natural history and collaborative efforts are essential to define disease manifestations, prevent known complications, and ensure new and targeted therapies to ameliorate and prevent malignant transformation.

INTRODUCTION

Shwachman-Diamond syndrome (SDS) is an autosomal-recessive inherited bone marrow failure (BMF) disorder characterized by exocrine pancreatic dysfunction, BMF, and predisposition toward myelodysplasia syndrome (MDS) or acute leukemia, particularly acute myeloid leukemia (AML). SDS is rare, with an estimated incidence of 1/76,000.[1] Many different body systems are affected, including the skeletal, cardiac, endocrine, nervous, hepatic, and immune systems, although these are not universally affected in all patients, or even within family cohorts.

SDS is a disorder of ribosomal biogenesis, with approximately 90% of individuals having biallelic mutations in the Shwachman-Bodian-Diamond Syndrome (SBDS) gene located on chromosome 7q11. Although the role of the SBDS protein is yet to be fully established, it is thought to play an integral part in ribosomal maturation,

The authors have no commercial or financial conflicts of interest.
Division of Bone Marrow Transplantation and Immune Deficiency, Cincinnati Children's Hospital Medical Center, 3333 Burnet Avenue, Cincinnati, OH 45229, USA
* Corresponding author. Cincinnati Children's Hospital Medical Center, 3333 Burnet Avenue, MLC 11027, Cincinnati, OH 45229.
E-mail address: Kasiani.myers@cchmc.org

and cellular proliferation and the hematopoietic microenvironment. Recently three additional genes associated with ribosome assembly or protein translation (DNAJC21, ELF1, and SRP54) were reported in association with an SDS phenotype.[2–4]

There is great phenotypic diversity among individuals with SDS, despite most sharing one or more common allelic mutations within *SBDS*. Given its rarity, the understanding of the pathogenesis, phenotype, treatment, and outcomes has been limited to case series and reports from new registry studies. Similarly, guidelines on management and treatment are based primarily on expert consensus and small cohort studies. Ongoing large collaborative studies are needed to further define the pathogenesis, treatment, and natural history of SDS to improve clinical practice and promote investigation in novel therapeutic approaches.

This article focuses on the diagnosis, treatment, and molecular pathology of SDS and recent insights into this disease.

CLINICAL MANIFESTATIONS

Bone marrow and pancreatic dysfunction as described in the most recent consensus guidelines (**Box 1**) are the classic clinical features of SDS. In the North American SDS registry, however, only 51% (19 of 37) of those with biallelic *SBDS* mutations presented with classic findings of neutropenia with steatorrhea.[5] In fact, 14% had no

---

Box 1
Clinical and molecular diagnostic features of Shwachman-Diamond syndrome

Diagnostic Criteria

Biallelic SBDS mutations known or predicted to be pathogenic, or mutations in other SDS-associated genes DNAJC21, ELF1, SRP54 (autosomal dominant)

Clinical Diagnosis
  Hematologic features (present on at least two occasions)
  • Neutropenia (absolute neutrophil count <1500)
  • Anemia or macrocytosis (unexplained by other causes, such as iron/B_{12} deficiency)
  • Thrombocytopenia (platelet count <150,000) on at least two occasions
  • Bone marrow findings
    ○ Hypocellularity for age
    ○ Myelodysplasia
    ○ Leukemia
    ○ Cytogenetic abnormalities
  Pancreatic features
  • Reduced levels of pancreatic enzyme relevant to age
    ○ Trypsinogen <3 years
    ○ Isoamylase >3 years
  • Low levels of fecal elastase
  • Supportive features
    ○ Abnormal pancreatic imaging with lipomatosis
    ○ Elevated fecal fat excretion >72 hours
  Additional supportive features
  • Skeletal abnormalities including thoracic dystrophy
  • Neurocognitive/behavioral problems
  • Unexplained height less than third percentile
  • First-degree family member with SDS

Adapted from Dror Y, Donadieu J, Koglmeier J, et al. Draft consensus guidelines for diagnosis and treatment of Shwachman-Diamond syndrome. Ann N Y Acad Sci 2011;1242(1):43; with permission.

history of cytopenias at initial evaluation. Similarly, the diagnosis of SDS could not be ruled out in this cohort by absence of pancreatic lipomatosis on imaging, normal fecal elastase levels, or normal skeletal imaging.

HEMATOLOGIC MANIFESTATIONS

Although the hematologic phenotype of SDS typically manifests with neutropenia other cytopenias are also frequently present. Neutropenia, defined as an absolute neutrophil count less than 1500/μL, is a classic finding in SDS. Neutropenia typically presents in the first year of life, although it can present late (adulthood) or may be absent in a small number of individuals.[5] It is of unpredictable severity and may be intermittent or persistent. Neutrophils may exhibit chemotaxis and migration defects; however, individuals with SDS maintain the ability to form empyema and abscesses in contrast to other disorders of neutrophil chemotaxis.[6–8] Anemia and reticulocytopenia occur in up to 80% of patients, with a normochromic, normocytic appearance, although occasional macrocytosis has been noted.[9] Thrombocytopenia is variably seen.

Progression to trilineage cytopenia and resulting severe aplastic anemia is a lifelong risk for patients with SDS. The French Severe Chronic Neutropenia Registry reported 41 of 102 SDS patients (40%) developed transient severe cytopenias, with half of these developing progressive severe cytopenias with either hemoglobin less than 7 g/dL or platelets less than 20×10^9/L.[10]

There are varying reports of malignant transformation to MDS or AML in SDS. The Canadian Inherited Marrow Failure Registry reported a 20% risk (n = 40) of hematologic disease progression (including malignant or clonal myeloid transformation, acquisition of new or additional cytogenetic clones, or worsening of cytopenias) by age 18 years.[11] The Severe Congenital Neutropenia International Registry reported an incidence of 1% per year of MDS/AML in SDS patients and an overall incidence of 8.1% of MDS/AML over 10 years in 37 patients.[12] Risk of malignant transformation may, however, increase with age.

Risk of solid tumor development in patients with SDS remains to be ascertained, with case reports of solid tumors in patients ages 18 to 38, including bilateral breast cancer, central nervous system large B-cell lymphoma, pancreatic adenocarcinoma, and slow progressive dermatofibrosarcoma.[13,14]

Cytogenetic changes are common in SDS, in the absence of MDS or AML. Common cytogenetic abnormalities associated with SDS include del(20) (q11) and isochromosome 7q (i[7] [q10]).[15] These changes may be transient or persist over time, and may not portend impending malignant transformation to MDS or AML.[16–18] Whether the maternal or paternal allele bears the del(20) (q) abnormality may affect the hematologic phenotype. Higher hemoglobin levels and red cell counts were observed in patients with paternal deletion of 20(q).[19] The exact mechanism is yet to be elucidated, but may be related to bystander gene loss involving *L3MBTL1* and loss of transcriptional repressor activity.

Novel cytogenetic abnormalities in the presence and absence of del(20) (q11) and isochromosome 7q (i[7] [q10]) anomalies were recently reported in a cohort of 91 Italian patients with SDS, including unbalanced structural anomalies of chromosome 7, complex rearrangements of del(20) (q) involving duplicated and deleted portions and unbalanced translocation t(3;6) with partial trisomy of the long arm of chromosome 3 and partial monosomy of the long arm of chromosome 6.[20] Some of these subjects did progress to MDS/AML both with i(7) (q10) or del(20) (q11) (2 of 5) and without (6 of 13). Although significance of infrequent acquired chromosomal changes in SDS remains unclear, additional acquired cytogenetic abnormalities may preempt development of MDS or AML.

The understanding of immune function in SDS is not clear. Individuals with SDS are at risk of a diverse range of infections, including bacterial, viral, and fungal infections, generally believed to be beyond that expected in patients with neutropenia. Defects in humoral (decreased B cell numbers, low IgG levels) and cellular (decreased T-cell proliferation) have been reported in SDS individuals.

GASTROINTESTINAL MANIFESTATIONS

Depletion of pancreatic acinar cells results in the hallmark exocrine pancreatic dysfunction observed in SDS.[21] Disorder of pancreatic function is typically seen within the first 6 to 12 months of life, although the spectrum of disease presentation remains varied. Some patients present with severe pancreatic dysfunction manifested by failure to thrive and malabsorption, whereas others are asymptomatic.[5,22]

Many patients with SDS and exocrine pancreatic dysfunction spontaneously improve over time, with almost half of patients no longer requiring supplemental pancreatic enzyme therapy despite persistent native secretory enzyme deficiency.[23]

The acinar defect in SDS may be generalized to pancreatic and parotid glands. Serum pancreatic and parotid isoamylase levels are lower in patients with SDS,[24] and compared with other disorders involving pancreatic dysfunction, such as cystic fibrosis, ductal function is normal in SDS.[25] Beyond acinar dysfunction, histologic evidence of duodenal inflammation has been demonstrated on mucosal biopsy of 50% of SDS patients.[26] This enteropathy may contribute to vitamin and mineral deficiencies observed in SDS, with vitamin A, E, selenium, zinc, and copper noted to be low in some patients despite supplemental nutrition and enzymatic replacement.[27] Monitoring of trace elements is essential to maximize nutritional benefit in individuals with SDS.

Other gastrointestinal abnormalities associated with SDS include abnormalities of the liver. Elevation of transaminases and hepatomegaly of unclear cause are often present in early life and resolve spontaneously.[28] Elevated bile acids were reported in one Finnish study in 7 of 12 SDS individuals.[28] There are also reports of hepatic failure of uncertain cause in older individuals with SDS including a 15 year old with cholestasis and fibrosis[29] and one individual in the North American SDS registry in their sixth decade.

SKELETAL MANIFESTATIONS

Classical skeletal manifestations of SDS include short stature; progressive metaphyseal dysplasia/thickening of the long bones and costochondral junctions; thoracic abnormalities, such as pectus, asphyxiating thoracic dystrophy, and flared ribs; and delayed development of normally shaped epiphyses and wormian appearance of skull bones.[30] These abnormalities may evolve over time.

SDS is also associated with a low-turnover osteoporosis, and abnormalities of bone health,[31] including low z scores and vertebral compression fractures. Other markers of bone health were abnormal, including vitamin D and K deficiency and associated secondary hyperparathyroidism. It is important to ensure accurate measurement of bone mineral density, because patients with SDS have short stature and may have an incorrectly reported low bone mineral density because of low height z score.[32]

NEUROLOGIC MANIFESTATIONS

A wide range of cognitive defects have been noted in individuals with SDS. Areas of limitation have been observed in higher-order language, intellectual reasoning, visual-motor skills, and academic achievement with approximately 20% of SDS individuals meeting the diagnostic criteria for intellectual disability.[33] Attention deficits were also more common in SDS individuals and their siblings than control subjects. Recently Perobelli and colleagues[34] performed questionnaire-based quality-of-life and psychological assessments and showed cognitive impairment varied widely in 65% of younger individuals and 76% of adults from mild to severe and was increased compared with control subjects with cystic fibrosis. Individuals with SDS also reported more social problems, attention deficits, and somatic complaints.

Toiviainen-Salo and coworkers[35] showed decreased brain volume globally in white and gray matter (1.74 L vs 1.94 L; $P = .019$) in nine individuals with SDS. Booij and colleagues[36] demonstrated a dysregulated dopaminergic system and comparably decreased brain volumes, most evident posteriorly and caudally. Additionally, Perobelli[37] and colleagues were recently able to combine cognitive assessments and MRI neuroimaging in nine individuals with SDS to show cognitive impairment associated with diffuse changes in gray and white matter. Whether these changes signify a static change, a delay in neurocognitive development, or will continue to advance is unknown.

Rarely SDS may mimic neuromuscular disorders, with reports of infants presenting with asphyxia, narrow thorax, and severe hypotonia.[38] Myopathic changes were demonstrated on muscle biopsy with prominent variability in muscle fiber size and abnormal expression of developmental isoforms of myosin.

OTHER MANIFESTATIONS

Other phenotypes of SDS have been described, including those of the endocrine and cardiac systems. SDS may present with unique endocrine manifestations, including neonatal hypoglycemia, micropenis, and congenital hypopituitarism.[39] Other reports of endocrine dysfunction in SDS describe type I diabetes or growth hormone deficiency.[23,40–46] Short stature, however, is a classic finding associated with SDS.[47] Short stature with height z scores less than −1.8, was found in 56% of biallelic SBDS mutation carrying individuals in a small retrospective study (n = 25).

Cardiac abnormalities were seen in 11% of SDS individuals in the French Severe Chronic Neutropenia Registry[48] including congenital heart defects, most of which required clinical intervention. Other abnormalities included cardiomyopathy, occasionally associated with radiation/cyclophosphamide treatments or viral infection.

Patients with SDS may also present in infancy with an eczematous-like rash that does not respond to topical treatments. Less commonly, other skin manifestations may be present, including ichthyosis.

Case reports of sensorineural hearing loss and congenital ear malformations have been reported in children with SDS[49]

DIAGNOSIS AND CLINICAL MANAGEMENT

The diagnosis of SDS early within the first year of life is often by classic criteria of failure to thrive and feeding difficulties, along with cytopenias and recurrent infections. A high index of suspicion is required in those with nonclassical phenotypes, who may present later in childhood or adulthood. Diagnostic criteria for SDS are summarized in **Box 1**.[15] Approximately 90% of SDS individuals carry biallelic mutations in SBDS.

Recently described mutations in ribosomal biogenesis and protein translation involving DNAJC21,[4] EFL1,[3] and SRP54[2] suggest novel genetic mutations in small numbers of patients with an SDS phenotype, and the need for continued genetic evaluation for BMF disorders including SDS.

A high index of suspicion is needed in patients who fit the clinical phenotype of SDS yet lack a classical SBDS gene mutation.[50] Marrow dysfunction in the setting of other causes of pancreatic dysfunction, such as Pearson marrow-pancreas syndrome or cystic fibrosis, should be considered. A recent analysis of 1514 patients transplanted for MDS demonstrated 4% of young adults harbored compound heterozygote mutations in SBDS with concurrent TP53 mutations and a poor prognosis.[51]

Comprehensive screening for known disease complications should be pursued in individuals with SDS at diagnosis and regular intervals thereafter (**Table 1**).

Monitoring blood counts and bone marrow evaluations is vital to assess for malignant transformation. Neutropenia is common and often intermittent. Most individuals with SDS do not need chronic granulocyte colony–stimulating factor (G-CSF) therapy. Persistent severe neutropenia with severe or recurrent bacterial or fungal infections is

Table 1
Clinical evaluation for patients with Shwachman-Diamond Syndrome

	Frequency
Hematology	
CBC	Diagnosis, every 3–6 mo or as indicated
Bone marrow aspirate and biopsy	Diagnosis, every 1–3 y or as indicated
Iron, folate, B$_{12}$	Diagnosis, as clinically indicated
Immunoglobulins and lymphocyte subpopulations	Diagnosis, as clinically indicated
HLA testing	As clinically indicated, impending BMT
Gastroenterology	
Pancreatic enzyme measurement	Diagnosis, as clinically indicated
Fat-soluble vitamins and prothrombin time	Diagnosis, 1 mo after commencement of enzyme therapy, then 6–12 mo as indicated
Hepatic profile	Diagnosis, yearly or as clinically indicated
Pancreatic imaging	Diagnosis
Endoscopy	As clinically indicated
Skeletal system	
Growth evaluation: Height, weight, head circumference	Yearly (more frequently if on GH replacement)
Skeletal survey	Diagnosis, as clinically indicated
Bone densitometry	Adulthood, as clinically indicated
Other evaluations	
Neuropsychological testing	Diagnosis, regular assessment during school years 6–8, 11–13, 15–17 y
Endocrine evaluation (eg, TSH, GH)	As clinically indicated
Auditory testing	As clinically indicated

Abbreviations: BMT, bone marrow transplantation; CBC, complete blood count; GH, growth hormone; TSH, thyroid-stimulating hormone.

Adapted from Dror Y, Donadieu J, Koglmeier J, et al. Draft consensus guidelines for diagnosis and treatment of Shwachman-Diamond syndrome. Ann N Y Acad Sci 2011;1242(1):46–7; with permission.

an indication for G-CSF therapy. Most SDS individuals have adequate response with low-dose G-CSF but may range from intermittent to continuous daily dosing. A marrow evaluation including cytogenetics and fluorescence in situ hybridization studies are recommended before starting G-CSF whenever feasible, to avoid potentially promoting abnormal clone growth.

Hematopoietic stem cell transplant remains the only curative therapy for SDS individuals with severe aplastic anemia or malignant transformation. Historically outcomes were poor with high treatment-related mortality using standard myeloablative preparative regimens.[52] Transplant outcomes in the setting of severe aplastic anemia or MDS have significantly improved with the introduction of reduced-intensity regimens.[53,54] Outcomes for SDS individuals with AML, however, remain poor, highlighting the importance of systematic blood and marrow surveillance. Achieving sustained remission with chemotherapy in the setting of SDS and AML has been challenging, leading to significant toxicity and increased transplant risk. Timely use of hematopoietic stem cell transplant in this setting is essential.

Growth, nutrition, neurodevelopment, and bone health should be monitored regularly for early recognition of areas of concern for prompt intervention. All siblings of an individual with SDS are at risk for SDS regardless of clinical symptoms,[5] and genetic counseling should be offered to patients and family members.

MOLECULAR PATHOGENESIS

The SBDS protein is involved in multiple important pathways including ribosomal maturation,[55,56] the stromal microenvironment,[57,58] and mitosis.[59,60] The crucial role of the SBDS protein in ribosome biogenesis was demonstrated by Finch and colleagues[55] in murine models. EIF6 release from the pre-60S ribosomal subunit results from coupling of GTPase elongation factor-like 1(EFL1) in an SBDS-dependent manner. Association of the 60S ribosomal subunit to the 40S subunit is sterically blocked by EIF6. EIF6 release permits joining of the 60S and 40S subunits and formation of the translationally active 80S ribosome.[61,62] Mutations in *Tif6*, the eIF6 yeast ortholog, reverse the slow growth phenotype of yeast lacking *Sdo1*, the *SBDS* ortholog.[61] In humans SBDS associates with the large 60S subunit but not mature polysomal ribosomes.[63] Half-mers are present in polysome profiles of SBDS-deficient animal models, a pattern caused by defective ribosome joining of the 40S and 60S subunits.[55] These half-mer patterns are not seen in cells from SDS individuals, likely because of low level residual SBDS expression, but they do show impaired ribosome association *in vitro*.[64] EIF6 knockdown improves ribosome association but not hematopoietic colony formation of SBDS-deficient CD34$^+$ cells from SDS individuals. Additionally, *SBDS* may have a surveillance role in monitoring conformational maturation of the ribosomal P-site in addition to regulating departure of eIF6.[65]

Biallelic mutations in *EFL1* clinically manifest as an SDS-like phenotype and present a novel mutation that may be present in SDS patients without typical mutations in *SBDS*. Four patients with infantile pancytopenia, exocrine pancreatic insufficiency, and skeletal anomalies were found to have homozygous mutations in *EFL1*; further study of the yeast EFL1 homologue showed that mutations prevent release of cytoplasmic Tif6 from the 60s subunit and prevent the formation of mature ribosomes.[3]

Mutations in *DNAJC21*, first reported in four children with BMF and short stature,[66] have also been recently reported in four subjects with a clinical phenotype of BMF, pancreatic dysfunction, and skeletal manifestations.[4] *DNAJC21* is ubiquitously expressed and its yeast homolog *Jjj1* is also required for ribosome biogenesis through the DnaJ domain and is involved in release of maturation factors from the pre-60S ribosomal subunit, via Arx1/Alb1, with dysfunction of 60S ribosomal subunit biogenesis on deletion of the homologs in yeast.

In and colleagues[67] report their findings that *SBDS* is required for translation of mRNAs responsible for granulocytic differentiation. Specifically, *SBDS* is required for efficient translation and reinitiation of C/EBPalpha and C/EBPbeta mRNAs. Furthermore, deregulated mRNA translation results in decreased *MYC* expression, which may result in loss of hematopoietic progenitor proliferation and contribute to the hematologic phenotype of SDS.

Similarly, novel mutations in *SRP54*, a key member of the cotranslation protein-targeting pathway, lead to an SDS-like phenotype.[2] A trio of patients with an SDS phenotype were found to have de novo missense variants in *SRP54*, resulting in neutropenia and other SDS features. GTPase activity of the mutated proteins was impaired and the level of SRP54 mRNA in the bone marrow was 3.6-fold lower in patients with *SRP54* mutations compared with healthy control subjects. The SDS phenotype with neutropenia was observed in a zebrafish *srp54*-knockdown model, indicating this may be a novel mutation in previously SBDS-negative SDS patients.

Additional roles outside of ribosomal maturation have been demonstrated for *SBDS*. Austin and colleagues[59] demonstrated localization of SBDS to mitotic spindles of primary human marrow stromal cells. Fibroblasts and lymphocytes from individuals with SDS have increased quantities of multipolar spindles, leading to increased genomic instability that is rescued with addition of purified SBDS protein.[59] Addition of the microtubule stabilizing agent taxol improved primary SDS bone marrow hematopoietic progenitor colony formation. Polymerization of purified microtubules was also increased with addition of recombinant SBDS protein, supporting a direct effect of SBDS on microtubule stabilization. Colocalization of SBDS with centromeres and microtubules of the mitotic spindle and the microtubule organizing center in neutrophils in interphase has also been demonstrated.[60,68]

In vitro neutrophil proliferation and differentiation are different in SDS compared with control subjects, suggesting an important role for SBDS in myeloid lineage proliferation and division. This was noted in a preleukemic mouse model of SDS, where mesenchymal inflammation resulted in mitochondrial dysfunction, oxidative stress, and activation of DNA damage response systems (particularly toll-like receptor inflammatory signaling) leading to genotoxic stress and evolution of leukemia.[69] These findings suggest inflammatory modulators may present a potential therapeutic approach for prevention of progression to leukemia in susceptible individuals.

SBDS may play a role in energy metabolism within the cell. Ribosomal biogenesis is a high-energy cellular process requiring finely coordinated complex cellular energy production. Ravera and colleagues[70] show impaired oxygen consumption, defective complex IV activity and electron transport defects, and increased cytoplasmic calcium levels in SDS cells. These changes led to an oxidative phosphorylation defect with decreased ATP production. Increased phosphorylation of mTOR was observed in SDS cells, affecting 60s maturation and binding of *SBDS* and *EIF6* possibly to modulate defective ribosome biogenesis through increased cytoplasmic calcium concentration to drive nuclear import of *EIF6*. Finally, addition of leucine resulted in improved erythropoiesis, which may represent a therapeutic adjuvant to be tested in future trials.

Bezzerri and colleagues[71] demonstrate loss of SBDS expression is associated with hyperactivation of mTOR and STAT3 pathways. SDS derived EBV-immortalized B cells show constitutive increased activation of mTOR and STAT3 pathways. STAT3 is a key regulator of many cellular processes, and the dysregulation of the mTOR and STAT3 pathways observed in this model may represent putative targets for investigation of commercially available mTOR and STAT pathway inhibitors, which theoretically may benefit neutrophil development and reduce progression to BMF.

SBDS has also been implicated in a variety of other cellular functions including increased reactive oxygen species production,[72] intensified cellular stress responses,[73] Fas-ligand induced apoptosis,[74] and mitochondrial insufficiency.[75] SBDS may also be involved in marrow stromal function.[76,77] Increased expression of vascular endothelial growth factor-A and osteoprotegerin are seen in SBDS knockdown cell lines, which are known to influence monocyte and macrophage migration, osteoclast differentiation, and angiogenesis.[58] Targeted deletion of SBDS in murine osteoprogenitors resulted in significant marrow abnormalities including lymphopenia, leukopenia, and myelodysplasia in the setting of bony changes.[57] Targeted deletion of Sbds in murine osteoprogenitor cells results in mitochondrial dysfunction and oxidative stress in hematopoietic cells leading to genotoxic stress. This process is driven through p53-S100A8/9-TLR4 signaling and was predictive of evolution to MDS/AML in non-SDS individuals with low risk MDS.[69] Together this suggests that decreased expression of SBDS in stromal cells may alter the hematopoietic microenvironment and favor development of BMF and/or malignant transformation. Normal in vitro function of SBDS-deficient mesenchymal stem cells, however, has been demonstrated by others.[77]

The early embryonic lethality of targeted deletion of murine Sbds results has limited use of this animal model of SDS.[78] Delayed in vitro myeloid differentiation, impaired homing of hematopoietic progenitors, and decreased short-term engraftment is seen after knockdown of murine Sbds with RNA interference in murine bone marrow followed by transplantation.[79] Sbds knockdown in zebrafish morpholinos demonstrated neutrophil loss, skeletal changes, and pancreatic hypoplasia, similar to clinical SDS phenotype.[80] Organ-specific models in mice have shown findings similar to human disease. A pancreas-specific murine knock-in model, created by introducing a missense mutation in Sbds, was smaller overall, with smaller pancreata that show hypoplastic acini and fatty infiltration with decreased zymogen granules but intact islet cells, which is similar to the phenotype of SDS individuals.[81] Zambetti and colleagues[82] most recently developed a conditional Sbds murine knockout under control of a CEBPα-Cre recombinase, allowing for transplantation of Sbds-deficient fetal liver cells into lethally irradiated wild-type recipients. Recipients subsequently developed hypocellular bone marrow and neutropenia similar to the human phenotype. These mice demonstrate activation of p53 with arrest in myeloid differentiation at the myelocyte stage suggesting this phenotype may be mediated by apoptotic pathways. In the short 4-month follow-up, no malignant transformation was observed. Knockdown of SBDS in human embryonic stem cells has been used to develop induced pluripotent stem cells derived from SDS individuals that show enhanced apoptosis with defective hematopoietic differentiation and exocrine pancreatic dysfunction.[83]

Novel gene discovery along with development of animal and induced pluripotent stem cells models allows further evolution in the understanding of the pathogenesis of SDS further elucidating the role of SBDS and other novel proteins in critical cellular pathways, such as ribosome biogenesis, mitosis, and stress response. These exciting scientific advances may lead to putative therapeutic targets and strategies to improve clinical care of individuals with SDS.

REFERENCES

1. Goobie S, Popovic M, Morrison J, et al. Shwachman-Diamond syndrome with exocrine pancreatic dysfunction and bone marrow failure maps to the centromeric region of chromosome 7. Am J Hum Genet 2001;68(4):1048–54.

2. Carapito R, Konantz M, Paillard C, et al. Mutations in signal recognition particle SRP54 cause syndromic neutropenia with Shwachman-Diamond–like features. J Clin Invest 2017;127(11):4090–103.
3. Stepensky P, Chacón-Flores M, Kim KH, et al. Mutations in EFL1, an SBDS partner, are associated with infantile pancytopenia, exocrine pancreatic insufficiency and skeletal anomalies in a Shwachman-Diamond like syndrome. J Med Genet 2017;54(8):558–66.
4. Dhanraj S, Matveev A, Li H, et al. Biallelic mutations in DNAJC21 cause Shwachman-Diamond syndrome. Blood 2017;129(11):1557–62.
5. Myers KC, Bolyard AA, Otto B, et al. Variable clinical presentation of Shwachman-Diamond syndrome: update from the North American Shwachman-Diamond Syndrome Registry. J Pediatr 2014;164(4):866–70.
6. Aggett PJ, Harries JT, Harvey BA, et al. An inherited defect of neutrophil mobility in Shwachman syndrome. J Pediatr 1979;94(3):391–4.
7. Rothbaum RJ, Williams DA, Daugherty CC. Unusual surface distribution of concanavalin A reflects a cytoskeletal defect in neutrophils in Shwachman's syndrome. Lancet 1982;2(8302):800–1.
8. Grinspan ZM, Pikora CA. Infections in patients with Shwachman-Diamond syndrome. Pediatr Infect Dis J 2005;24(2):179–81.
9. Woods WG, Krivit W, Lubin BH, et al. Aplastic anemia associated with the Shwachman syndrome. In vivo and in vitro observations. Am J Pediatr Hematol Oncol 1981;3(4):347–51.
10. Donadieu J, Fenneteau O, Beaupain B, et al. Classification of and risk factors for hematologic complications in a French national cohort of 102 patients with Shwachman-Diamond syndrome. Haematologica 2012;97(9):1312–9.
11. Cada M, Segbefia CI, Klaassen R, et al. The impact of category, cytopathology and cytogenetics on development and progression of clonal and malignant myeloid transformation in inherited bone marrow failure syndromes. Haematologica 2015;100(5):633–42.
12. Dale DC, Bolyard AA, Schwinzer BG, et al. The severe chronic neutropenia international registry: 10-year follow-up report. Support Cancer Ther 2006;3(4):220–31.
13. Singh SA, Vlachos A, Morgenstern NJ, et al. Breast cancer in a case of Shwachman Diamond syndrome. Pediatr Blood Cancer 2012;59(5):945–6.
14. Sack JE, Kuchnir L, Demierre MF. Dermatofibrosarcoma protuberans arising in the context of Shwachman-Diamond syndrome. Pediatr Dermatol 2011;28(5):568–9.
15. Dror Y, Donadieu J, Koglmeier J, et al. Draft consensus guidelines for diagnosis and treatment of Shwachman-Diamond syndrome. Ann N Y Acad Sci 2011;1242:40–55.
16. Crescenzi B, La Starza R, Sambani C, et al. Totipotent stem cells bearing del(20q) maintain multipotential differentiation in Shwachman Diamond syndrome. Br J Haematol 2009;144(1):116–9.
17. Maserati E, Pressato B, Valli R, et al. The route to development of myelodysplastic syndrome/acute myeloid leukaemia in Shwachman-Diamond syndrome: the role of ageing, karyotype instability, and acquired chromosome anomalies. Br J Haematol 2009;145(2):190–7.
18. Cunningham J, Sales M, Pearce A, et al. Does isochromosome 7q mandate bone marrow transplant in children with Shwachman-Diamond syndrome? Br J Haematol 2002;119(4):1062–9.

19. Nacci L, Valli R, Maria Pinto R, et al. Parental origin of the deletion del(20q) in Shwachman-Diamond patients and loss of the paternally derived allele of the imprinted L3MBTL1 gene. Genes Chromosomes Cancer 2017;56(1):51–8.
20. Valli R, De Paoli E, Nacci L, et al. Novel recurrent chromosome anomalies in Shwachman-Diamond syndrome. Pediatr Blood Cancer 2017;64(8):e26454.
21. Hill RE, Durie PR, Gaskin KJ, et al. Steatorrhea and pancreatic insufficiency in Shwachman syndrome. Gastroenterology 1982;83(1 Pt 1):22–7.
22. Andolina JR, Morrison CB, Thompson AA, et al. Shwachman-Diamond syndrome: diarrhea, no longer required? J Pediatr Hematol Oncol 2013;35(6):486–9.
23. Mack DR, Forstner GG, Wilschanski M, et al. Shwachman syndrome: exocrine pancreatic dysfunction and variable phenotypic expression. Gastroenterology 1996;111(6):1593–602.
24. Stormon MO, Ip WF, Ellis L, et al. Evidence of a generalized defect of acinar cell function in Shwachman-Diamond syndrome. J Pediatr Gastroenterol Nutr 2010; 51(1):8–13.
25. Uc A, Fishman DS. Fishman, pancreatic disorders. Pediatr Clin North Am 2017; 64(3):685–706.
26. Shah N, Cambrook H, Koglmeier J, et al. Enteropathic histopathological features may be associated with Shwachman-Diamond syndrome. J Clin Pathol 2010; 63(7):592–4.
27. Pichler J, Meyer R, Köglmeier J, et al. Nutritional status in children with Shwachman-Diamond syndrome. Pancreas 2015;44(4):590–5.
28. Toiviainen-Salo S, Durie PR, Numminen K, et al. The natural history of Shwachman-Diamond syndrome-associated liver disease from childhood to adulthood. J Pediatr 2009;155(6):807–11.e2.
29. Schaballie H, Renard M, Vermylen C, et al. Misdiagnosis as asphyxiating thoracic dystrophy and CMV-associated haemophagocytic lymphohistiocytosis in Shwachman-Diamond syndrome. Eur J Pediatr 2013;172(5):613–22.
30. McLennan TW, Steinbach HL. Schwachman's syndrome: the broad spectrum of bony abnormalities. Radiology 1974;112(1):167–73.
31. Toiviainen-Salo S, Mäyränpää MK, Durie PR, et al. Shwachman-Diamond syndrome is associated with low-turnover osteoporosis. Bone 2007;41(6):965–72.
32. Shankar RK, Giri N, Lodish MB, et al. Bone mineral density in patients with inherited bone marrow failure syndromes. Pediatr Res 2017;82(3):458–64.
33. Kerr EN, Ellis L, Dupuis A, et al. The behavioral phenotype of school-age children with Shwachman Diamond syndrome indicates neurocognitive dysfunction with loss of Shwachman-Bodian-Diamond syndrome gene function. J Pediatr 2010; 156(3):433–8.
34. Perobelli S, Nicolis E, Assael BM, et al. Further characterization of Shwachman-Diamond syndrome: psychological functioning and quality of life in adult and young patients. Am J Med Genet A 2012;158A(3):567–73.
35. Toiviainen-Salo S, Mäkitie O, Mannerkoski M, et al. Shwachman-Diamond syndrome is associated with structural brain alterations on MRI. Am J Med Genet A 2008;146A(12):1558–64.
36. Booij J, Reneman L, Alders M, et al. Increase in central striatal dopamine transporters in patients with Shwachman-Diamond syndrome: additional evidence of a brain phenotype. Am J Med Genet A 2013;161(1):102–7.
37. Perobelli S, Alessandrini F, Zoccatelli G, et al. Diffuse alterations in grey and white matter associated with cognitive impairment in Shwachman–Diamond syndrome: Evidence from a multimodal approach. Neuroimage Clin 2015;7:721–31.

38. Topa A, Tulinius M, Oldfors A, et al. Novel myopathy in a newborn with Shwachman-Diamond syndrome and review of neonatal presentation. Am J Med Genet A 2016;170A(5):1155–64.

39. Jivani N, Torrado-Jule C, Vaiselbuh S, et al. A unique case of Shwachman-Diamond syndrome presenting with congenital hypopituitarism. J Pediatr Endocrinol Metab 2016;29(11):1325–7.

40. Kamoda T, Saito T, Kinugasa H, et al. A case of Shwachman-Diamond syndrome presenting with diabetes from early infancy. Diabetes Care 2005;28(6):1508–9.

41. Rosendahl J, Teich N, Mossner J, et al. Compound heterozygous mutations of the SBDS gene in a patient with Shwachman-Diamond syndrome, type 1 diabetes mellitus and osteoporosis. Pancreatology 2006;6(6):549–54.

42. Gana S, Sainati L, Frau MR, et al. Shwachman-Diamond syndrome and type 1 diabetes mellitus: more than a chance association? Exp Clin Endocrinol Diabetes 2011;119(10):610–2.

43. Akdogan MF, Altay M, Denizli N, et al. A rare case: Shwachman-Diamond syndrome presenting with diabetic ketoacidosis. Endocrine 2011;40(1):146–7.

44. Goeteyn M, Oranje AP, Vuzevski VD, et al. Ichthyosis, exocrine pancreatic insufficiency, impaired neutrophil chemotaxis, growth retardation, and metaphyseal dysplasia (Shwachman syndrome). Report of a case with extensive skin lesions (clinical, histological, and ultrastructural findings). Arch Dermatol 1991;127(2): 225–30.

45. Kawashima H, Ushio M, Aritaki K, et al. Discordant endocrinopathy in a sibling with Shwachman-Diamond syndrome. J Trop Pediatr 2006;52(6):445–7.

46. Terlizzi V, Zito E, Mozzillo E, et al. Can continuous subcutaneous insulin infusion improve health-related quality of life in patients with Shwachman-Bodian-Diamond syndrome and diabetes? Diabetes Technol Ther 2014;17(1):64–7.

47. Ginzberg H, Shin J, Ellis L, et al. Shwachman syndrome: phenotypic manifestations of sibling sets and isolated cases in a large patient cohort are similar. J Pediatr 1999;135(1):81–8.

48. Hauet Q, Beaupain B, Micheau M, et al. Cardiomyopathies and congenital heart diseases in Shwachman-Diamond syndrome: a national survey. Int J Cardiol 2013;167(3):1048–50.

49. Kalejaiye A, Giri N, Brewer CC, et al. Otologic manifestations of Fanconi anemia and other inherited bone marrow failure syndromes. Pediatr Blood Cancer 2016; 63(12):2139–45.

50. Fadus MC, Rush ET, Lettieri CK. Syndrome of progressive bone marrow failure and pancreatic insufficiency remains cryptic despite whole exome sequencing: variant of Shwachman-Diamond syndrome or new condition? Clin Case Rep 2017;5(6):748–52.

51. Lindsley RC, Saber W, Mar BG, et al. Prognostic mutations in myelodysplastic syndrome after stem-cell transplantation. N Engl J Med 2017;376(6):536–47.

52. Myers KC, Davies SM. Hematopoietic stem cell transplantation for bone marrow failure syndromes in children. Biol Blood Marrow Transplant 2009;15(3):279–92.

53. Burroughs LM, Shimamura A, Talano JA, et al. Allogeneic hematopoietic cell transplantation using treosulfan-based conditioning for treatment of marrow failure disorders. Biol Blood Marrow Transplant 2017;23(10):1669–77.

54. Bhatla D, Davies SM, Shenoy S, et al. Reduced-intensity conditioning is effective and safe for transplantation of patients with Shwachman-Diamond syndrome. Bone Marrow Transplant 2008;42(3):159–65.

55. Finch AJ, Hilcenko C, Basse N, et al. Uncoupling of GTP hydrolysis from eIF6 release on the ribosome causes Shwachman-Diamond syndrome. Genes Dev 2011;25(9):917–29.
56. Wegman-Ostrosky T, Savage SA. The genomics of inherited bone marrow failure: from mechanism to the clinic. Br J Haematol 2017;177(4):526–42.
57. Raaijmakers MH, Mukherjee S, Guo S, et al. Bone progenitor dysfunction induces myelodysplasia and secondary leukaemia. Nature 2010;464(7290):852–7.
58. Nihrane A, Sezgin G, Dsilva S, et al. Depletion of the Shwachman-Diamond syndrome gene product, SBDS, leads to growth inhibition and increased expression of OPG and VEGF-A. Blood Cells Mol Dis 2009;42(1):85–91.
59. Austin KM, Gupta ML Jr, Coats SA, et al. Mitotic spindle destabilization and genomic instability in Shwachman-Diamond syndrome. J Clin Invest 2008; 118(4):1511–8.
60. Orelio C, Verkuijlen P, Geissler J, et al. SBDS expression and localization at the mitotic spindle in human myeloid progenitors. PLoS One 2009;4(9):e7084.
61. Menne TF, Goyenechea B, Sánchez-Puig N, et al. The Shwachman-Bodian-Diamond syndrome protein mediates translational activation of ribosomes in yeast. Nat Genet 2007;39(4):486–95.
62. Wong CC, Traynor D, Basse N, et al. Defective ribosome assembly in Shwachman-Diamond syndrome. Blood 2011;118(16):4305–12.
63. Ganapathi KA, Austin KM, Lee CS, et al. The human Shwachman-Diamond syndrome protein, SBDS, associates with ribosomal RNA. Blood 2007;110(5): 1458–65.
64. Burwick N, Coats SA, Nakamura T, et al. Impaired ribosomal subunit association in Shwachman-Diamond syndrome. Blood 2012;120(26):5143–52.
65. Ma C, Yan K, Tan D, et al. Structural dynamics of the yeast Shwachman-Diamond syndrome protein (Sdo1) on the ribosome and its implication in the 60S subunit maturation. Protein Cell 2016;7(3):187–200.
66. Tummala H, Walne AJ, Williams M, et al. DNAJC21 mutations link a cancer-prone bone marrow failure syndrome to corruption in 60S ribosome subunit maturation. Am J Hum Genet 2016;99(1):115–24.
67. In K, Zaini MA, Müller C, et al. Shwachman-Bodian-Diamond syndrome (SBDS) protein deficiency impairs translation re-initiation from C/EBPalpha and C/EBP-beta mRNAs. Nucleic Acids Res 2016;44(9):4134–46.
68. Orelio C, Kuijpers TW. Shwachman-Diamond syndrome neutrophils have altered chemoattractant-induced F-actin polymerization and polarization characteristics. Haematologica 2009;94(3):409–13.
69. Zambetti NA, Ping Z, Chen S, et al. Mesenchymal inflammation drives genotoxic stress in hematopoietic stem cells and predicts disease evolution in human pre-leukemia. Cell Stem Cell 2016;19(5):613–27.
70. Ravera S, Dufour C, Cesaro S, et al. Evaluation of energy metabolism and calcium homeostasis in cells affected by Shwachman-Diamond syndrome. Sci Rep 2016;6:25441.
71. Bezzerri V, Vella A, Calcaterra E, et al. New insights into the Shwachman-Diamond Syndrome-related haematological disorder: hyper-activation of mTOR and STAT3 in leukocytes. Sci Rep 2016;6:33165.
72. Ambekar C, Das B, Yeger H, et al. SBDS-deficiency results in deregulation of reactive oxygen species leading to increased cell death and decreased cell growth. Pediatr Blood Cancer 2010;55(6):1138–44.

73. Ball HL, Zhang B, Riches JJ, et al. Shwachman-Bodian Diamond syndrome is a multi-functional protein implicated in cellular stress responses. Hum Mol Genet 2009;18(19):3684–95.

74. Rujkijyanont P, Watanabe K, Ambekar C, et al. SBDS-deficient cells undergo accelerated apoptosis through the Fas-pathway. Haematologica 2008;93(3): 363–71.

75. Kanprasoet W, Jensen LT, Sriprach S, et al. Deletion of mitochondrial porin alleviates stress sensitivity in the yeast model of Shwachman-Diamond syndrome. J Genet Genomics 2015;42(12):671–84.

76. Dror Y, Freedman MH. Shwachman-Diamond syndrome: an inherited preleukemic bone marrow failure disorder with aberrant hematopoietic progenitors and faulty marrow microenvironment. Blood 1999;94(9):3048–54.

77. Andre V, Longoni D, Bresolin S, et al. Mesenchymal stem cells from Shwachman-Diamond syndrome patients display normal functions and do not contribute to hematological defects. Blood Cancer J 2012;2:e94.

78. Zhang S, Shi M, Hui CC, et al. Loss of the mouse ortholog of the Shwachman-Diamond syndrome gene (SBDS) results in early embryonic lethality. Mol Cell Biol 2006;26(17):6656–63.

79. Rawls AS, Gregory AD, Woloszynek JR, et al. Lentiviral-mediated RNAi inhibition of SBDS in murine hematopoietic progenitors impairs their hematopoietic potential. Blood 2007;110(7):2414–22.

80. Provost E, Wehner KA, Zhong X, et al. Ribosomal biogenesis genes play an essential and p53-independent role in zebrafish pancreas development. Development 2012;139(17):3232–41.

81. Tourlakis ME, Zhong J, Gandhi R, et al. Deficiency of SBDS in the mouse pancreas leads to features of Shwachman-Diamond syndrome, with loss of zymogen granules. Gastroenterology 2012;143(2):481–92.

82. Zambetti NA, Bindels EM, Van Strien PM, et al. Deficiency of the ribosome biogenesis gene SBDS in hematopoietic stem and progenitor cells causes neutropenia in mice by attenuating lineage progression in myelocytes. Haematologica 2015;100(10):1285–93.

83. Tulpule A, Kelley JM, Lensch MW, et al. Pluripotent stem cell models of Shwachman-Diamond syndrome reveal a common mechanism for pancreatic and hematopoietic dysfunction. Cell Stem Cell 2013;12(6):727–36.

Critical Issues in Diamond-Blackfan Anemia and Prospects for Novel Treatment

Hojun Li, MD, PhD[a], Harvey F. Lodish, PhD[b],
Colin A. Sieff, MB,BCh, FRCPath[a],*

KEYWORDS

- Diamond-Blackfan anemia • Ribosomal protein gene mutation • GATA1
- Ribosome function • Red cell aplasia

KEY POINTS

- Diamond-Blackfan anemia is a congenital red cell aplasia caused by ribosomal protein gene and rarely GATA1 mutations.
- The erythroid specificity is caused by reduced ribosome numbers that decrease translation of complex structured mRNAs.
- Treatment with steroids is successful long term in approximately 40% of patients and those that fail require hematopoietic stem cell transplantation or red cell transfusions.
- Treatment-related issues include steroid toxicity, risks associated with transplantation, and transfusion hemosiderosis.
- Several novel treatments for DBA are in trial or under preclinical development.

INTRODUCTION

Diamond-Blackfan anemia (DBA) is a congenital red blood cell aplasia that usually presents during the first year of life. Only 10% of patients are anemic at birth and 80% by 6 months. Although DBA may present at any age, it is considered a disease affecting infants.

The main hematologic features of DBA are severe normochromic and macrocytic anemia, reticulocytopenia, an increase in erythrocyte adenosine deaminase, and erythroid hypoplasia in the bone marrow, with preservation of other lineages. Other

Disclosure Statement: None of the authors have any disclosures to report.
[a] Division of Hematology/Oncology, Dana Farber and Boston Children's Cancer and Blood Disorders Center, 450 Brookline Avenue, Boston, MA 02215, USA; [b] Whitehead Institute for Biomedical Research, 455 Main Street, Cambridge, MA 02142, USA
* Corresponding author.
E-mail address: Colin.Sieff@childrens.harvard.edu

developmental abnormalities, most commonly affecting the head, upper limb, kidneys, heart, and eyes, are present in about 40% of cases.

Erythroid failure is characterized by a marked reduction in erythroid precursors and their progenitors, the erythroid burst-forming unit (BFU-E) and colony-forming unit (CFU-E).[1] Persistent macrocytosis and increased HbF and erythrocyte "i" antigen expression in patients are features of stress erythropoiesis that is more fetal than adult in nature.[2,3] The disease has been associated with point mutations and large deletions in 18 ribosomal protein (RP) genes in about 60% to 65% of patients.[4–7] Mutations are also rarely present in two non-RP genes (GATA1, an essential erythroid transcription factor, and TSR2).[7]

RP haploinsufficiency accounts for most cases of DBA, and an intriguing question is why deficiency of RPs, structural components of ribosomes expressed in all nucleated cells, leads to the specific erythroid and other congenital defects characteristic of DBA. There is good evidence that ribosomal stress leads to free RPs sequestering MDM2, resulting in p53 stabilization and consequent cell cycle arrest or apoptosis, but this does not explain the tissue specificity of disease manifestations. There are two leading hypotheses: the first postulates the importance of specialized (tissue specific) ribosomes that comprise different subsets of RPs that are critical for the translation of specific mRNAs. Support for this theory comes from tissue-specific expression of eL38 in Ts mice that show surprising patterning defects caused by perturbed translation of specific homeobox mRNAs of eL38-deficient tissues. However,[8] there is no evidence to date that indicates different ribosome composition in erythroid compared with nonerythroid cells. The second hypothesis posits that ribosome deficiency adversely affects the translation of complex structured mRNAs that have low initiation rates (**Fig. 1**). Compelling evidence for this theory comes from the demonstration that GATA1 translation is impaired in DBA patients with different RP gene mutations because ribosomes are limiting,[9] and that cells in which DBA-associated genes have been knocked down do not have altered ribosome composition compared with their wild-type counterparts, but do have overall decreased levels of ribosomes.[10] GATA1 has a complex 5′ UTR that predicts poor translation initiation rates, and such mRNAs are more sensitive to ribosome deficiency than mRNAs with high initiation rates (for an excellent review see[11]).

This article focuses on current issues in the management of patients with DBA and on prospects for novel treatment approaches.

STEROIDS

It is sobering to realize that treatment of DBA with corticosteroids, observed by Gasser in 1951,[12] is still the only medication effective in clinical practice. Approximately 75% of patients respond to treatment with an increase in reticulocytes and hemoglobin. Although some patients remain steroid dependent and can be maintained on a tolerably low dose (usually a maximum of 0.5 mg/kg/d prednisone), others require too high a dose of steroids and have to be maintained on regular blood transfusions to avoid steroid toxicity, which includes pathologic fractures, avascular necrosis, cataracts, growth retardation, hypertension, and diabetes. Close monitoring is necessary to avoid these complications because their detection requires a steroid taper and switch to transfusion therapy.[13] Although the molecular mechanism of action of corticosteroids in DBA patients has not been completely elucidated, studies of normal mouse erythroid development demonstrate that corticosteroids are able to increase BFU-E cell numbers by stimulating self-renewal, thereby expanding the progenitor cell population first lost in DBA.[14] Approximately 40% of patients remain steroid

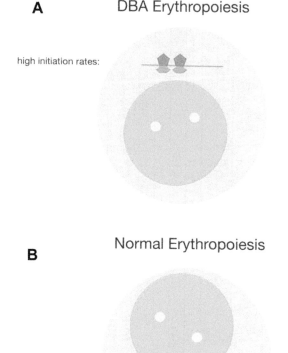

A   DBA Erythropoiesis

high initiation rates:

B   Normal Erythropoiesis

mRNAs
high initiation rates:

low initiation rates:
(structured mRNAs)

5'_____3'

LSU
SSU

Fig. 1. Effect of ribosome availability on mRNA translation. (*A*) In DBA ribosome structure is normal but ribosomes are reduced (haploinsufficiency), and these cells only translate mRNAs with high initiation rates, such as RPs and hemoglobin, but not mRNAs with low initiation rates, such as those with a structured 5' open reading frame, such as GATA1, an upstream AUG, or an internal ribosome entry site. LSU, large subunit; SSU, small subunit. (*B*) Normal erythroid progenitors with a full complement of ribosomes can translate mRNAs with high and low initiation rates (k_is).

responsive; 40% become steroid refractory, require blood transfusions and are eligible for a hematopoietic stem cell transplant (HSCT); and 20% remit and do not require medication.[15]

HEMATOPOIETIC STEM CELL TRANSPLANTATION

The only cure for DBA is stem cell transplantation, and excellent results have been obtained for patients aged less than 10 years with HLA-matched allogeneic sibling donors (>90% survival).[16] Published results for unrelated HLA-matched transplants have not been as good, in particular for patients transplanted before 2000 and for those older than 10 years.[17,18] However, advances in molecular tissue typing and transplantation of young patients to avoid the deleterious effects of iron overload have led to improved results. **Table 1** shows several recently published single center

Table 1
Unrelated donor transplantation for Diamond-Blackfan anemia

#	Age (mo)	Conditioning	HSCT Source	Acute GVHD	Chronic GVHD	Cx	FU (mo)	Ref
MAC								
1.1	24	BU/CY/ATG	MUD/PBSC	II	No	CMV react	A,7	Li et al,[45] 2017
1.2	42	"	MMSD-9/10/PBSC	No	Ltd	Infection	A,14	
1.3	72	"	MUD/PBSC	No	No	HC, VOD	A,31	
1.4	10	"	UCB-6/6	II	No	VOD	A,31	
1.5	18	"	UCB-5/6	II	No	No	A,33	
1.6	18	"	UCB-6/6	II	No	No	A,76	
1.7	20	"	MUD/PBSC	III	Ltd	ICH, OVD	A,130	
RIC								
2.1	74	Treo/Flu/rATG	MUD/BM	+	+	AIHA	A,54	Burroughs et al,[46] 2017
2.2	146	"	MUD/BM	+	No		A,48	
2.3	263	"	MUD/BM	No	No		A,36	
2.4	27	"	MUD/BM	+	No		A,3	
3.1	9	Treo/Flu/Thio	MSD	II+12	No		A,48	Crazzolara et al,[47] 2016
3.2	7	"	MUD	I			A,37	
3.3	13	Flu/Thio	MUD				A,124	
4	14	Al/Flu/M	MUD	I			A,21	Asquith et al,[48] 2015

Abbreviations: A, alive; AIHA, autoimmune hemolytic anemia; BM, bone marrow; CMV, cytomegalovirus; Cx, Complications; FU, follow-up; GVHD, graft-versus-host disease; HC, hemorrhagic cystitis; ICH, intracranial hemorrhage; Ltd, Limited; MUD, matched unrelated donor; MMSD, mismatched sibling donor; MSD, matched sibling donor; OVD, obstructive ventilation disorder; PBSC, peripheral blood stem cells; UCB, umbilical cord blood; VOD, veno-occlusive disease.

Myeloablative Conditioning (MAC): Busufan (BU) 16 mg/kg, Cyclophosphamide 200 mg/kg, rabbit antithymocyte globulin (rATG) 10 mg/kg. Reduced Intensity Conditioning (RIC): Treosulfan 42 mg/m2 (Treo), Fludarabine (Flu) 150 mg/m2, rabbit Antithymocyte Globulin (rATG) 6 mg/kg, Treosulfan (Treo) 56 g/m2, Flu 8mg/m2, Thiotepa (Thio) 160 mg/m2, Alemtuzumab (Al) 45 mg, Flu 150 mg/m2, Melphalan (M) 140 mg/m.

studies. Although numbers are still low and length of follow-up limited, all patients were alive at the time of reporting after either myeloablative or reduced intensity conditioning without undue infectious, graft-versus-host disease complications, or failure of engraftment.

TRANSFUSIONAL HEMOSIDEROSIS

One critical and controversial question is whether DBA patients are more susceptible to early and more severe iron toxicity than other chronically transfused patients. Most patients with DBA are diagnosed during the first few months of life. They frequently present with severe anemia and require an immediate blood transfusion after diagnostic tests have been obtained. The standard of care is to continue blood transfusions for 1 year, because the early use of steroids can impair growth, which is already a concern in patients with DBA. Although 70% to 80% of patients respond to steroids, only half are maintained long term on sufficiently low doses to avoid toxicity. Patients who fail to respond and those who become resistant to steroids require monthly blood transfusions. They are eligible for HSCT if a suitable donor is available and parents choose to pursue this path.

Few studies have compared the effects of chronic transfusions in DBA with other transfused patients, such as those with β-thalassemia major (TM) and sickle cell disease (SCD). A case control study of 31 transfusion-dependent DBA patients and a comparable group of β-thalassemia patients on deferoxamine showed a significantly increased liver iron concentration with a high rate of organ toxicity in DBA, and raised the possibility that DBA patients may be more susceptible to organ toxicity than those with thalassemia.[3] However, compliance with the chelation regime was poor, so it was impossible to determine whether these results might have been caused by a difference in biology or by poor compliance. To evaluate the rate of iron loading in 124 children with transfusion-dependent anemias including DBA, TM, congenital dyserythropoietic anemia (CDA), and SCD, Berdoukas and colleagues[19] retrospectively evaluated initial MRIs, done before or soon after the start of chelation, and subsequent liver, cardiac, and pancreas R2* MRIs. All initial MRI R2* values for liver iron concentration in patients younger than 10 years were increased and showed no significant differences among diseases. Strikingly, initial and subsequent pancreatic MRIs showed that 50% of subjects with DBA developed pancreatic R2* greater than 100 Hz, compared with 25% CDA or TM and 2.5% with SCD, predicting a risk of glucose intolerance. Similarly, 25% of DBA and CDA patients developed increased cardiac iron (R2* >50 Hz), compared with 10% of those with TM; 2 of the 17 DBA children in the study showed the increase at the young ages of 2.5 and 3.7 years.

Extrahepatic iron deposition is related to an increase in nontransferrin bound iron (NTBI), which includes the toxic redox reactive labile plasma iron component. NTBI levels increase when transferrin saturation exceeds 60% to 70%. Mechanisms of NTBI generation were examined in DBA, TM, and SCD patients with matched transfusion histories by comparing the key parameters of iron metabolism.[20] A comparison of hepcidin levels in transfusion-dependent DBA, TM, and SCD shows that hepcidin levels are high in DBA. Does the regulation of hepcidin play a critical role in the extrahepatic iron deposition seen at an early age in DBA?

Although there is no physiologic mechanism for excreting the excess iron acquired by repeated red cell transfusions, hepcidin plays a critical role in iron transport regulation by controlling iron absorption and recirculation through binding to ferroportin, which exports iron into plasma from the basolateral side of duodenal enterocytes and from macrophages and hepatocytes. This leads to ferroportin ubiquitination and degradation. Hepcidin synthesis is regulated by three pathways, iron availability, inflammation, and erythropoiesis:

1. Iron availability: when iron levels are high, excess transferrin-bound iron (Tf-Fe2) displaces the hemochromatosis protein HFE from the high affinity TFR1 to a complex with the lower affinity TFR2 and hemojuvelin. This complex mediates BMP6 signaling through ALK3 and BMPR2 to activate R-SMAD, SMAD4, and an increase in hepcidin transcription (**Fig. 2**). Ferroportin is also important for cells that do not contribute to plasma iron, such as cardiomyocytes.[8]
2. Inflammation is characterized by increased levels of cytokines, such as interleukin-6 and activin B. Interleukin-6 leads to high hepcidin expression through the interleukin-6 receptor, which activates JAK and STAT3 to increase hepcidin transcription. Activin B can stimulate hepcidin through the BMP6 pathway (see **Fig. 2**).
3. When erythropoiesis is increased the requirement for iron is met by an increase in dietary absorption from enterocytes and release of iron from hepatic and reticuloendothelial stores through inhibition of hepcidin transcription and stabilization of ferroportin. Hepcidin repression depends on erythropoietin (EPO) and a functional bone marrow.[21] In mice there is good evidence that EPO induces erythroid cells via

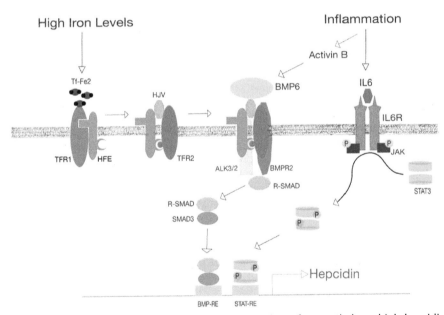

Fig. 2. Regulation of hepcidin transcription. DBA patients frequently have high hepcidin levels, higher than other transfusion-dependent anemias, and can load iron rapidly, including the liver, heart, and endocrine organs, such as the pancreas. Increased hepcidin transcription occurs through high concentrations of Tf-Fe2, which displaces HFE from TFR1. HFE forms a complex TFR2 and hemojuvelin, which augments BMP6 activation of serine threonine kinase receptors ALK3/2 and BMPR2 leading to phosphorylation of receptor-activated SMAD (R-SMAD) and hepcidin transcription. Inflammation can lead to increased activin B mediated BMP6 signaling and interleukin (IL)-6 expression, activation of the IL-6 receptor (IL6R), and recruitment/phosphorylation of JAK tyrosine kinase, which in turn phosphorylates STAT3 to augment hepcidin transcription. Hepcidin binds to ferroportin, leading to ubiquitination and degradation of this iron transporter expressed on hepatocytes, macrophages, and cardiomyocytes.

JAK2/STAT5 to secrete a long sought erythroid regulator named erythroferrone, because $Erfe^{-/-}$ animals, in contrast to wild-type, fail to inhibit hepcidin in response to hemorrhage or EPO injections.[22] Ablation of Erfe in thalassemic mice leads to restoration of hepcidin mRNA and reduction in liver and spleen iron content.[23] The role of erythroferrone in human erythropoiesis is uncertain, as is the signaling pathway. Growth differentiation factor-15 has also been implicated as a protein secreted by erythroblasts in the ineffective erythropoiesis that characterizes TM[24] and CDA type 1,[25] although these data are controversial.[26]

In DBA, hepcidin synthesis is most likely increased through excessive Tf-Fe2 stimulation of the BMP6 signaling pathway, but the downregulation of ferroportin is insufficient to significantly limit transfusional iron overload. High hepcidin levels could also decrease cardiomyocyte expression of ferroportin, thus trapping iron within these cells. Indeed, conditional deletion of ferroportin in cardiomyocytes leads to severe compromise of cardiac function caused by iron accumulation in these cells.[8] Although EPO levels are high, suppression of hepcidin does not occur in the absence of erythropoiesis. Most importantly, the absence of erythropoieisis results in lack of iron uptake by erythroblasts, thus accounting for the high transferrin saturation and high levels of NTBI and labile plasma iron. This is most likely the explanation for the increased iron toxicity in DBA.

With respect to clinical practice, chronic transfusion alone in DBA is not a satisfactory long-term management strategy and it is essential that chelation is included early in the treatment plan. DBA patients tolerate deferasirox (Exjade, Jaydenu) and deferoxamine (Desferal) well; however, prolonged subcutaneous administration of deferoxamine is more difficult to manage and to achieve good compliance, especially in older children. DBA patients may be uniquely susceptible to the toxic effects of the other oral agent deferiprone (Ferriprox), which is useful in removing cardiac iron. Indeed, the first case of septic agranulocytosis was reported in a DBA patient and others have been reported.[27,28] In summary, because of efficacy, safety, and ease of administration, oral deferasirox is usually tried first; in severely overloaded patients deferoxamine is added either subcutaneously or intravenously, and deferiprone is reserved and used cautiously only in patients with cardiac iron overload.

PROSPECTS FOR NOVEL TREATMENT OF DIAMOND-BLACKFAN ANEMIA
Gene Therapy

For those cases of DBA with an identifiable underlying genetic mutation, gene therapy is an attractive potential therapy to cure DBA. Similar to the goal of allogeneic HSCT, gene therapy for DBA aims to replace DBA HSCs, and their diseased erythroid progeny, with HSCs able to produce adequate numbers of number erythroid progenitors that ultimately give rise to normal mature red blood cells. The difference between allogeneic HSCT and gene therapy is that the source of normal HSCs in gene therapy does not come from an outside donor but from the patient's own HSCs into which a normal copy of the mutated gene has been inserted.

Given that 25% of DBA cases are associated with a mutation in the *RPS19* gene,[15] there has been significant interest in the development of gene therapy to deliver a normal copy of *RPS19* to *RPS19*-mutated DBA HSCs. In a series of studies, Karlsson and colleagues have demonstrated that retroviral gene therapy vectors carrying the wild-type *RPS19* gene can transduce human DBA patient CD34$^+$ cells, the cell population that contains human HSCs. This results in an erythroid engraftment advantage in immunocompromised mice compared with mock-transduced DBA CD34$^+$ cells.[29] They have also shown that lentiviral gene therapy vectors carrying wild-type *RPS19* can transduce mouse HSCs and correct the anemia found in a mouse model of DBA that depletes RPS19 protein levels using shRNA knockdown.[30] Future studies are needed to determine if the newer lentiviral vectors are also able to efficiently transduce human CD34$^+$ cells. Additionally, CRISPR/Cas9-mediated genome editing has recently been shown to be highly efficient in human HSCs.[31] This genome editing paradigm physically corrects a disease-causing mutation within the genome, and may mediate cure without the use of an integrating viral vector.

Novel Drug Therapeutics

To find treatment alternatives to corticosteroids, there has been great interest in identifying novel drug candidates for the management of DBA. Although no other effective medications have been discovered for DBA in the last 60 years, the last decade has seen a substantial increase in the number of candidates with therapeutic potential.

After observing that decreased protein synthesis in lymphoid cells from DBA patients could be increased with high concentrations of L-leucine,[32] Pospisilova and colleagues[33] treated a single DBA patient with high levels of dietary L-leucine and observed an approximately 50% increase in hemoglobin levels 6 months after L-leucine initiation. Subsequently, Payne and colleagues[34] and Jaako and colleagues[35] demonstrated that high-levels of L-leucine were able to improve the anemia in RP knockdown DBA models in the zebrafish and mouse, respectively. A clinical trial is currently underway to evaluate L-leucine in DBA patients, but there have been no report of efficacy to date.

To address one of the underlying pathophysiologic mechanisms of disease in DBA, Zon and colleagues (unpublished data) identified through a chemical screen in RPS19-deficient zebrafish that calmodulin inhibition rescued hemoglobin levels. In human cell culture models, the calmodulin inhibitor trifluoperazine blocked nuclear accumulation and transcriptional activity of p53 by inhibiting calmodulin-dependent kinase phosphorylation of the p53 c-terminal domain. Trifluoperazine also increased hemoglobin levels in a RPS19 knockdown mouse model of DBA. Although unpublished, this work has been presented in abstract form at the American Society of Hematology annual meeting in 2015, and a clinical trial will begin soon to evaluate calmodulin inhibition in DBA.

Additional preclinical investigations have focused on finding therapeutic targets that may have a synergistic therapeutic effect with corticosteroids, which would ideally allow DBA patients to either maintain the same level of disease control with less steroid toxicity or maintain disease control when patients become less steroid-responsive. Lodish and colleagues[14] probed promoter regions of genes activated in mouse BFU-Es that were stimulated with glucocorticoids and found many promoters contained hypoxia-induced factor 1-α binding sites. Because degradation of hypoxia-induced factor 1-α is mediated by intracellular prolyl hydroxylase activity, they then tested the effect of the prolyl hydroxylase inhibitor dimethyloxalylglycine on mouse BFU-E expansion, with the rationale that increased BFU-E expansion would address the initial underlying deficiency in early erythroid progenitor cells in DBA. They found that although dimethyloxalylglycine treatment by itself did not increase BFU-E expansion, treatment with both dimethyloxalylglycine and corticosteroids resulted in increased BFU-E expansion compared with corticosteroids alone. To date, no clinical trial of prolyl hydroxylase inhibitors in DBA patients have been initiated, but there are currently several prolyl hydroxylase inhibitors being evaluated for EPO induction in chronic kidney disease.[36] These studies will be invaluable in defining the toxicity profile of prolyl hydroxylase inhibitors before trials in DBA patients can be undertaken.

Another therapeutic target that potentially synergizes with corticosteroids is the transcription factor peroxisome proliferator activated receptor (PPAR)-α. Lee and colleagues[37] identified PPAR-α as the nuclear receptor with the greatest increase in expression on treatment of mouse BFU-Es with corticosteroids, and also determined that the glucocorticoid receptor and PPAR-α share similar sites of chromatin occupancy in mouse BFU-Es. Further experiments with mouse and human BFU-Es demonstrated that the addition of either of the PPAR-α agonists GW7647 or fenofibrate to corticosteroid treatment resulted in increased BFU-E expansion in vitro when compared with corticosteroids alone. This could potentially lower the concentration of corticosteroids needed to increase output of red cells from earlier progenitors. Additionally, GW7647 treatment resulted in a less severe hemoglobin nadir in a mouse model of phenylhydrazine-induced acute hemolytic anemia, and an improvement in hemoglobin levels of a mouse model of chronic anemia caused by heterozygous mutation of the transcription factor erythroid Kruppel-like factor. Further work is still under way to evaluate the efficacy of PPAR-α agonists in preclinical models of DBA.

There have also been recent efforts to use unbiased large-scale chemical screens to identify candidate drugs for DBA therapy. Using induced pluripotent stem cells (iPSCs) generated from DBA patients with RPS19 or RPL5 haploinsufficiency, Doulatov and colleagues[38] demonstrated DBA iPSCs have multiple erythropoietic defects in vitro, and in vivo. These DBA iPSCs were then used in an unbiased screen that not only identified corticosteroids as a mediator of erythroid phenotype rescue, but also independently identified the compound SMER28, which is a quinazolinamine derivative previously shown to induce autophagy. They then went on to demonstrate SMER28 is able to alleviate anemia in a zebrafish RP knockdown model of DBA and in a mouse model of DBA with inducible single copy loss of the Rpl11 gene. Given the recent reporting of these findings, clinical translation of SMER28 as a potential DBA therapeutic is still pending.

Lastly, several recent lines of evidence have pointed to inhibition of transforming growth factor (TGF)-β signaling as a potential therapy for DBA. Ge and colleagues[39] recently found that iPSCs from DBA patients, with RPS19 or RPL5 haploinsufficiency, are characterized by increased TGF-β receptor signaling and increased expression of TGF-β target genes. Gao and colleagues[40] also recently found that the type 3 TGF-β receptor increases in expression during the transition from developmentally early to late BFU-Es, and that treatment with a TGF-β inhibitor increases in vitro expansion of mouse and human BFU-Es. Because the type 3 TGF-β receptor does not possess a signaling domain, the hypothesis is that increasing surface expression of the type 3 TGF-β receptor binds TGF-β signaling molecules and sequesters them at the late BFU-E cell surface, allowing greater opportunity for binding the type 1 and 2 TGF-β receptors. Type 1 and 2 TGF-β receptor activation may then mediate signaling that results in differentiation of BFU-Es as opposed to continued BFU-E cell proliferation, whereas inhibition of TGF-β signaling may lead to increased output of red blood cells by increasing BFU-E cell proliferation.

Ear and colleagues[41] also reported additional evidence for the therapeutic potential of inhibiting signaling of TGF-β superfamily receptors, recently showing that the activin receptor trap RAP-011 improves erythropoiesis in a RPL11 knockdown zebrafish model of DBA. Activin receptor traps were first proposed as therapy for correcting ineffective erythropoiesis associated with β-thalassemia,[42] but activin receptor traps, such as RAP-011, or the humanized version ACE-011, additionally have the potential for binding other members of the TGF-β superfamily of ligands, such as growth differentiation factor-11. Interestingly, ACE-011 has been observed to increase hemoglobin in nonanemic postmenopausal women[43] and in oncology patients experiencing chemotherapy-induced anemia.[44] Neither of these two patient populations were affected by β-thalassemia and did not demonstrate signs of ineffective erythropoiesis. Given the existing clinical experience with ACE-011, there is now an active clinical trial evaluating the safety and efficacy of ACE-011 in DBA.

REFERENCES

1. Nathan DG, Clarke BJ, Hillman DG, et al. Erythroid precursors in congenital hypoplastic (Diamond-Blackfan) anemia. J Clin Invest 1978;61:489–98.
2. Xiang J, Wu D-CC, Chen Y, et al. In vitro culture of stress erythroid progenitors identifies distinct progenitor populations and analogous human progenitors. Blood 2015;125(11):1803–12.
3. Roggero S, Quarello P, Vinciguerra T, et al. Severe iron overload in Blackfan-Diamond anemia: a case-control study. Am J Hematol 2009;84(11):729–32.
4. Mirabello L, Khincha PP, Ellis SR, et al. Novel and known ribosomal causes of Diamond-Blackfan anaemia identified through comprehensive genomic characterisation. J Med Genet 2017;54:417–25.
5. Mirabello L, Macari ER, Jessop L, et al. Whole-exome sequencing and functional studies identify RPS29 as a novel gene mutated in multicase Diamond-Blackfan anemia families. Blood 2014;124(1):24–32.
6. Farrar JE, Quarello P, Fisher R, et al. Exploiting pre-rRNA processing in Diamond Blackfan anemia gene discovery and diagnosis. Am J Hematol 2014;89(10):985–91.
7. Gripp KW, Curry C, Olney AH, et al. Diamond-Blackfan anemia with mandibulofacial dystostosis is heterogeneous, including the novel DBA genes TSR2 and RPS28. Am J Med Genet A 2014;164A(9):2240–9.
8. Lakhal-Littleton S, Wolna M, Carr CA, et al. Cardiac ferroportin regulates cellular iron homeostasis and is important for cardiac function. Proc Natl Acad Sci U S A 2015;112(10):3164–9.
9. Ludwig LS, Gazda HT, Eng JC, et al. Altered translation of GATA1 in Diamond-Blackfan anemia. Nat Med 2014;20(7):748–53.
10. Khajuria RK, Munschauer M, Ulirsch JC, et al. Ribosome levels selectively regulate translation and lineage commitment in human hematopoiesis. Cell 2018;173(1):90–103.e19.
11. Mills EW, Green R. Ribosomopathies: there's strength in numbers. Science 2017;358(6363) [pii:eaan2755].
12. Gasser C. Aplastiche Anamie (chronische Erythroblastophthise) und Cortison. Schweiz Med Wochenschr 1951;81:1241.
13. Vlachos A, Muir E. How I treat Diamond-Blackfan anemia. Blood 2010;116(19):3715–23.
14. Flygare J, Rayon Estrada V, Shin C, et al. HIF1alpha synergizes with glucocorticoids to promote BFU-E progenitor self-renewal. Blood 2011;117(12):3435–44.
15. Vlachos A, Ball S, Dahl N, et al. Diagnosing and treating Diamond Blackfan anaemia: results of an international clinical consensus conference. Br J Haematol 2008;142(6):859–76.
16. Fagioli F, Quarello P, Zecca M, et al. Haematopoietic stem cell transplantation for Diamond Blackfan anaemia: a report from the Italian Association of Paediatric Haematology and Oncology Registry. Br J Haematol 2014;165(5):673–81.
17. Lipton JM, Atsidaftos E, Zyskind I, et al. Improving clinical care and elucidating the pathophysiology of Diamond Blackfan anemia: an update from the Diamond Blackfan Anemia Registry. Pediatr Blood Cancer 2006;46(5):558–64.

18. Roy V, Perez WS, Eapen M, et al. Bone marrow transplantation for Diamond-Blackfan anemia. Biol Blood Marrow Transplant 2005;11(8):600–8.
19. Berdoukas V, Nord A, Carson S, et al. Tissue iron evaluation in chronically transfused children shows significant levels of iron loading at a very young age. Am J Hematol 2013;88(11):5.
20. Porter JB, Walter PB, Neumayr LD, et al. Mechanisms of plasma non-transferrin bound iron generation: insights from comparing transfused Diamond Blackfan anaemia with sickle cell and thalassaemia patients. Br J Haematol 2014;167(5):692–6.
21. Pak M, Lopez MA, Gabayan V, et al. Suppression of hepcidin during anemia requires erythropoietic activity. Blood 2006;108(12):3730–5.
22. Kautz L, Jung G, Valore EV, et al. Identification of erythroferrone as an erythroid regulator of iron metabolism. Nat Genet 2014;46(7):678–84.
23. Kautz L, Jung G, Du X, et al. Erythroferrone contributes to hepcidin suppression and iron overload in a mouse model of β-thalassemia. Blood 2015;126(17):2031–7.
24. Tanno T, Bhanu NV, Oneal PA, et al. High levels of GDF15 in thalassemia suppress expression of the iron regulatory protein hepcidin. Nat Med 2007;13(9):1096–101.
25. Tamary H, Shalev H, Perez-Avraham G, et al. Elevated growth differentiation factor 15 expression in patients with congenital dyserythropoietic anemia type I. Blood 2008;112(13):5241–4.
26. Casanovas G, Swinkels DW, Altamura S, et al. Growth differentiation factor 15 in patients with congenital dyserythropoietic anaemia (CDA) type II. J Mol Med 2011;89(8):811–6.
27. Henter J II, Karlén J. Fatal agranulocytosis after deferiprone therapy in a child with Diamond-Blackfan anemia. Blood 2007;109(12):5157–9.
28. Hoffbrand AV, Bartlett AN, Veys PA, et al. Agranulocytosis and thrombocytopenia in patient with Blackfan-Diamond anaemia during oral chelator trial. Lancet 1989;2(8660):457.
29. Flygare J, Olsson K, Richter J, et al. Gene therapy of Diamond Blackfan anemia CD34(+) cells leads to improved erythroid development and engraftment following transplantation. Exp Hematol 2008;36(11):1428–35.
30. Jaako P, Debnath S, Olsson K, et al. Gene therapy cures the anemia and lethal bone marrow failure in a mouse model of RPS19-deficient Diamond-Blackfan anemia. Haematologica 2014;99(12):1792–8.
31. Dever DP, Bak RO, Reinisch A, et al. CRISPR/Cas9 beta-globin gene targeting in human haematopoietic stem cells. Nature 2016;539(7629):384–9.
32. Cmejlova J, Dolezalova L, Pospisilova D, et al. Translational efficiency in patients with Diamond-Blackfan anemia. Haematologica 2006;91(11):1456–64.
33. Pospisilova D, Cmejlova J, Hak J, et al. Successful treatment of a Diamond-Blackfan anemia patient with amino acid leucine. Haematologica 2007;92(5):7.
34. Payne EM, Virgilio M, Narla A, et al. L-Leucine improves the anemia and developmental defects associated with Diamond-Blackfan anemia and del(5q) MDS by activating the mTOR pathway. Blood 2012;120(11):2214–24.
35. Jaako P, Debnath S, Olsson K, et al. Dietary L-leucine improves the anemia in a mouse model for Diamond-Blackfan anemia. Blood 2012;120(11):2225–8.
36. Gupta N, Wish JB. Hypoxia-inducible factor prolyl hydroxylase inhibitors: a potential new treatment for anemia in patients with CKD. Am J Kidney Dis 2017;69(6):815–26.

37. Lee HY, Gao X, Barrasa MI, et al. PPAR-alpha and glucocorticoid receptor synergize to promote erythroid progenitor self-renewal. Nature 2015;522(7557):474–7.

38. Doulatov S, Vo LT, Macari ER, et al. Drug discovery for Diamond-Blackfan anemia using reprogrammed hematopoietic progenitors. Sci Transl Med 2017;9(376) [pii: eaah5645].

39. Ge J, Apicella M, Mills JA, et al. Dysregulation of the transforming growth factor beta pathway in induced pluripotent stem cells generated from patients with Diamond Blackfan anemia. PLoS One 2015;10(8):e0134878.

40. Gao X, Lee HY, da Rocha EL, et al. TGF-beta inhibitors stimulate red blood cell production by enhancing self-renewal of BFU-E erythroid progenitors. Blood 2016;128(23):2637–41.

41. Ear J, Huang H, Wilson T, et al. RAP-011 improves erythropoiesis in zebrafish model of Diamond-Blackfan anemia through antagonizing lefty1. Blood 2015; 126(7):880–90.

42. Dussiot M, Maciel TT, Fricot A, et al. An activin receptor IIA ligand trap corrects ineffective erythropoiesis in beta-thalassemia. Nat Med 2014;20(4):398–407.

43. Ruckle J, Jacobs M, Kramer W, et al. Single-dose, randomized, double-blind, placebo-controlled study of ACE-011 (ActRIIA-IgG1) in postmenopausal women. J Bone Miner Res 2009;24(4):744–52.

44. Raftopoulos H, Laadem A, Hesketh PJ, et al. Sotatercept (ACE-011) for the treatment of chemotherapy-induced anemia in patients with metastatic breast cancer or advanced or metastatic solid tumors treated with platinum-based chemotherapeutic regimens: results from two phase 2 studies. Support Care Cancer 2016; 24(4):1517–25.

45. Li Q, Luo C, Luo C, et al. Disease-specific hematopoietic stem cell transplantation in children with inherited bone marrow failure syndromes. Ann Hematol 2017; 96(8):1389–97.

46. Burroughs LM, Shimamura A, Talano J-A, et al. Allogeneic hematopoietic cell transplantation using treosulfan-based conditioning for treatment of marrow failure disorders. Biol Blood Marrow Transpl 2017;23(10):1669–77.

47. Crazzolara R, Kropshofer G, Haas OA, et al. Reduced-intensity conditioning and stem cell transplantation in infants with Diamond Blackfan anemia. Haematologica 2016;102(3):e73–5.

48. Asquith JM, Copacia J, Mogul MJ, et al. Successful use of reduced-intensity conditioning and matched-unrelated hematopoietic stem cell transplant in a child with Diamond-Blackfan anemia and cirrhosis. Pediatr Transplant 2015;19(6): E157–9.

Germline *GATA2* Mutation and Bone Marrow Failure

Lisa J. McReynolds, MD, PhD[a],*, Katherine R. Calvo, MD, PhD[b],
Steven M. Holland, MD[c]

KEYWORDS

- GATA2 • Monocytopenia • Micromegakaryocytes • MDS

KEY POINTS

- GATA2 deficiency has variable clinical presentations including warts, mycobacterial infections, fungal infections, lymphedema, pulmonary alveolar proteinosis, aplastic anemia, myelodysplastic syndrome, or acute myeloid leukemia.
- Bone marrow histology in symptomatic GATA2 deficiency is hypocellular with characteristic abnormal megakaryocytes, separated nuclear lobes, micromegakaryocytes with hypolobated nuclei, loss of monocytes and hematogones, and an inverted CD4:CD8 ratio.
- Historical features that suggest underlying GATA2 deficiency include persistent warts, lymphedema, pulmonary alveolar proteinosis or disseminated, and/or unusual infections.
- Bone marrow transplantation can reverse the infectious, hematopoietic, and pulmonary complications. Without bone marrow transplantation, there is a significant risk of transformation.

INTRODUCTION

GATA2 encodes a zinc finger transcription factor necessary for normal hematopoiesis located on chromosome 3q21.2. The protein contains 2 zinc fingers and a nuclear localization signal. GATA2 binds to the consensus sequence W/GATA/R (W = A or T and R = A or G) in promoter/enhancer regions of target genes including *SPI1* (PU.1), *LMO2*, *TAL1*, *FLI1*, and *RUNX1* to regulate endothelial to hematopoietic transition in the early embryo, the formation of hematopoietic stem cells (HSCs) and definitive hematopoiesis.[1] In the adult, GATA2 is critical for maintenance of the stem cell

Disclosure Statement: None of the authors have any disclosures to report.
[a] Clinical Genetics Branch, Division of Cancer Epidemiology and Genetics, National Cancer Institute, National Institutes of Health, 9609 Medical Center Drive, Bethesda, MD 20892, USA;
[b] Hematology Section, Department of Laboratory Medicine, Clinical Center, National Institutes of Health, 9000 Rockville Pike, Bethesda, MD 20892, USA; [c] Laboratory of Clinical Immunology and Microbiology, National Institute of Allergy and Infectious Diseases, National Institutes of Health, 9000 Rockville Pike, Bethesda, MD 20892, USA
* Corresponding author.
E-mail address: lisa.mcreynolds@nih.gov

Hematol Oncol Clin N Am 32 (2018) 713–728
https://doi.org/10.1016/j.hoc.2018.04.004
0889-8588/18/Published by Elsevier Inc.

hemonc.theclinics.com

pool through HSC survival and self-renewal. GATA2 is also important for production of megakaryocytes, mast cells, natural killer (NK) cells and monocytes.[2]

In mice, $Gata2^{-/-}$ leads to embryonic lethality at embryonic day 9.5 owing to a lack of definitive hematopoiesis, whereas $Gata2^{+/-}$ mice have decreased progenitor cell numbers and reduced transplant repopulation.[3,4] The level of functional GATA2 protein is critical for HSC survival and normal hematopoiesis, as shown by conditional $Gata2$ mouse models.[5]

Pathogenic germline variants in $GATA2$ affect exons and critical regulatory intronic regions of the gene, as well as deletions. Several groups described constellations of symptoms, each giving them different names: MonoMAC[6,7]; familial myelodysplastic syndrome (MDS)/acute myeloid leukemia (AML)[8]; DCML deficiency (dendritic cell, monocyte, B, and NK lymphoid deficiency)[9]; and Emberger syndrome (MDS with lymphedema).[10] In 2011, it was recognized that underlying all of these autosomal-dominant disorders were heterozygous germline mutations in $GATA2$, hence, this syndrome is best referred to as GATA2 deficiency.

Germline pathogenic variants include deletions, missense, nonsense, frameshift, and splice site changes and alterations of intronic regulatory elements. Mechanistically, all variants seem to lead to haploinsufficiency.[11] Most pathogenic variants cluster in the 2 zinc fingers, leading to a nonfunctional protein unable to bind DNA or other transcription factor partners.[12,13] Whole or partial gene deletions produce haploinsufficiency by hemizygosity.[14] Mutations in the intron 5 enhancer lead to reduced transcription of the cis allele.[15] Frameshift mutations lead to nonsense mediated decay, premature stop codons, or splice site alterations.[2]

Since gene identification in 2011, the number of cases identified has increased steadily, with associated phenotypic expansion. We briefly review the clinical manifestations with a focus on the bone marrow failure aspects, discuss management, and bone marrow transplantation.

CLINICAL MANIFESTATIONS
Hematologic

Patients molecularly diagnosed with germline $GATA2$ mutations at birth, owing to an affected family member, are immunologically and hematologically normal. Over time, the majority evolve cytopenias, including deficiencies in monocytes, B-lymphocytes, dendritic cells, and NK cells. However, there is significant variability in this presentation (**Box 1**). Profound monocytopenia is one of the most consistent features, but only later in the development of disease. Unlike other marrow failure syndromes, anemia and thrombocytopenia are uncommon early presentations, except in those patients who present with aplastic anemia (AA), MDS, or AML. Lymphocyte subset evaluation may identify B and NK cell cytopenias. Pediatric MDS with germline $GATA2$ mutation can present without recognized immunodeficiency.[16,17]

Bone marrow is typically hypocellular (**Fig. 1A**) with characteristic features, including atypical megakaryocytes, ranging from large abnormal forms with separated nuclear lobes (osteoclast-like), to smaller forms with separated nuclear lobes, micromegakaryocytes, to small hypolobated or mononuclear megakaryocytes[18] (**Fig. 1B–E**). In some cases, the marrow is very hypocellular with very few megakaryocytes. Immunohistochemistry for CD61 performed on core biopsies may help to identify megakaryocytic atypia (see **Fig. 1E**); immunohistochemistry for CD34 can help to identify increased blasts (**Fig. 1L**). Patients with disseminated nontuberculous mycobacterial infections (NTM) may have granulomata in the marrow with mycobacteria. Review of aspirate smears is critical for assessing progression to MDS, which can be subtle or hindered

---

Box 1
Diagnostic clues

Medical history/physical examination

Human papilloma virus—persistent warts

Nontuberculous mycobacterial infection, disseminated

Aspergillosis

Lymphedema

Hearing loss

Panniculitis

Erythema nodosum

Thrombosis

Miscarriage/preterm labor

Epstein–Barr virus viremia

Peripheral blood

Monocytopenia

Dendritic cell cytopenia

Natural killer cell cytopenia

B-Cell cytopenia

Neutropenia

Bone marrow

Hypocellular for age

Megakaryocytic atypia/dysplasia: large megakaryocytes with separated nuclear lobes, monolobated megakaryocytes, micromegakaryocytes

BM Flow cytometry: Marked decrease to absence of monocytes, B-cell precursors, B-cells, dendritic cells, NK-cells; inverted CD4:CD8 ratio

Radiologic

Crazy paving on chest computed tomography scanning

Subpleural blebs

Paraseptal emphysema

Ground glass opacities

Splenomegaly

---

by paucicellular specimens. GATA2 deficiency-associated hypocellular MDS may display multilineage dysplastic changes (**Fig. 1**F–H) involving erythroid precursors (nuclear budding, binucleation, megaloblastic changes), myeloid precursors (nuclear hyposegmentation, hypogranularity, nuclear to cytoplasmic maturation asynchrony), and markedly dysplastic megakaryocytes.

Bone marrow flow cytometry often shows hypogranular granulocytes, absent monocytes and hematogones (B cells progenitors), reduced mature B cells, and NK cells and inverted CD4:CD8 ratios with relatively increased CD57[+] T cells (**Fig. 2**). Absent hematogones, inverted CD4:CD8 ratio with monocytopenia, NK cell cytopenia, and B-cell cytopenia differentiate GATA2 deficiency from idiopathic AA.[19] In pediatric patients with MDS, a lack of B cells and B-cell progenitors predicts GATA2

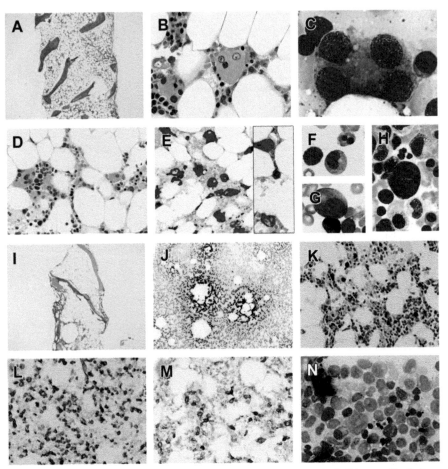

Fig. 1. The range of bone marrow pathologies seen in GATA2 deficiency. (*A–C*) Bone marrow and immunodeficiency disorder with germline *GATA2* mutation. (*A*) Hypocellular marrow for age (late adolescent patient with history of warts and infections) with characteristic atypical megakaryocytes with separated nuclear lobes present on (*B*) core biopsy and (*C*) aspirate. No overt morphologic dysplastic changes are present in myeloid and erythroid precursors. Cytogenetic analysis showed a normal karyotype. A complete blood count (CBC) with differential and peripheral blood flow cytometric analysis revealed severe monocytopenia, B/natural killer (NK)-cell lymphopenia. (*D–H*) Myelodysplastic syndrome with multilineage dysplasia and germline *GATA2* mutation. The bone marrow is hypocellular for age (young adult in third decade) with (*D*) increased atypical megakaryocytes with separated nuclear lobes, hypolobated and mononuclear forms. (*E*) Megakaryocytes are highlighted by immunohistochemistry stain for CD61 (*E*, inset small positive cell in center) revealing micromegakaryocytes. Aspirate smear shows (*F*) dyserythropoiesis with nuclear budding and (*H*) binucleation; myeloid maturation asynchrony with (*G*) nuclear hyposegmentation and (*H*) hypogranular myeloid cells. Cytogenetic analysis showed monosomy 7. A CBC with differential and peripheral blood flow cytometric analysis revealed moderate pancytopenia with severe monocytopenia, and B/NK-cell lymphopenia. (*I, J*) Aplastic anemia, with unrecognized germline *GATA2* mutation at diagnosis. The bone marrow is markedly hypocellular with trilineage hypoplasia. The aspirate is paucicellular with insufficient cells to evaluate for dysplastic changes. Cytogenetic analysis failed owing to poor mitotic index. Bone marrow flow cytometry analysis was not performed. The patient later evolved to

deficiency.[17] Decreased or absent intron RSS-Kde recombination excision circles are also common in pediatric MDS owing to GATA2 deficiency.[17] Within the bone marrow compartment, there is a loss of CD34$^+$, CD38 multilymphoid or lymphoid-primed multipotent progenitors and depletion of CD38$^+$ granulocytic monocytic progenitors.[2] Increased serum FLT3 ligand tracks with worsening of bone marrow failure and clinical disease in patients with GATA2 deficiency.[20]

Because GATA2 deficiency can present as AA (**Figs. 1I, J and 2**), it is critical to differentiate it from idiopathic AA.[21] One report identified 5 patients who presented with AA who had *GATA2* regulatory region mutations.[22] Mild chronic neutropenia with monocytopenia can also be a presentation of GATA2 deficiency, 10 such patients were found in a French registry of patients with severe congenital neutropenia.[23]

Hematopoietic malignancies

GATA2 deficiency predisposes to leukemia: an original description was familial AML.[8,24,25] Myeloid neoplasms of any type eventually develop in up to 75% of patients.[26] The average age of onset for myeloid neoplasms varies, depending on the cohort studied, but overall has been shown to be 12 to 35 years old with a median age of 19.7 years.[27] However, myeloid neoplasms owing to this germline predisposition can develop into late adulthood, as late as the eighth decade has been reported and should be recognized.[26] The development of myeloid neoplasms is remarkably inconsistent within families. The underlying biology of these differences is not understood.[28]

MDS is very common in GATA2 deficiency, often accompanied by cytogenetic changes, most commonly monosomy 7 (41% of cases), trisomy 8 (15%), and trisomy 1q.[7,19,29] Interestingly, del5q has not been reported in GATA2 deficiency, nor have ringed sideroblasts. One study found 7% of primary pediatric MDS and 15% of children with advanced MDS to have GATA2 deficiency. Of those with pediatric MDS and monosomy 7, there were 37% with germline *GATA2* mutations; in adolescents with MDS plus monosomy 7, there were 72% with underlying germline GATA2 mutations, suggesting that GATA2 deficiency may be the most common genetic defect predisposing to pediatric MDS.[16] Therefore, it is critical for all pediatric patients with MDS and all patients with AML with a somatic *GATA2* mutation to be screened for germline mutations.[16,30]

The mechanisms behind the development of MDS in GATA2 deficiency are only partially understood. It is hypothesized that the combination of HSC loss, bone marrow stress, and clonal evolution drive the development of dysplasia and transformation to leukemia (**Fig. 3**).[27,31,32] Bone marrow stress occurs owing the progressive cytopenias and recurrent infections.[33] Clonal evolution can occur through

---

myelodysplastic syndrome (MDS) and a *GATA2* mutation was identified. (*K–N*) Acute myeloid leukemia with myelodysplasia related changes and germline *GATA2* mutation. (*K*) Hypocellular marrow from a man (early third decade) previously diagnosed with aplastic anemia that had evolved to MDS with monosomy 7. Marrow shows background hemosiderin laden macrophages from red cell transfusions. (*L*) Immunohistochemistry stain for CD34 reveals (*M*) numerous CD34 positive blasts that are also positive for CD117. (*N*) Aspirate smear showed increased blasts (35% on differential count) indicative of progression to acute myeloid leukemia. Cytogenetic analysis showed monosomy 7. The stain and magnification for *A* (Hematoxylin and eosin [H&E], original magnification ×40); *B* (H&E, original magnification ×1000); *C* (WG, original magnification ×1000 [cropped]); *D* (H&E, original magnification ×500); *E* (CD61 IHC, original magnification ×500); *F* (WG, original magnification ×1000 [cropped]); *G* (WG, original magnification ×1000 [cropped]); *H* (WG, original magnification ×1000 [cropped]); *I* (H&E, original magnification ×40); *J* (WG, original magnification ×40); *K* (H&E, original magnification ×500); *L* (CD34 IHC, original magnification ×500); *M* (CD117 IHC, original magnification ×500); *N* (WG, original magnification ×1000).

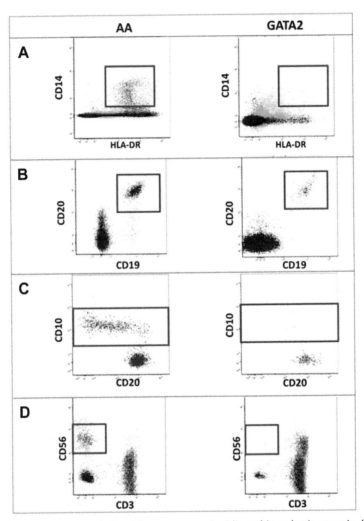

Fig. 2. Flow cytometry analysis of bone marrow in idiopathic aplastic anemia (AA) and GATA2 deficiency. (*A*) Monocytic cells, designated by positivity for CD14 and HLA-DR (within *red box*) are typically present in the bone marrow of AA and disproportionately decreased to absent in GATA2 deficiency; all nucleated cells in the marrow are gated. (*B*) Mature B-cells, marked by positivity for CD19 and CD20 (within *red box*), are typically present in AA and reduced to absent in GATA2 deficiency; lymphocytes in the marrow are gated. (*C*) B-cell precursors (hematogones; within *red box*) are often reduced but detectable in AA, but in GATA2 deficiency there is an absence of B-cell precursors. CD19+ cells in the bone marrow are gated; the cells outside of the red box are mature B-cells, which are CD20+ and CD10-. (*D*) Natural killer cells, positive for CD56 and negative for CD3, are present in AA and are often absent in GATA2 deficiency; the bone marrow lymphocyte gate is displayed.

development of cytogenetic clones and progression to MDS/AML (**Fig. 1**K–N). The most common gene with somatic mutation in hematopoietic clones is *ASXL1*, found in 29% in one series.[34] Wang and colleagues[35] identified *ASXL1* mutations in 2 of 6 patients screened within 3 families. Bodor and colleagues[24] identified a family with a pair of siblings with a *GATA2* mutation, one with a concurrent *ASXL1* mutation

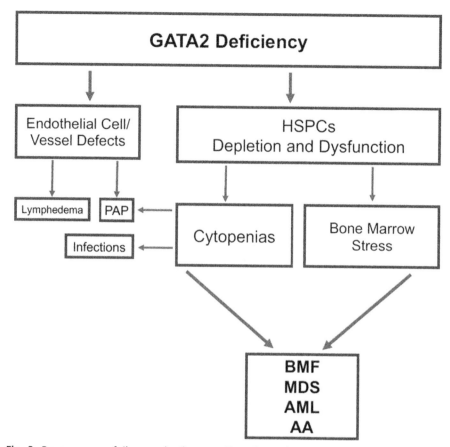

Fig. 3. Bone marrow failure and other manifestations of GATA2 deficiency. GATA2 deficiency syndrome is caused by gene mutations in both the exonic and intronic regulatory regions of the gene leading to haploinsufficiency. Loss of GATA2 protein leads to hematopoietic stem and progenitor cell (HSPC) loss and dysfunction. This depletion leads to a combination of cytopenias—B cells, dendritic cells, natural killer cells, and monocytes. The resultant immunodeficiency drives infections such as human papilloma virus and nontuberculous mycobacterial infections, and pulmonary alveolar proteinosis (PAP). Overall, these factors lead to bone marrow stress, hypocellularity and the ultimate development of bone marrow failure (BMF), aplastic anemia (AA) myelodysplastic syndrome (MDS), and acute myeloid leukemia (AML).

and MDS and the other without either. Acquisition of *ASXL1* mutations may cooperate with germline *GATA2* mutations to drive the hypoplastic bone marrow to a proleukemic hyperplastic state.[36]

Other somatic mutations have also been reported. In the families described by Wang and colleagues,[35] 2 members had *NRAS* mutations, and others had mutations in *RUNX1*, *TP53*, *STAG2*, and *SETBP1*. Ding and colleagues[37] described a father–son pair, both of whom had *STAG2* mutations, but in different genomic locations. Fujiwara and colleagues[38] described a patient who progressed to MDS/AML with somatic mutations in *EZH2*, *HECW1* and *GATA1*. Loyola and colleagues[39] screened 60 GATA2 deficiency patients with MDS and found recurrent mutations in *SETBP1*, *ASXL1*, *STAG2*, *RUNX1*, *CBL*, *EZH2*, *NRAS*, *JAK3*, and *PTPN11*. Fisher and colleagues[40] described 2 pediatric patients with GATA2 deficiency MDS, one with *RUNX1, SETBP1*, and *IKZF1* somatic mutations, and the other with a *CRLF2* mutation.

MDS and AML are the best described myeloid neoplasms in GATA2 deficiency. However, chronic myelomonocytic leukemia in GATA2 deficiency has been associated with monocytosis and often have *ASXL1* somatic mutations.[27,29,34]

A single case of pre–B-cell acute lymphoblastic leukemia occurred in an adolescent girl who developed disseminated *Mycobacterium kansasii* after chemotherapy.[41] She also had other features of GATA2 deficiency, including warts as a young child, megakaryocyte dysplasia, monosomy 7, disseminated fungal disease, pulmonary alveolar proteinosis (PAP), and long-standing monocytopenia.

GATA2 plays an important role in germline predisposition to AML, but also in de novo AML, when *GATA2* is somatically altered. A unique mechanism is involved in the pathogenesis of inv(3) AML, which repositions a *GATA2* binding element upstream of *EVI1*, an oncogene, increasing *EVI1* expression and decreasing *GATA2* expression, thus creating somatic haploinsufficiency within the leukemic blasts.[42,43] Epigenetic alterations also lead to decreased *GATA2* expression in normal karyotype AML.[44] GATA2 levels are tightly regulated throughout hematopoiesis, and dysregulation of the level of GATA2 promotes stem cell loss, dysfunction, and leukemogenesis.

Immunologic

Much of the immune dysregulation in GATA2 deficiency is attributed to cytopenias and the underlying loss of stem cells.[45] However, quantitative cytopenia does not fully explain the breadth of immune dysregulation seen. Low numbers and dysfunction of NK cells is a key feature of GATA2 deficiency. GATA2 is required for normal and complete maturation of NK cells, maintenance of the CD56[bright] population, and full cytotoxicity.[46] Schlums and colleagues[47] found that GATA2 deficiency leads to loss of NK cell progenitors, thus decreasing canonical NK cell differentiation. Adaptive NK cells may persist in GATA2-deficient patients, even after these patients have lost their canonical NK cells. The remaining NK cells have decreased CXCL12/CXCR4-dependent chemotaxis, and the B cells have increased CXCL12-induced chemotaxis.[48] Ruiz-Garcia and associates[49] studied 4 patients and showed that those with worse clinical phenotype had increased T-cell senescence.

GATA2-deficient patients also get panniculitis, erythema nodosum, and arthritis. Autoimmune hepatitis in GATA2 deficiency has been reported.[50] It is important to keep the infection predisposition in mind, because erythema nodosum is more common in patients with active mycobacterial disease. There may also be a T-regulatory cell, dendritic cell, and CD38⁻CD21⁻ B-cell deficiency.[2] These autoimmune complaints may present initially to rheumatologists.[51] Hypogammaglobulinemia clinically consistent with common variable immunodeficiency also occurs.[52]

Infectious

NTM infections were found in up to in 53% of patients in 1 study,[29] often disseminated and difficult to control, owing to slow (*Mycobacterium avium* complex, *M kansasii*, and *M szulgai*) and rapid growing (*M fortuitum*, *M abscessus*, and *M chelonae*) organisms.[29,53,54] *M kansasii* can cause a characteristic necrotizing mediastinal lymphadenitis.[55] Disseminated NTM disease correlates with cytopenias in adolescents or young adults; it is uncommon in childhood when the cell numbers are intact. Smoking may increase the risk for the dissemination of NTM in the setting of already compromised alveolar macrophage function.[55]

Other severe bacterial infections include *Clostridium difficile* and group *C* streptococcal infections.[29] One case of *Pneumocystis jiroveci* pneumonia was reported.[56]

Approximately 16% of patients had fungal infections including aspergillosis, disseminated histoplasmosis, and candidiasis.[29]

Human papilloma virus (HPV) infections occur in two-thirds as recalcitrant warts, condylomata, and/or cervical dysplasia. Persistent warts in a patient with cytopenias or bone marrow failure suggests GATA2 deficiency.

Epstein–Barr virus (EBV) viremia was found in 11% of patients in 1 study,[29] including a variety of EBV-associated pathologies such as mononucleosis, chronic active EBV, hydroa vacciniforme-like lymphoma with hemophagocytic lymphohistiocytosis, and smooth muscle cell tumors.[57] EBV-associated spindle cell tumor and demyelinating sensorimotor polyradiculoneuropathy have been reported.[58,59] Severe disseminated herpes simplex infections are also important to watch for, because they can lead to dire complications.[60,61] Overall, approximately 80% of patients will have infectious complications of their disease leading to significant morbidity and mortality.

Dermatologic

Warts are seen on extremities and genitalia (common or flat type) in about 50% of patients and are difficult to treat.[62,63] Neutrophilic pustulosis (Sweet syndrome) can be seen in patients who go on to develop MDS or AML. Panniculitis, erythema nodosum, and cellulitis have also been described.[64]

Vascular

Kazenwadel and colleagues[65] showed that GATA2 is expressed in lymphatic vessels and is a critical regulator of development of lymphatic vessel valves. Patients with gene deletions and stop codons seem to be at especially increased risk of lymphedema. Lymphedema, particularly in an adolescent or young adult with cytopenias, suggests GATA2 deficiency. GATA2 is also expressed in the vascular epithelium and platelets, and thrombosis occurs in a significant number of patients. The risk for thrombosis is likely multifactorial, because GATA2-deficient patients often have other risk factors, including infection and malignancy. Maternal-related preterm labor has been observed, as well as frequent miscarriage.

Pulmonary

PAP is a common and life-threatening complication of GATA2 deficiency caused by the overaccumulation of surfactant in alveoli impairing gas exchange. It is typically suspected on computed tomography scan and confirmed on PAS staining or electron microscopy of bronchoalveolar lavage specimens.[66] PAP in GATA2 deficiency is likely owing to alveolar macrophage dysfunction, in part from abnormal granulocyte macrophage colony stimulating factor-related signaling. Griese and colleagues[67] identified 2 patients with GATA2 deficiency in a cohort of patients with negative granulocyte macrophage colony stimulating factor autoantibody PAP. Svobodova and colleagues[68] identified a GATA2-deficient patient who presented with persistent diffuse parenchymal lung disease in childhood. Pulmonary hypertension has been seen in GATA2 deficiency, both before and after the development of severe PAP.[69,70] Subpleural and paraseptal emphysematous changes in the lung may be seen long before overt clinical manifestations.

Eye and Ear

Congenital deafness has been observed in GATA2 deficiency, probably more often in those with gene deletions or stop codon mutations. Using conditional mouse models, Haugas and colleagues[71] showed that GATA2 is required for proliferation of the epithelium in the semicircular duct and for clearance of mesenchymal cells to generate the vestibular perilymphatic space. Berry and Fekrat[72] reported a case of central retinal vein occlusion in GATA2 deficiency, which may have represented underlying hypercoagulability owing to cellular or vascular defects.

Oncologic: Solid Tumors

A variety of solid malignancies have been reported, most related to HPV infection, such as genital dysplasias and invasive squamous cell carcinomas. HPV-associated head and neck squamous cell carcinoma have also been seen.[20,29] EBV-related tumors, such as leiomyosarcomas occur. Crall and colleagues[73] reported a case of Merkel cell carcinoma in an adult with both GATA2 deficiency and neurofibromatosis type 1. Last, in the National Institutes of Health cohort, there is significant frequency of breast cancer in (approximately 20% in women older than 35 years of age), for unclear reasons.[29]

Hematopoietic Stem/Progenitor Cell Transplantation

Hematopoietic stem/progenitor cell transplantation (HSCT) is highly effective in the treatment of GATA2 deficiency. HSCT restores normal hematopoiesis, resolves MDS, clears long-standing underlying infections, and resolves PAP and pulmonary hypertension in patients with GATA2 deficiency.[74] The optimal timing of transplantation is unclear. Our institutional strategy has been to proceed with transplant when cytopenias are present, if life-threatening infections have occurred, or if PAP or other significant organ dysfunction develops. However, the disease course is often difficult to predict, and patients may be diagnosed only in the later stages of the disease.

The best choices for preparative regimen, donor source and graft-versus-host disease (GVHD) prophylaxis are areas of current investigation. Cuellar-Rodriguez and colleagues[74] reported successful transplantation for GATA2 deficiency in 6 patients. Since that time, multiple other groups have reported good outcomes with HSCT for GATA2 deficiency. Both myeloablative and reduced intensity preparative regimens have been successful. Matched related and unrelated peripheral blood stem cells, matched and haploidentical bone marrows, and umbilical cord grafts have all been reported.

Ciullini Mannurita and colleagues[75] reported a young patient who received a transplant from his matched brother using an ablative regimen. Ramzan and colleagues[76] reported a very young patient with Emberger syndrome and MDS who underwent successful myeloablative HSCT with resolution of MDS. Lubking and colleagues[77] described an adult with MDS and *ASXL1* somatic mutation who underwent successful HSCT from an unrelated peripheral blood stem cell donor with resolution of MDS and condylomata. Maeurer and colleagues[78] described a young adult with severe disseminated HPV skin disease treated with matched related HSCT. After HSCT, her condylomata disappeared and her cervical cancer in situ resolved. These authors suggested preharvest donor HPV vaccination if not previously vaccinated. Mallhi and colleagues[79] reported 2 pediatric cases of HSCT using cord blood; the first patient had AML with MDS-related changes and received a myeloablative regimen and the other had MDS and received reduced intensity conditioning. Saida and colleagues[80] reported a pediatric patient with successful reduced intensity HSCT.

Following up Cuellar-Rodriguez and colleagues, Grossman and colleagues[81] reported 8 more patients (a total of 14) from an open HSCT trial specifically for GATA2 deficiency. This group included both matched and haploidentical donors. The authors currently use a myeloablative regimen to improve engraftment and reduce the risk of relapse, beyond what was seen in the prior cohort.

GVHD has been seen in GATA2 HSCT at typical or increased rates, but different prophylaxis regimens make it difficult to generalize rates. Shah and colleagues[82] reported a pair of monozygotic twins who both underwent HSCT for GATA2 deficiency from the same donor with the same conditioning regimen one twin developed severe acute GVHD of the skin and gastrointestinal tract requiring immunosuppression for 1.5 years, the other twin only had grade 1 GVHD of skin not requiring systemic corticosteroids. This unique report highlights the nonheritable factors affecting GVHD outcomes. It is hypothesized that prior and peritransplant exposures, especially infectious, may contribute to such differences.

PATIENT MONITORING AND SCREENING

Currently, there are no guidelines for patient care and monitoring. However, expert opinion in the literature and our practice are given in **Box 2**. Once a *GATA2* mutation has been identified and cytopenias of any degree are noted we start daily azithromycin prophylaxis for NTM. HPV vaccination should be given on the full schedule, as well as other childhood vaccines. We have not seen problems with live virus vaccines in children with normal counts or marrows. BCG vaccination has also not been a problem in GATA2 deficiency as long as counts are normal. Baseline bone marrow aspiration, biopsy, and cytogenetics should be performed. We follow at least biannual complete blood count with differential, and yearly lymphocyte subset evaluation, bone marrow biopsy and aspiration, pulmonary function testing, comprehensive skin examinations, and, for females, gynecologic examinations. Good oral hygiene and regular dental visits are recommended, especially for surveillance for HPV-related oral disease. If MDS develops, prompt referral to an HSCT team with disease specific knowledge is advisable. Likewise, if a patient with GATA2 deficiency develops AA, prompt HSCT is advisable because immunosuppressive therapy seems to increase risk and delays definitive treatment.

Overall, HSCT is the only curative option for patients with GATA2 deficiency; gene therapy is unlikely to be available any time soon. Screening of potential donor family members for *GATA2* mutation, in addition to HLA typing, is absolutely essential, given the wide variation in GATA2 deficiency phenotype and age at presentation. Although the timing of transplantation is hard to precisely prescribe, the consequences of waiting until after major infections, organ dysfunction or malignancy develop are dire and baleful.

Box 2
Screening recommendations

Twice yearly complete blood count with differential

Yearly lymphocyte subset evaluation—monitor monocyte loss or outgrowth

Yearly bone marrow biopsy and aspiration with mycobacterial culture, flow cytometry and cytogenetics; consider somatic mutation panel testing

Yearly pulmonary function testing

Yearly comprehensive skin examination

Yearly gynecologic examination

Recommendations for testing and frequency listed herein are only based on expert opinion and are not evidence based at this time.

REFERENCES

1. Crispino JD, Horwitz MS. GATA factor mutations in hematologic disease. Blood 2017;129(15):2103–10.
2. Collin M, Dickinson R, Bigley V. Haematopoietic and immune defects associated with GATA2 mutation. Br J Haematol 2015;169(2):173–87.
3. Tsai FY, Keller G, Kuo FC, et al. An early haematopoietic defect in mice lacking the transcription factor GATA-2. Nature 1994;371(6494):221–6.
4. Rodrigues NP, Janzen V, Forkert R, et al. Haploinsufficiency of GATA-2 perturbs adult hematopoietic stem-cell homeostasis. Blood 2005;106(2):477–84.
5. Lim KC, Hosoya T, Brandt W, et al. Conditional Gata2 inactivation results in HSC loss and lymphatic mispatterning. J Clin Invest 2012;122(10):3705–17.
6. Hsu AP, Sampaio EP, Khan J, et al. Mutations in GATA2 are associated with the autosomal dominant and sporadic monocytopenia and mycobacterial infection (MonoMAC) syndrome. Blood 2011;118(10):2653–5.
7. Vinh DC, Patel SY, Uzel G, et al. Autosomal dominant and sporadic monocytopenia with susceptibility to mycobacteria, fungi, papillomaviruses, and myelodysplasia. Blood 2010;115(8):1519–29.
8. Hahn CN, Chong CE, Carmichael CL, et al. Heritable GATA2 mutations associated with familial myelodysplastic syndrome and acute myeloid leukemia. Nat Genet 2011;43(10):1012–7.
9. Bigley V, Haniffa M, Doulatov S, et al. The human syndrome of dendritic cell, monocyte, B and NK lymphoid deficiency. J Exp Med 2011;208(2):227–34.
10. Ostergaard P, Simpson MA, Connell FC, et al. Mutations in GATA2 cause primary lymphedema associated with a predisposition to acute myeloid leukemia (Emberger syndrome). Nat Genet 2011;43(10):929–31.
11. Hsu AP, Johnson KD, Falcone EL, et al. GATA2 haploinsufficiency caused by mutations in a conserved intronic element leads to MonoMAC syndrome. Blood 2013;121(19):3830–7, s1–7.
12. Chong CE, Venugopal P, Stokes PH, et al. Differential effects on gene transcription and hematopoietic differentiation correlate with GATA2 mutant disease phenotypes. Leukemia 2018;32(1):194–202.
13. Cortes-Lavaud X, Landecho MF, Maicas M, et al. GATA2 germline mutations impair GATA2 transcription, causing haploinsufficiency: functional analysis of the p.Arg396Gln mutation. J Immunol 2015;194(5):2190–8.
14. Dorn JM, Patnaik MS, Van Hee M, et al. WILD syndrome is GATA2 deficiency: a novel deletion in the GATA2 gene. J Allergy Clin Immunol Pract 2017;5(4):1149–52.e1.
15. Johnson KD, Hsu AP, Ryu MJ, et al. Cis-element mutated in GATA2-dependent immunodeficiency governs hematopoiesis and vascular integrity. J Clin Invest 2012;122(10):3692–704.
16. Wlodarski MW, Hirabayashi S, Pastor V, et al. Prevalence, clinical characteristics, and prognosis of GATA2-related myelodysplastic syndromes in children and adolescents. Blood 2016;127(11):1387–97 [quiz: 1518].
17. Novakova M, Zaliova M, Sukova M, et al. Loss of B cells and their precursors is the most constant feature of GATA-2 deficiency in childhood myelodysplastic syndrome. Haematologica 2016;101(6):707–16.
18. Calvo KR, Vinh DC, Maric I, et al. Myelodysplasia in autosomal dominant and sporadic monocytopenia immunodeficiency syndrome: diagnostic features and clinical implications. Haematologica 2011;96(8):1221–5.

19. Ganapathi KA, Townsley DM, Hsu AP, et al. GATA2 deficiency-associated bone marrow disorder differs from idiopathic aplastic anemia. Blood 2015;125(1): 56–70.
20. Dickinson RE, Milne P, Jardine L, et al. The evolution of cellular deficiency in GATA2 mutation. Blood 2014;123(6):863–74.
21. Calvo KR, Hickstein DD, Holland SM. MonoMAC and GATA2 deficiency: overlapping clinical and pathological features with aplastic anemia and idiopathic CD4+ lymphocytopenia. Haematologica 2012;97(4):e12–3.
22. Townsley DMHA, Dumitriu B, Holland SM, et al. Regulatory mutations in GATA2 associated with aplastic anemia. Blood 2014;120(21):3488.
23. Pasquet M, Bellanne-Chantelot C, Tavitian S, et al. High frequency of GATA2 mutations in patients with mild chronic neutropenia evolving to MonoMac syndrome, myelodysplasia, and acute myeloid leukemia. Blood 2013;121(5):822–9.
24. Bodor C, Renneville A, Smith M, et al. Germ-line GATA2 p.THR354MET mutation in familial myelodysplastic syndrome with acquired monosomy 7 and ASXL1 mutation demonstrating rapid onset and poor survival. Haematologica 2012;97(6): 890–4.
25. Hyde RK, Liu PP. GATA2 mutations lead to MDS and AML. Nat Genet 2011; 43(10):926–7.
26. Wlodarski MW, Collin M, Horwitz MS. GATA2 deficiency and related myeloid neoplasms. Semin Hematol 2017;54(2):81–6.
27. Hirabayashi S, Wlodarski MW, Kozyra E, et al. Heterogeneity of GATA2-related myeloid neoplasms. Int J Hematol 2017;106(2):175–82.
28. Brambila-Tapia AJL, Garcia-Ortiz JE, Brouillard P, et al. GATA2 null mutation associated with incomplete penetrance in a family with Emberger syndrome. Hematology 2017;22(8):467–71.
29. Spinner MA, Sanchez LA, Hsu AP, et al. GATA2 deficiency: a protean disorder of hematopoiesis, lymphatics, and immunity. Blood 2014;123(6):809–21.
30. Stieglitz E, Loh ML. Pediatric MDS: GATA screen the germline. Blood 2016; 127(11):1377–8.
31. Hsu AP, McReynolds LJ, Holland SM. GATA2 deficiency. Curr Opin Allergy Clin Immunol 2015;15(1):104–9.
32. Rodrigues NP, Tipping AJ, Wang Z, et al. GATA-2 mediated regulation of normal hematopoietic stem/progenitor cell function, myelodysplasia and myeloid leukemia. Int J Biochem Cell Biol 2012;44(3):457–60.
33. Matatall KA, Jeong M, Chen S, et al. Chronic infection depletes hematopoietic stem cells through stress-induced terminal differentiation. Cell Rep 2016; 17(10):2584–95.
34. West RR, Hsu AP, Holland SM, et al. Acquired ASXL1 mutations are common in patients with inherited GATA2 mutations and correlate with myeloid transformation. Haematologica 2014;99(2):276–81.
35. Wang X, Muramatsu H, Okuno Y, et al. GATA2 and secondary mutations in familial myelodysplastic syndromes and pediatric myeloid malignancies. Haematologica 2015;100(10):e398–401.
36. Micol JB, Abdel-Wahab O. Collaborating constitutive and somatic genetic events in myeloid malignancies: ASXL1 mutations in patients with germline GATA2 mutations. Haematologica 2014;99(2):201–3.
37. Ding LW, Ikezoe T, Tan KT, et al. Mutational profiling of a MonoMAC syndrome family with GATA2 deficiency. Leukemia 2017;31(1):244–5.

38. Fujiwara T, Fukuhara N, Funayama R, et al. Identification of acquired mutations by whole-genome sequencing in GATA-2 deficiency evolving into myelodysplasia and acute leukemia. Ann Hematol 2014;93(9):1515–22.

39. Pastor Loyola VB, Hirabayashi S, Pohl S, et al. Somatic genetic and epigenetic architecture of myelodysplastic syndromes arising from GATA2 deficiency. American Society of Hematology Meeting Abstracts 2015;126(23):299.

40. Fisher KE, Hsu AP, Williams CL, et al. Somatic mutations in children with GATA2-associated myelodysplastic syndrome who lack other features of GATA2 deficiency. Blood Adv 2017;1(7):443–8.

41. Koegel AK, Hofmann I, Moffitt K, et al. Acute lymphoblastic leukemia in a patient with MonoMAC syndrome/GATA2 haploinsufficiency. Pediatr Blood Cancer 2016; 63(10):1844–7.

42. Groschel S, Sanders MA, Hoogenboezem R, et al. A single oncogenic enhancer rearrangement causes concomitant EVI1 and GATA2 deregulation in leukemia. Cell 2014;157(2):369–81.

43. Yamazaki H, Suzuki M, Otsuki A, et al. A remote GATA2 hematopoietic enhancer drives leukemogenesis in inv(3)(q21;q26) by activating EVI1 expression. Cancer Cell 2014;25(4):415–27.

44. Celton M, Forest A, Gosse G, et al. Epigenetic regulation of GATA2 and its impact on normal karyotype acute myeloid leukemia. Leukemia 2014;28(8):1617–26.

45. Dotta L, Badolato R. Primary immunodeficiencies appearing as combined lymphopenia, neutropenia, and monocytopenia. Immunol Lett 2014;161(2):222–5.

46. Mace EM, Hsu AP, Monaco-Shawver L, et al. Mutations in GATA2 cause human NK cell deficiency with specific loss of the CD56(bright) subset. Blood 2013; 121(14):2669–77.

47. Schlums H, Jung M, Han H, et al. Adaptive NK cells can persist in patients with GATA2 mutation depleted of stem and progenitor cells. Blood 2017;129(14): 1927–39.

48. Maciejewski-Duval A, Meuris F, Bignon A, et al. Altered chemotactic response to CXCL12 in patients carrying GATA2 mutations. J Leukoc Biol 2016;99(6): 1065–76.

49. Ruiz-Garcia R, Rodriguez-Vigil C, Marco FM, et al. Acquired senescent T-Cell phenotype correlates with clinical severity in GATA binding protein 2-deficient patients. Front Immunol 2017;8:802.

50. Webb G, Chen YY, Li KK, et al. Single-gene association between GATA-2 and autoimmune hepatitis: a novel genetic insight highlighting immunologic pathways to disease. J Hepatol 2016;64(5):1190–3.

51. Johnson JA, Yu SS, Elist M, et al. Rheumatologic manifestations of the "Mono-MAC" syndrome. a systematic review. Clin Rheumatol 2015;34(9):1643–5.

52. Chou J, Lutskiy M, Tsitsikov E, et al. Presence of hypogammaglobulinemia and abnormal antibody responses in GATA2 deficiency. J Allergy Clin Immunol 2014;134(1):223–6.

53. Vila A, Dapas JI, Rivero CV, et al. Multiple opportunistic infections in a woman with GATA2 mutation. Int J Infect Dis 2017;54:89–91.

54. Camargo JF, Lobo SA, Hsu AP, et al. MonoMAC syndrome in a patient with a GATA2 mutation: case report and review of the literature. Clin Infect Dis 2013; 57(5):697–9.

55. Lovell JP, Zerbe CS, Olivier KN, et al. Mediastinal and disseminated mycobacterium kansasii disease in GATA2 deficiency. Ann Am Thorac Soc 2016;13(12): 2169–73.

56. Gonzalez-Lara MF, Wisniowski-Yanez A, Perez-Patrigeon S, et al. Pneumocystis jiroveci pneumonia and GATA2 deficiency: expanding the spectrum of the disease. J Infect 2017;74(4):425–7.

57. Cohen JI, Dropulic L, Hsu AP, et al. Association of GATA2 deficiency with severe primary Epstein Barr virus (EBV) infection and EBV-associated cancers. Clin Infect Dis 2016;63(1):41–7.

58. Parta M, Cuellar-Rodriguez J, Freeman AF, et al. Resolution of multifocal Epstein-Barr virus-related smooth muscle tumor in a patient with GATA2 deficiency following hematopoietic stem cell transplantation. J Clin Immunol 2017;37(1): 61–6.

59. Kazamel M, Klein CJ, Benarroch EE, et al. Subacute demyelinating polyradiculoneuropathy complicating Epstein-Barr virus infection in GATA2 haploinsufficiency. Muscle Nerve 2018;57(1):150–6.

60. Spinner MA, Ker JP, Stoudenmire CJ, et al. GATA2 deficiency underlying severe blastomycosis and fatal herpes simplex virus-associated hemophagocytic lymphohistiocytosis. J Allergy Clin Immunol 2016;137(2):638–40.

61. Delgado-Marquez AM, Zarco C, Ruiz R, et al. Severe disseminated primary herpes simplex infection as skin manifestation of GATA2 deficiency. J Eur Acad Dermatol Venereol 2016;30(7):1248–50.

62. West ES, Kingsbery MY, Mintz EM, et al. Generalized verrucosis in a patient with GATA2 deficiency. Br J Dermatol 2014;170(5):1182–6.

63. Muszynski MA, Zerbe CS, Holland SM, et al. A woman with warts, leg swelling, and deafness. J Am Acad Dermatol 2014;71(3):577–80.

64. Polat A, Dinulescu M, Fraitag S, et al. Skin manifestations among GATA2-deficient patients. Br J Dermatol 2018;178(3):781–5.

65. Kazenwadel J, Secker GA, Liu YJ, et al. Loss-of-function germline GATA2 mutations in patients with MDS/AML or MonoMAC syndrome and primary lymphedema reveal a key role for GATA2 in the lymphatic vasculature. Blood 2012; 119(5):1283–91.

66. Ballerie A, Nimubona S, Meunier C, et al. Association of pulmonary alveolar proteinosis and fibrosis: patient with GATA2 deficiency. Eur Respir J 2016;48(5): 1510–4.

67. Griese M, Zarbock R, Costabel U, et al. GATA2 deficiency in children and adults with severe pulmonary alveolar proteinosis and hematologic disorders. BMC Pulm Med 2015;15:87.

68. Svobodova T, Mejstrikova E, Salzer U, et al. Diffuse parenchymal lung disease as first clinical manifestation of GATA-2 deficiency in childhood. BMC Pulm Med 2015;15:8.

69. Sanges S, Prevotat A, Fertin M, et al. Haemodynamically proven pulmonary hypertension in a patient with GATA2 deficiency-associated pulmonary alveolar proteinosis and fibrosis. Eur Respir J 2017;49(5) [pii:1700178].

70. Jouneau S, Ballerie A, Kerjouan M, et al. Haemodynamically proven pulmonary hypertension in a patient with GATA2 deficiency-associated pulmonary alveolar proteinosis and fibrosis. Eur Respir J 2017;49(5) [pii:1700407].

71. Haugas M, Lillevali K, Hakanen J, et al. Gata2 is required for the development of inner ear semicircular ducts and the surrounding perilymphatic space. Dev Dyn 2010;239(9):2452–69.

72. Berry D, Fekrat S. Central retinal vein occlusion in Gata2 deficiency. Retin Cases Brief Rep 2017;1–4.

73. Crall C, Morley KW, Rabinowits G, et al. Merkel cell carcinoma in a patient with GATA2 deficiency: a novel association with primary immunodeficiency. Br J Dermatol 2016;174(1):169–71.
74. Cuellar-Rodriguez J, Gea-Banacloche J, Freeman AF, et al. Successful allogeneic hematopoietic stem cell transplantation for GATA2 deficiency. Blood 2011; 118(13):3715–20.
75. Ciullini Mannurita S, Vignoli M, Colarusso G, et al. Timely follow-up of a GATA2 deficiency patient allows successful treatment. J Allergy Clin Immunol 2016; 138(5):1480–3.e4.
76. Ramzan M, Lowry J, Courtney S, et al. Successful myeloablative matched unrelated donor hematopoietic stem cell transplantation in a young girl with GATA2 deficiency and Emberger syndrome. J Pediatr Hematol Oncol 2017;39(3):230–2.
77. Lubking A, Vosberg S, Konstandin NP, et al. Young woman with mild bone marrow dysplasia, GATA2 and ASXL1 mutation treated with allogeneic hematopoietic stem cell transplantation. Leuk Res Rep 2015;4(2):72–5.
78. Maeurer M, Magalhaes I, Andersson J, et al. Allogeneic hematopoietic cell transplantation for GATA2 deficiency in a patient with disseminated human papillomavirus disease. Transplantation 2014;98(12):e95–6.
79. Mallhi K, Dix DB, Niederhoffer KY, et al. Successful umbilical cord blood hematopoietic stem cell transplantation in pediatric patients with MDS/AML associated with underlying GATA2 mutations: two case reports and review of literature. Pediatr Transplant 2016;20(7):1004–7.
80. Saida S, Umeda K, Yasumi T, et al. Successful reduced-intensity stem cell transplantation for GATA2 deficiency before progression of advanced MDS. Pediatr Transplant 2016;20(2):333–6.
81. Grossman J, Cuellar-Rodriguez J, Gea-Banacloche J, et al. Nonmyeloablative allogeneic hematopoietic stem cell transplantation for GATA2 deficiency. Biol Blood Marrow Transplant 2014;20(12):1940–8.
82. Shah NN, Parta M, Baird K, et al. Monozygotic twins with GATA2 deficiency: same haploidentical-related donor, different severity of GvHD. Bone Marrow Transplant 2017;52(11):1580–2.

Monosomy 7 in Pediatric Myelodysplastic Syndromes

Marcin W. Wlodarski, MD[a,b,c],*, Sushree S. Sahoo, MSc[a,d,e],
Charlotte M. Niemeyer, MD[a,b]

KEYWORDS

• Monosomy 7 • GATA2 • SAMD9L • SAMD9 • Pediatric MDS

KEY POINTS

• Complete (monosomy 7) or partial (del7q) loss of chromosome 7 is the most common cytogenetic aberration in pediatric myelodysplastic syndromes (MDS).
• Most children with primary MDS and chromosome 7 loss carry an underlying genetic defect: GATA2 deficiency or SAMD9/SAMD9L disease.
• In patients with germline SAMD9/SAMD9L mutations, the evolution of monosomy 7 or del7q is nonrandom and selects for clones retaining wild-type alleles.
• MDS with monosomy 7 is associated with a high risk of clonal progression and therefore necessitates early hematopoietic stem cell transplantation.

INTRODUCTION

Pediatric myelodysplastic syndromes (MDS) are a rare group of clonal hematopoietic stem cell (HSC) disorders accounting for less than 5% of hematopoietic neoplasia in childhood. The main hallmarks are morphologic dysplasia, ineffective hematopoiesis, and PB cytopenias.[1] The first World Health Organization (WHO) classification for pediatric MDS in 2001 recognized the categories of refractory cytopenia of childhood (RCC) characterized by peripheral blood (PB) blasts less than 2% and bone marrow (BM) blasts less than 5%, refractory anemia with excess blasts (RAEB) with PB blasts 2% to 19% and/or BM blasts 5% to 19%, and RAEB in transformation (RAEB-T) with PB and/or BM blasts 20% to 29%.[1] This straightforward approach was incorporated into the next WHO classification in 2008.[2] In the latest WHO classification from 2016, the criteria for RCC remained the same; however, MDS with excess of blasts is now referred to as MDS-EB and would encompass both pediatric categories RAEB and RAEB-T.[3]

Disclosures: none.
[a] Department of Pediatrics and Adolescent Medicine, Division of Pediatric Hematology and Oncology, Faculty of Medicine, Medical Center, University of Freiburg, Mathildenstr.1, Freiburg 79106, Germany; [b] German Cancer Consortium (DKTK), Freiburg, Germany; [c] Department of Hematology, St. Jude Children's Research Hospital, Memphis, TN, USA; [d] Faculty of Biology, University of Freiburg, Freiburg, Germany; [e] Spemann Graduate School of Biology and Medicine, University of Freiburg, Albertstr.19A, Freiburg 79104, Germany
* Corresponding author. Mathildenstr. 1, Freiburg 79106, Germany.
E-mail address: marcin.wlodarski@uniklinik-freiburg.de

Hematol Oncol Clin N Am 32 (2018) 729–743
https://doi.org/10.1016/j.hoc.2018.04.007
0889-8588/18/© 2018 Elsevier Inc. All rights reserved.

There are several important differences between pediatric and adult MDS. In children, the findings of ringed sideroblasts or del(5q) cytogenetic aberration are exceedingly rare; instead, loss of chromosome 7 is the most common cytogenetic aberration. Although anemia is frequently the main initial symptom in adults with MDS, thrombocytopenia and neutropenia are more prominent in children.[4] The somatic mutational landscape also differs according to the age at diagnosis. The typical adult-type mutations in *TET2*, *DNMT3A*, and the spliceosome complex are generally not present in children. Instead, somatic driver mutations in *SETBP1*, *ASXL1*, *RUNX1*, and the *RAS* oncogenes define the clonal mutational landscape in pediatric MDS.[5,6]

MDS secondary to chemo- or radiation therapy differs in biology, clinical course and outcome from MDS developing in the presence of a preceding classical inherited bone marrow failure syndrome (IBMFS) such as Fanconi anemia (FA) or severe congenital neutropenia (SCN), or MDS with prior acquired aplastic anemia (AA). All other cases of MDS are conventionally referred to as "primary" MDS, although it has to be assumed that these cases have an underlying yet unknown predisposition. In fact, the recently reported MDS predisposition syndromes GATA2 deficiency and SAMD9/SAMD9L diseases account for a considerable proportion of these cases in pediatric cohorts. Monosomy 7 and partial deletion of the long arm of chromosome 7 (del7q) are common cytogenetic lesions encountered across all ages in myeloid malignancies.[7] The heterogeneous nature and rapid clonal progression of −7 MDS pose a challenge to clinical management.

In this article, the authors provide a summary of their understanding of pediatric MDS with monosomy 7, with a specific focus on MDS predisposition syndromes associated with monosomy 7.

FREQUENCY OF MONOSOMY 7 IN PEDIATRIC MYELODYSPLASTIC SYNDROMES

Among patients with loss of chromosome 7 aberrations, a complete loss of one copy of chromosome 7 (monosomy 7, -7) accounts for the majority of cases. Some patients may however acquire only a partial deletion of genomic material on 7q (del7q), or the unbalanced translocation der(1;7)(q10;p10), resulting in monosomy for 7q. For clarity, all aforementioned cytogenetic aberrations are referred to as monosomy 7 or −7 in this article. Isochromosome 7q [i (7)(q10)] is a rare and nonrandom cytogenetic aberration that is fairly specific to patients with Shwachman-Diamond syndrome (SDS).[8] Although karyotypes involving −7 are very common in pediatric MDS, they are generally rare in pediatric patients with acute myeloid leukemia (AML), accounting for less than 5% of cases.[9]

Primary Myelodysplastic Syndromes

The overall incidence of monosomy 7 in pediatric MDS can be assessed from several studies investigating heterogenous patient cohorts. Within primary MDS (combining both RCC and MDS-EB), monosomy 7 occurs in up to ~20% of patients.[4,10,11] RCC is the most common subtype of pediatric MDS (>2/3 of cases). Most RCC patients (~80%) have hypocellular marrow, and in this patient group, monosomy 7 is found in 9% of cases. In the remaining ~20% of RCC patients with normal or increased cellularity, the incidence of monosomy 7 increases to 19%.[1] Among patients with MDS predisposition syndromes, a strong association can be seen with GATA2 deficiency and SAMD9/SAMD9L disorders.[6,10] As of today, it can be assumed that both genetic syndromes explain the hereditary cause in at least half of patients with "primary" pediatric MDS and −7 (**Fig. 1**). These syndromes are discussed in detail in the later discussion. Monosomy 7 has also been reported, albeit at considerably lower frequencies in MDS arising from germline *RUNX1* and *ERCC6L2* mutations.[12,13]

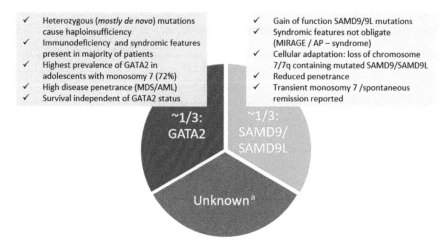

Fig. 1. Underlying causes of primary childhood MDS with monosomy 7. In patients with primary MDS and monosomy 7, underlying GATA2 deficiency can be found in approximately one-third of patients. Germline mutations in *SAMD9/SAMD9L* account for roughly another one-third of cases. AP, ataxia pancytopenia syndrome; MIRAGE, myelodysplasia, infection, restriction of growth, adrenal hypoplasia, genital phenotypes, and enteropathy. [a] Single cases of monosomy 7 in patients with germline *RUNX1* and *ERCC6L2* mutations had been reported.

Myelodysplastic Syndromes After Inherited Bone Marrow Failure Syndromes

The prevalence of −7 is very high in secondary MDS, with approximately one-third of patients developing −7 mostly in the context of a structurally complex karyotype[11,14] (**Table 1**). Based on the current knowledge, the association between −7 and IBMFS can be summarized as follows:

- FA: A recent study that investigated cytogenetic aberrations in FA-related MDS established that almost all patients acquire cytogenetic aberrations in the course of their disease.[15] Aberrations −7/del7q along with gains of 1q and 3q were the most common, accounting for more than half of the reported cases.
- SCN: A recent comprehensive review of 96 patients with SCN who develop MDS/AML showed that 12 (12.5%) acquired −7 karyotypes.[16]
- SDS: Isochromosome 7q is a fairly specific cytogenetic marker present in up to 44% of SDS patients. Altogether, chromosome 7 aberrations occur in approximately two-thirds of patients with SDS; monosomy 7/del7q are detected in approximately one-third of patients.[8]
- Dyskeratosis congenita: MDS is rare in dyskeratosis congenita with only a few cases reported. Out of 552 reviewed cases, Alter and colleagues[17] reported 2 patients with MDS and monosomy 7.
- Diamond-Blackfan anemia (DBA): Similarly, the occurrence of MDS is very rare in DBA. According to literature, only one patient with *GATA1*-mutated DBA developed MDS with a −7/complex karyotype.[18]

Myelodysplastic Syndromes After Severe Aplastic Anemia

It is well known that secondary MDS can develop in patients with AA who received immunosuppressive therapy. The evolution rates in adult cohorts are in the range of 10% to 15% in 10 years, and −7 karyotype is most common.[19,20] In children with MDS after severe AA, these numbers are much lower, likely owing to a clear

Table 1
Types of childhood myelodysplastic syndromes associated with monosomy 7

Condition	Occurrence of Monosomy 7
"Primary MDS", including MDS predisposition syndromes	~20% of cases
GATA2	+++[a]
SAMD9 & SAMD9L	++[b]
RUNX1	+
ERCC6L2	+
MDS after inherited BM failure	
FA	+++[c,d]
SCN	++[c]
SDS	+++[c]
Dyskeratosis congenita	(+)[e]
Amegakaryocytic thrombocytopenia/RUSAT	-
DBA	_[f]
MDS after therapy or AA	~33% of cases
Therapy related	+++[c]
After severe AA	(+)[g]

Abbreviation: RUSAT, radioulnar synostosis with amegakaryocytic thrombocytopenia.
[a] Several cases reported with unbalanced translocation der(1;7)(q10;p10).
[b] Transient monosomy 7 reported in young children. Often del7q or UPD7q present. Whole or partial deletion of chromosome 7 is associated with loss of germline mutant SAMD9/SAMD9L allele.
[c] Frequently in context of complex karyotype.
[d] Often in association with gains of 1q and 3q.
[e] Not reported in children.
[f] One patient with DBA due to GATA1 mutation and monosomy 7 had been reported.
[g] Clonal evolution is rare in children with severe AA.

differentiation between severe AA and RCC (RCC seems to have a higher propensity for clonal evolution) at presentation. In the German severe AA study, 123 patients diagnosed after the implementation of centralized hematopathology review had a 10-year probability of developing clonal disease of only 3%.[21]

Myelodysplastic Syndromes After Cytotoxic Therapy

Children with MDS secondary to cytotoxic therapies (radiation or chemotherapy) generally have a poor prognosis.[22,23] Monosomy 7 often occurs as part of structurally complex karyotypes (characterized by ≥3 chromosomal aberrations and including at least 1 structural change). Monosomy 7 is not a prognostic factor in MDS secondary to cytotoxic therapies, but rather structural complex abnormalities are associated with a very poor outcome.[11]

HISTORICAL PERSPECTIVE

One of the first descriptions of −7 in MDS dates back to 1964, when 3 cases with refractory anemia, granulocytic hyperplasia, and a missing "group C" chromosome were reported.[24] The recurrent interstitial microdeletions on the q-arm of chr7, that is, bands 7q22 and 7q34-q36 in patients with MDS and AML, implicated a critical role of genes mapped to those regions.[25–27] Candidate genes such as *PLANH1*, *MET*, and *CUTL1* were proposed as possible putative tumor suppressor genes required for the development of MDS −7; however, no experimental evidence exists to support this notion. In a more recent study, *SAMD9* (Sterile Alpha Motif Domain-containing 9), its paralogue *SAMD9L* (SAMD9-like), and *Miki/HEPACAM2*, all located within a 7q21 cluster in patients with myeloid neoplasia, were discussed as potential genes driving the clonal evolution in −7[28,29] (**Fig. 2**). Experimental studies elucidating *SAMD9/SAMD9L* gene function convincingly assign a mechanistic role as tumor suppressors in the development of myeloid neoplasia associated with −7 karyotypes (discussed in detail in later discussion).

The inherited basis underlying the development of MDS with −7 persisted as an uncharted subject. For many years, the IBMFS had been established as the only known germline cause predisposing to the acquisition of −7 in the BM, whereas the hereditary factors in primary MDS remained undetermined.[30] More recently, inherited diseases predisposing to MDS −7 such as GATA2 deficiency and the SAMD9/SAMD9L diseases have been described (see **Fig. 1**). The underlying genetic mechanisms are discussed in detail in the respective paragraphs.

GATA2 DEFICIENCY: MONOSOMY 7 AS A MOST COMMON CYTOGENETIC ABERRATION

The initial description of GATA2 deficiency dates back to 2011, when several groups described different phenotypic manifestations of the same disease, which included monocytopenia and Mycobacterium avium complex/dendritic cell, monocyte, B and NK lymphoid deficiency (MIM #614172), primary lymphedema with AML predisposition, Emberger syndrome (MIM #614038), and familial MDS/AML (MIM #601626 and #614286).[31–35] The common denominator for all these patients is the high risk for the development of MDS/AML, and the association with monosomy

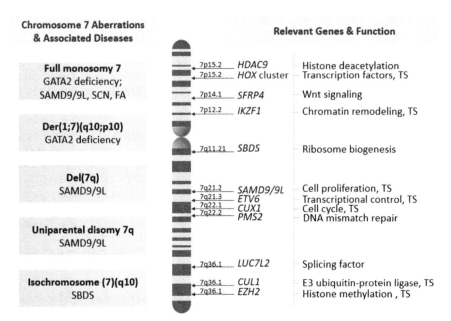

Fig. 2. Relevant neoplasia-related genes located on chromosome 7. Chromosome 7 is a medium-sized submetacentric autosome that accounts for 160 Mb or ~5% of the human genome. On the left, various types of chromosome 7 aberrations and predisposing diseases are shown. On the right, relevant genes, mostly tumor suppressors (TS), are shown.

7 karyotype. To date, approximately 400 patients had been reported in several case series.[36]

Gene Function

GATA2 plays a crucial role in hematopoietic development because it controls the transition from hemogenic endothelium to HSCs and is essential for HSC survival and self-renewal. In this process, it is involved in a tightly regulated network involving other important hematopoietic transcription factors, for example, FLI1, SCL/TAL1, LYL1, PU1, RUNX1.[36–38] Heterozygous Gata2 knockout mice have reduced numbers of progenitor cells, whereas homozygous knockouts are embryonically lethal.[39] GATA2 protein contains 2 highly conserved zinc finger domains (ZF1 and ZF1) responsible for its DNA-binding ability and interaction with other proteins. All germline pathogenic mutations in GATA2 are thought to cause loss of function, or alteration of transactivation/DNA binding ability, and can be categorized into protein-truncating mutations, missense mutations in ZF1, mutations in intron 4 regulatory site, and whole gene deletions.

Association with Pediatric Myelodysplastic Syndromes and – 7

In a study investigating 426 children and adolescents with primary MDS, germline GATA2 mutations were established as the most common germline defect present in 37% of patients with primary MDS and −7 (see **Fig. 1**), 16% of trisomy 8 cases, and were absent in patients with secondary MDS.[10] Stratified by age, 72% of adolescents with −7 were GATA2 mutation carriers. Some patients with GATA2-related MDS carried the translocation der(1;7)(q10;p10) leading to monosomy 7q. Concomitant cytogenetic aberrations in patients with −7 include trisomy 8, or trisomy 21, whereas complex karyotypes were not observed. Isolated trisomy 8 is the second most common cytogenetic lesion. Overall, although −7 karyotype is by far the most common genetic lesion encountered in the pediatric population,[10,40] in adults the incidence of monosomy 7 seems to be evenly balanced with isolated trisomy 8.[41] Recurrent somatic mutations in patients with GATA2-related MDS affect SETBP1, RUNX1, and ASXL1 genes.[5,6,42–44] The authors investigated somatic mutations in larger cohorts of children with primary MDS and −7 and did not observe a significant difference between GATA2-mutated and wild-type patients, suggesting that the somatic mutational landscape correlates with the −7 karyotype and is not directly determined by GATA2 germline mutational status (unpublished data). One can speculate that the monosomy 7 clone arises as the first somatic lesion and is followed by the acquisition of other somatic mutation or mutations[5]; however, additional studies are warranted.

In studies of the European Working Group of MDS in Childhood (EWOG-MDS) the overall survival and outcome of HSCT were not affected by the presence of germline GATA2 mutations in children with MDS and −7, indicating that the MDS subtype was the relevant prognostic factor.[10] However, the underlying immunodeficiency has to be taken into consideration because the overall prognosis and survival after HSCT might deteriorate in older individuals with GATA2 deficiency and in the presence of severe preceding infections.[41]

SAMD9 AND SAMD9L GERMLINE DISEASES: NONRANDOM LOSS OF CHROMOSOME 7

SAMD9 and its paralogue gene SAMD9L are recently identified constitutional genetic factors responsible for the development of monosomy 7.[45] Overall, both SAMD9 and SAMD9L disorders are the most common entities predisposing to childhood MDS, accounting for as many as 17% to 19% of patients with pediatric BM failure/primary

MDS.[6,13] Based on first estimates in the literature and the authors' unpublished observations, the incidence of SAMD9/9L disorders among primary MDS with 7 can be estimated to be nearly as high as GATA2 deficiency.

Gene Function

Evolutionarily, both *SAMD9/9L* are the result of a common ancestral gene duplication event, thereby sharing similar gene structures that encode proteins with 60% amino acid identity.[45,46] However, absence of *SAMD9* in mice and *SAMD9L* in cows indicates a partial functional redundancy between the 2 genes. Although limited, knowledge of cellular function assigns both genes as negative regulators of cellular proliferation, thus functioning as tumor suppressors.[46] The identification of a common microdeletion cluster in 7q21.3 subband, containing 3 poorly characterized genes, that is, *SAMD9*, *SAMD9L*, and *Miki/HEPACAM2*, in patients with myeloid neoplasia was the primary association of *SAMD9/9L* with MDS.[28] Notably, *Samd9l*-haploinsufficient mice were shown to develop myeloid malignancies characterized by cytopenias and mimicking human MDS with −7.[29] The functional elucidation implicated that SAMD9L protein localizes in early endosomes, and *SAMD9L*-deficient cells showed delays in endosome fusion. The insufficiency of SAMD9L results in the inability of endosome transition and degradation in lysosomes leading to persistence of ligand-bound cytokine receptors. The enhanced colony-forming and in vivo reconstitution potential of *SAMD9L*-deficient HSCs supported the notion that *SAMD9L* is a tumor suppressor gene. Deleterious (loss-of-function) homozygous germline mutations in *SAMD9* in humans lead to normophosphatemic familial tumoral calcinosis, with massive deposition of calcified tumors, suggesting a crucial role of SAMD9 in extraosseous calcification.[47]

Phenotypes of Human Disease

Germline heterozygous missense mutations in both *SAMD9* and *SAMD9L* genes were reported in individuals with varying nonhematologic phenotypes, cytopenias, and a high propensity to develop MDS with −7. Based on cellular studies, these mutations are thought to be gain of function. The clinical spectrum of constitutional *SAMD9L* mutations extends from ataxia pancytopenia syndrome, with variable degrees of neurologic symptoms (ataxia, balance impairment, hyperreflexia, dysarthria, nystagmus, dysmetria) and hematologic abnormalities (single to trilineage cytopenias, MDS/−7)[48,49] to de novo and familial MDS without preexisting neurologic impairment.[6,13,50] Similarly, the clinical spectrum of inherited SAMD9 mutations ranges from severe phenotypes manifesting with all features of the MIRAGE syndrome (myelodysplasia, infection, restriction of growth, adrenal hypoplasia, genital phenotypes, and enteropathy)[51–53] to solely hematologic phenotype presenting as MDS −7 without additional nonhematologic manifestations.[6,13,54]

The reported pathogenic missense mutations in SAMD9/9L exhibit an enhanced growth-restrictive phenotype in vitro and are referred to as gain of function.[49–52,55] It is not known, however, if these mutations lead to increased protein stability, change in the protein structure, enhanced functional domain, or if these mutations exert an unknown effect.[50]

Nonrandom Loss of Chromosome 7 Harboring the Germline SAMD9/9L Mutation

The interesting aspect of disease pathogenesis and a common denominator of both *SAMD9/9L* disorders is the nonrandom loss of the chromosome 7 copy containing the mutated *SAMD9* or *SAMD9L* allele (**Fig. 3**). The selection for clones containing either complete monosomy 7 or del7q further depicts the SAMD9/9L mutated allell

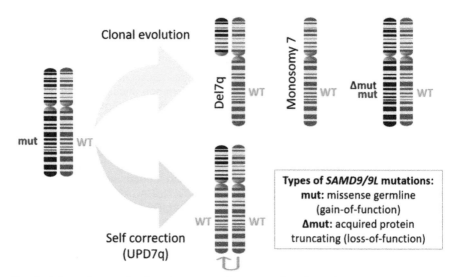

Fig. 3. Adaptation mechanisms to escape from germline SAMD9/9L mutations. Various mechanisms of adaptation to the growth-restrictive effect of germline *SAMD9/9L* mutations are depicted. Clonal escape from hematotoxic missense mutations can be attained by aneuploidy (monosomy 7, del7q) or by acquisition of in-cis truncating mutation in the respective gene. True genetic reversion occurs after reduplication of the wild-type (WT) allele in the setting of uniparental disomy.

loss.[49,50] Because the allelic frequency of the germline *SAMD9/9L* mutations decrease in hematopoiesis, these variants might erroneously be called somatic in next-generation sequencing studies, and therefore, germline validation is essential. Interestingly, another mechanism to counteract the growth-suppressive effect of germline *SAMD9/9L* mutations is the acquisition of true somatic, usually protein-truncating variants located on the same allele as the germline mutation. It seems however that these clones might not be potent enough to "take over" and repopulate the restricted hematopoiesis.[50] A true genetic reversion in *SAMD9/9L* genetic disorders is possible and was noted on several occasions in patients with transient monosomy 7 where the initial −7 karyotype vanished, PB cytopenias and BM picture normalized, and patients remained healthy until last follow-up, up to 20 years after initial diagnosis.[13,50] This genetic reversion occurs through the acquisition of segmental uniparental isodisomy of 7q (UPD7q), where 7q-arm-containing mutated *SAMD9/9L* is lost and replaced by the wild-type copy of 7q. Such revertant clones seem to be efficient in repopulating the marrow stem cell compartment and producing functional hematopoiesis. Interestingly, UPD7q is not only encountered in the myeloid compartment, because one study documented the development of UPD7q in long-term in vitro cultured lymphoblastoid cell lines of *SAMD9L* mutation carriers, pointing to the selective growth advantage of cells with the duplicated wild-type *SAMD9L* allele.[56]

Clonal Evolution to Myelodysplastic Syndromes

The attained loss −7 and del7q in the bone marrow can be understood as a cellular mechanism of adaptation to the hematotoxic growth-suppressive germline *SAMD9/9L* mutation, with various possible outcomes ranging from karyotype normalization with genetic reversion to clonal progression and development of advanced MDS. It is likely that additional somatic aberrations, for example, driver mutations, are required for MDS development. The authors and others observed somatic mutations in *SETBP1*, *KRAS*, *EZH2*, *PTPN11*, and *ETV6* arising from −7/7q background in patients with MDS.[6,50] This observation points to the need for sequential studies to determine potential somatic driver mutations in clinically stable patients.

POTENTIAL TUMOR SUPPRESSOR GENES LOCATED ON CHROMOSOME 7

Based on clinical data and functional studies, it seems that the loss of both tumor suppressor genes, *SAMD9* and *SAMD9L*, independent of the underlying germline cause, might explain the persistence and expansion of −7 clones haploinsufficient for these genes. However, several other genes with relevant tumor suppressor function are also lost in −7. A comprehensive analysis of chromosome 7 in 2003 disseminated a high degree of intrachromosomal duplication with large duplicons (>100 kb) identified at 7p22, 7p14-p15, the pericentromeric region, 7q11.21, 7q11.23, 7q22, and 7q36, which are also common microdeletion regions observed in myeloid neoplasia.[57] Chromosome 7 gene mapping decoded 1394 protein coding genes with 7.6% (n = 106) of them directly linked with cancer (http://www.cancerindex.org/geneweb/clinkc07.htm), and among these, some are shown to be associated with myeloid neoplasms. The functional annotation of the 13 depicted genes in **Fig. 2** groups them to histone modifiers (*HDAC9*, *EZH2*), tumor suppressors (*HOX* cluster, *IKZF1*, *SAMD9/9L*, *ETV6*, *CUX1*, *CUL1*), splicing factor (*LUC7L2*), Wnt signaling (*SFRP4*), DNA repair (*PMS2*), and ribosome biogenesis (*SBDS*).

EZH2, the catalytic subunit of the polycomb repressive complex 2 (PRC2/EED-EZH2), which catalyzes the dimethylation and trimethylation of the Lys-9 and 27 residues, is a commonly targeted epigenetic regulator in myeloid neoplasms.[58,59] Deactivating *EZH2* point and deletion mutations (7q36.1) account for 12% of adult cases with MDS/myeloproliferative disease.[60] EZH2 promoter hypermethylation was noted in T-ALL (T-cell Acute Lymphoblastic Leukemia) patients, resulting in similar functional consequences as that of the genetic haploinsufficiency.[61] HDAC9, a histone deacetylase involved in epigenetic repression, is shown to exhibit heterogeneous expression patterns in myeloid malignancies.[62] CUL1 protein is a critical component of the ubiquitin ligase system.[63] A study of 103 adult MDS cases depicted heterozygous somatic deletion of 7q36.1 encompassing both *EZH2* and *CUL1* in 12.7% cases, although singular involvement of *CUL1* is not reported to date.[59] *HOX* cluster genes are abundantly expressed in primitive HSCs, are downregulated upon differentiation, and show lineage-restrictive expression.[64] *HOXA* cluster is expressed in myeloid cells, and unlike *HOXB4*, prolonged overexpression of *HOXA9* causes HSC expansion with leukemia development.[65,66] Interestingly, loss of *ASXL1* (gene frequently mutated in pediatric MDS[5]) promotes myeloid transformation and causes overexpression of *HOXA9* in hematopoietic malignancies.[67] *IKZF1* is a known tumor suppressor gene implicated in acute lymphoid leukemia (ALL) and is also involved in myeloid differentiation. Although by themselves *IKZF1* deletions are not necessarily the leukemogenic driver, they might contribute as a secondary hit to disease progression in myeloid malignancy.[42,68] *CUX1* has been established as a tumor suppressor gene often inactivated in AML. Its location 7q22.1 is a frequently deleted region in adult MDS −7/del7q cases.[69] Haploinsufficiency of *CUX1* gives human HSC a significant engraftment advantage in a xenograft mouse model. Furthermore, Cux1-haploinsufficient mice develop MDS with anemia and trilineage dysplasia.[70] Point mutations in the *ETV6* gene have been reported in 2.7% cases of adult MDS[71] and are also associated with secondary transformation of MDS to CMML (Chronic Myelomonocytic

Leukemia).[72] Secondary *ETV6* hits account for 1.3% to 4.2% of adult MDS and display an association with the −7 karyotype.[71,73,74] Functionally, ETV6 serves as a transcriptional repressor binding to a particular DNA sequence, that is, 5-CCGGAAGT-3, and might play a role in malignant transformation. Strikingly, heterozygous germline mutations in *ETV6* are associated with thrombocytopenia, red cell macrocytosis, and predisposition to ALL. The mutations impair ETV6 nuclear localization and result in loss of transcriptional repression normally exerted by ETV6.[75] *SFRP4* is one of the 6 Wnt inhibitors (*Wif-1*, *SFRP1*, *SFRR2*, *SFRP4*, *SFRP5*, and *DKK1*) that undergoes promoter hypermethylation in approximately 1.5% of AML patients, described to be interacting with genetic alterations driving leukemogenesis.[76] A variant of Lynch syndrome featuring leukemia malignancy is caused by homozygous mutations in one of the 4 mismatch repair genes (MLH1, MSH2, MSH6, PMS2), with 7q-bound *PMS2* accounting for greater than 50% of documented cases.[77]

DIAGNOSTIC CONSIDERATIONS

Despite the advent of genomic and transcriptomic approaches allowing for copy-number analysis, conventional cytogenetics using metaphase G-banding is the gold standard in detection of chromosome 7 aberrations in pediatric MDS.[11] In particular, translocations, clonal progression with acquisition of new cytogenetic lesions, or the identification of independent cytogenetic clones can be ascertained by metaphase cytogenetics. Interphase fluorescence in situ hybridization does not rely on actively dividing cells. However, only losses/gains of chromosomal regions, for example, del7q, can be identified with this method. UPD7q is a copy-number neutral lesion that can be detected only by interrogation of many polymorphic markers.[20,50] Future studies are warranted to evaluate the diagnostic utility of whole genome/exome sequencing combined with RNA-seq to detect structural variations and UPD in MDS patients.

THERAPEUTIC APPROACHES

The therapeutic approach in children for MDS is generally curative and based on allo-geneic hematopoietic stem cell transplantation (HSCT). Because monosomy 7 in patients with RCC correlates with a high risk of rapid progression to advanced MDS (MDS-EB) and to MDS-related AML, these patients should be transplanted shortly after diagnosis. EWOG-MDS currently recommends HSCT from HLA-identical sibling or HLA-compatible unrelated donor following myeloablative (treosulfan or busulfan-based) conditioning for pediatric MDS with monosomy 7.[78] In a recent study, among a cohort of 100 patients with primary MDS and monosomy 7 enrolled in the EWOG-MDS registries, 91 had been transplanted. The 5-year Kaplan-Meier estimate of event-free survival was 60%, and the overall survival rate approached nearly 70%.[10] The use of unrelated cord blood as allograft seems inferior to BM and PB and therefore is generally restricted only to patients lacking a potential matched related or unrelated donor.[79] Monosomy 7 associated with complex karyotypes in context of MDS following radiotherapy/chemotherapy or IBMFS has an overall poor survival. Several retrospective observations pointed to an efficacy of reports it seems that the hypomethylating drug azacitidine in pediatric MDS prior to HSCT.[22,80–82] However, prospective trials are essential to investigate whether patients with −7 MDS might benefit from this type of therapy and to determine the effect of structurally complex karyotypes and/or *TP53* mutations.

There are anecdotal reports of very young children with transient monosomy 7. Some recent cases are linked do germline SAMD9/9L disorders.[13,50,54] For these patients, a watch-and-wait strategy might be implemented if the blood counts improve over time and the cytogenetic clone disappears.[50,54] The authors carefully monitor blood counts, BM morphology, and cytogenetics and perform serial quantitative genetic sequencing of *SAMD9/SAMD9L* and MDS-associated somatic mutations. The molecular screening using an SNP array or exome-based SNP/CNV analysis helps to identify patients with somatic revertant UPD7q clones that have the ability to "repopulate" the marrow stem cell niche and finally result in genetic reversion.

SUMMARY

Monosomy 7 is a common pathophysiologic denominator encountered in different subtypes of childhood MDS, irrespective of underlying genetic causes. Recent genomic discoveries establish GATA2 deficiency and SAMD9/9L disorders as common hereditary causes of primary MDS with −7, accounting for more than half of patients with this particular cytogenetic abnormality. The growth advantage and clonal evolution of HSC carrying monosomy 7 is likely a multifactorial process determined by loss of several tumor suppressors and the accumulation of somatic driver mutations in known oncogenes.

REFERENCES

1. Niemeyer CM, Baumann I. Classification of childhood aplastic anemia and myelodysplastic syndrome. Hematology Am Soc Hematol Educ Program 2011;2011: 84–9.
2. Vardiman JW, Thiele J, Arber DA, et al. The 2008 revision of the World Health Organization (WHO) classification of myeloid neoplasms and acute leukemia: rationale and important changes. Blood 2009;114(5):937–51.
3. Arber DA, Orazi A, Hasserjian R, et al. The 2016 revision to the World Health Organization classification of myeloid neoplasms and acute leukemia. Blood 2016; 127(20):2391–405.
4. Kardos G, Baumann I, Passmore SJ, et al. Refractory anemia in childhood: a retrospective analysis of 67 patients with particular reference to monosomy 7. Blood 2003;102(6):1997–2003.
5. Pastor V, Hirabayashi S, Karow A, et al. Mutational landscape in children with myelodysplastic syndromes is distinct from adults: specific somatic drivers and novel germline variants. Leukemia 2017;31(3):759–62.
6. Schwartz JR, Ma J, Lamprecht T, et al. The genomic landscape of pediatric myelodysplastic syndromes. Nat Commun 2017;8(1):1557.
7. Honda H, Nagamachi A, Inaba T. -7/7q- syndrome in myeloid-lineage hematopoietic malignancies: attempts to understand this complex disease entity. Oncogene 2015;34(19):2413–25.
8. Dror Y. Shwachman-Diamond syndrome. Pediatr Blood Cancer 2005;45(7): 892–901.
9. Hasle H, Alonzo TA, Auvrignon A, et al. Monosomy 7 and deletion 7q in children and adolescents with acute myeloid leukemia: an international retrospective study. Blood 2007;109(11):4641–7.
10. Wlodarski MW, Hirabayashi S, Pastor V, et al. Prevalence, clinical characteristics, and prognosis of GATA2-related myelodysplastic syndromes in children and adolescents. Blood 2016;127(11):1387–97 [quiz: 1518].
11. Gohring G, Michalova K, Beverloo HB, et al. Complex karyotype newly defined: the strongest prognostic factor in advanced childhood myelodysplastic syndrome. Blood 2010;116(19):3766–9.

12. Minelli A, Maserati E, Giudici G, et al. Familial partial monosomy 7 and myelodys-plasia: different parental origin of the monosomy 7 suggests action of a mutator gene. Cancer Genet Cytogenet 2001;124(2):147–51.

13. Bluteau O, Sebert M, Leblanc T, et al. A landscape of germ line mutations in a cohort of inherited bone marrow failure patients. Blood 2018;131(7):717–32.

14. Strahm B, Wlodarski MW, Pastor VB, et al. Impact of somatic mutations on the outcome of children and adolescents with therapy-related myelodysplastic syn-drome. ASH 2016.

15. Cioc AM, Wagner JE, MacMillan ML, et al. Diagnosis of myelodysplastic syn-drome among a cohort of 119 patients with Fanconi anemia: morphologic and cy-togenetic characteristics. Am J Clin Pathol 2010;133(1):92–100.

16. Pezeshki A, Podder S, Kamel R, et al. Monosomy 7/del (7q) in inherited bone marrow failure syndromes: a systematic review. Pediatr Blood Cancer 2017; 64(12).

17. Alter BP, Giri N, Savage SA, et al. Cancer in dyskeratosis congenita. Blood 2009; 113(26):6549–57.

18. Parrella S, Aspesi A, Quarello P, et al. Loss of GATA-1 full length as a cause of Diamond-Blackfan anemia phenotype. Pediatr Blood Cancer 2014;61(7):1319–21.

19. Afable MG 2nd, Tiu RV, Maciejewski JP. Clonal evolution in aplastic anemia. Hem-atol Am Soc Hematol Educ Program 2011;2011:90–5.

20. Afable MG 2nd, Wlodarski M, Makishima H, et al. SNP array-based karyotyping: differences and similarities between aplastic anemia and hypocellular myelodys-plastic syndromes. Blood 2011;117(25):6876–84.

21. Baumann I, Fuhrer M, Behrendt S, et al. Morphological differentiation of severe aplastic anaemia from hypocellular refractory cytopenia of childhood: reproduc-ibility of histopathological diagnostic criteria. Histopathology 2012;61(1):10–7.

22. Cseh AM, Niemeyer CM, Yoshimi A, et al. Therapy with low-dose azacitidine for MDS in children and young adults: a retrospective analysis of the EWOG-MDS study group. Br J Haematol 2016;172(6):930–6.

23. Hasle H, Niemeyer CM. Advances in the prognostication and management of advanced MDS in children. Br J Haematol 2011;154(2):185–95.

24. Freireich EJWJ, Tijo JH, Levin RH, et al. Refractory anemia, granulocytic hyper-plasia of bone marrow and a missing chromosome in marrow cells. A new clinical syndrome? Clin Res 1964;12:284.

25. Johnson E, Cotter FE. Monosomy 7 and 7q–associated with myeloid malignancy. Blood Rev 1997;11(1):46–55.

26. Lewis S, Abrahamson G, Boultwood J, et al. Molecular characterization of the 7q deletion in myeloid disorders. Br J Haematol 1996;93(1):75–80.

27. Kere J. Chromosome 7 long arm deletion breakpoints in preleukemia: mapping by pulsed field gel electrophoresis. Nucleic Acids Res 1989;17(4):1511–20.

28. Asou H, Matsui H, Ozaki Y, et al. Identification of a common microdeletion cluster in 7q21.3 subband among patients with myeloid leukemia and myelodysplastic syndrome. Biochem Biophys Res Commun 2009;383(2):245–51.

29. Nagamachi A, Matsui H, Asou H, et al. Haploinsufficiency of SAMD9L, an endo-some fusion facilitator, causes myeloid malignancies in mice mimicking human diseases with monosomy 7. Cancer Cell 2013;24(3):305–17.

30. Wlodarski MW, Niemeyer CM. Introduction: genetic syndromes predisposing to myeloid neoplasia. Semin Hematol 2017;54(2):57–9.

31. Hahn CN, Chong CE, Carmichael CL, et al. Heritable GATA2 mutations associ-ated with familial myelodysplastic syndrome and acute myeloid leukemia. Nat Genet 2011;43(10):1012–7.

32. Ostergaard P, Simpson MA, Connell FC, et al. Mutations in GATA2 cause primary lymphedema associated with a predisposition to acute myeloid leukemia (Emberger syndrome). Nat Genet 2011;43(10):929–31.
33. Bigley V, Haniffa M, Doulatov S, et al. The human syndrome of dendritic cell, monocyte, B and NK lymphoid deficiency. J Exp Med 2011;208(2):227–34.
34. Dickinson RE, Griffin H, Bigley V, et al. Exome sequencing identifies GATA-2 mutation as the cause of dendritic cell, monocyte, B and NK lymphoid deficiency. Blood 2011;118(10):2656–8.
35. Hsu AP, Sampaio EP, Khan J, et al. Mutations in GATA2 are associated with the autosomal dominant and sporadic monocytopenia and mycobacterial infection (MonoMAC) syndrome. Blood 2011;118(10):2653–5.
36. Wlodarski MW, Collin M, Horwitz MS. GATA2 deficiency and related myeloid neoplasms. Semin Hematol 2017;54(2):81–6.
37. Tsai FY, Keller G, Kuo FC, et al. An early haematopoietic defect in mice lacking the transcription factor GATA-2. Nature 1994;371(6494):221–6.
38. Gao X, Johnson KD, Chang YI, et al. Gata2 cis-element is required for hematopoietic stem cell generation in the mammalian embryo. J Exp Med 2013;210(13):2833–42.
39. Rodrigues NP, Janzen V, Forkert R, et al. Haploinsufficiency of GATA-2 perturbs adult hematopoietic stem-cell homeostasis. Blood 2005;106(2):477–84.
40. Novakova M, Zaliova M, Sukova M, et al. Loss of B cells and their precursors is the most constant feature of GATA-2 deficiency in childhood myelodysplastic syndrome. Haematologica 2016;101(6):707–16.
41. Spinner MA, Sanchez LA, Hsu AP, et al. GATA2 deficiency: a protean disorder of hematopoiesis, lymphatics, and immunity. Blood 2014;123(6):809–21.
42. Fisher KE, Hsu AP, Williams CL, et al. Somatic mutations in children with GATA2-associated myelodysplastic syndrome who lack other features of GATA2 deficiency. Blood Adv 2017;1(7):443–8.
43. West RR, Hsu AP, Holland SM, et al. Acquired ASXL1 mutations are common in patients with inherited GATA2 mutations and correlate with myeloid transformation. Haematologica 2014;99(2):276–81.
44. Bodor C, Renneville A, Smith M, et al. Germ-line GATA2 p.THR354MET mutation in familial myelodysplastic syndrome with acquired monosomy 7 and ASXL1 mutation demonstrating rapid onset and poor survival. Haematologica 2012;97(6):890–4.
45. Lemos de Matos A, Liu J, McFadden G, et al. Evolution and divergence of the mammalian SAMD9/SAMD9L gene family. BMC Evol Biol 2013;13:121.
46. Mekhedov SL, Makarova KS, Koonin EV. The complex domain architecture of SAMD9 family proteins, predicted STAND-like NTPases, suggests new links to inflammation and apoptosis. Biol Direct 2017;12(1):13.
47. Chefetz I, Ben Amitai D, Browning S, et al. Normophosphatemic familial tumoral calcinosis is caused by deleterious mutations in SAMD9, encoding a TNF-alpha responsive protein. J Invest Dermatol 2008;128(6):1423–9.
48. Chen DH, Below JE, Shimamura A, et al. Ataxia-pancytopenia syndrome is caused by missense mutations in SAMD9L. Am J Hum Genet 2016;98(6):1146–58.
49. Tesi B, Davidsson J, Voss M, et al. Gain-of-function SAMD9L mutations cause a syndrome of cytopenia, immunodeficiency, MDS, and neurological symptoms. Blood 2017;129(16):2266–79.
50. Pastor VB, Sahoo SS, Boklan J, et al. Constitutional SAMD9L mutations cause familial myelodysplastic syndrome and transient monosomy 7. Haematologica 2018;103(3):427–37.

51. Narumi S, Amano N, Ishii T, et al. SAMD9 mutations cause a novel multisystem disorder, MIRAGE syndrome, and are associated with loss of chromosome 7. Nat Genet 2016;48(7):792–7.

52. Buonocore F, Kuhnen P, Suntharalingham JP, et al. Somatic mutations and progressive monosomy modify SAMD9-related phenotypes in humans. J Clin Invest 2017;127(5):1700–13.

53. Sarthy J, Zha J, Babushok D, et al. Poor outcome with hematopoietic stem cell transplantation for bone marrow failure and MDS with severe MIRAGE syndrome phenotype. Blood Adv 2018;2(2):120–5.

54. Schwartz JR, Wang S, Ma J, et al. Germline SAMD9 mutation in siblings with monosomy 7 and myelodysplastic syndrome. Leukemia 2017;31(8):1827–30.

55. Li CF, MacDonald JR, Wei RY, et al. Human sterile alpha motif domain 9, a novel gene identified as down-regulated in aggressive fibromatosis, is absent in the mouse. BMC Genomics 2007;8:92.

56. Davidsson J, Puschmann A, Tedgard U, et al. SAMD9 and SAMD9L in inherited predisposition to ataxia, pancytopenia, and myeloid malignancies. Leukemia 2018;32(5):1106–15.

57. Scherer SW, Cheung J, MacDonald JR, et al. Human chromosome 7: DNA sequence and biology. Science 2003;300(5620):767–72.

58. Shiba N, Yoshida K, Shiraishi Y, et al. Whole-exome sequencing reveals the spectrum of gene mutations and the clonal evolution patterns in paediatric acute myeloid leukaemia. Br J Haematol 2016;175(3):476–89.

59. Nikoloski G, Langemeijer SM, Kuiper RP, et al. Somatic mutations of the histone methyltransferase gene EZH2 in myelodysplastic syndromes. Nat Genet 2010; 42(8):665–7.

60. Ernst T, Chase AJ, Score J, et al. Inactivating mutations of the histone methyltransferase gene EZH2 in myeloid disorders. Nat Genet 2010;42(8):722–6.

61. Schafer V, Ernst J, Rinke J, et al. EZH2 mutations and promoter hypermethylation in childhood acute lymphoblastic leukemia. J Cancer Res Clin Oncol 2016; 142(7):1641–50.

62. Yang H, Maddipoti S, Quesada A, et al. Analysis of class I and II histone deacetylase gene expression in human leukemia. Leuk Lymphoma 2015;56(12):3426–33.

63. O'Hagan RC, Ohh M, David G, et al. Myc-enhanced expression of Cul1 promotes ubiquitin-dependent proteolysis and cell cycle progression. Genes Dev 2000; 14(17):2185–91.

64. Seifert A, Werheid DF, Knapp SM, et al. Role of Hox genes in stem cell differentiation. World J Stem Cells 2015;7(3):583–95.

65. Alharbi RA, Pettengell R, Pandha HS, et al. The role of HOX genes in normal hematopoiesis and acute leukemia. Leukemia 2013;27(5):1000–8.

66. Huang Y, Sitwala K, Bronstein J, et al. Identification and characterization of Hoxa9 binding sites in hematopoietic cells. Blood 2012;119(2):388–98.

67. Inoue D, Kitaura J, Togami K, et al. Myelodysplastic syndromes are induced by histone methylation-altering ASXL1 mutations. J Clin Invest 2013;123(11):4627–40.

68. de Rooij JD, Beuling E, van den Heuvel-Eibrink MM, et al. Recurrent deletions of IKZF1 in pediatric acute myeloid leukemia. Haematologica 2015;100(9):1151–9.

69. McNerney ME, Brown CD, Wang X, et al. CUX1 is a haploinsufficient tumor suppressor gene on chromosome 7 frequently inactivated in acute myeloid leukemia. Blood 2013;121(6):975–83.

70. An N, Khan S, Imgruet MK, et al. Gene dosage effect of CUX1 in a murine model disrupts HSC homeostasis and controls the severity and mortality of MDS. Blood 2018. [Epub ahead of print].

71. Bejar R, Stevenson K, Abdel-Wahab O, et al. Clinical effect of point mutations in myelodysplastic syndromes. N Engl J Med 2011;364(26):2496–506.
72. Padron E, Yoder S, Kunigal S, et al. ETV6 and signaling gene mutations are associated with secondary transformation of myelodysplastic syndromes to chronic myelomonocytic leukemia. Blood 2014;123(23):3675–7.
73. Walter MJ, Shen D, Shao J, et al. Clonal diversity of recurrently mutated genes in myelodysplastic syndromes. Leukemia 2013;27(6):1275–82.
74. Bejar R, Stevenson KE, Caughey BA, et al. Validation of a prognostic model and the impact of mutations in patients with lower-risk myelodysplastic syndromes. J Clin Oncol 2012;30(27):3376–82.
75. Zhang MY, Churpek JE, Keel SB, et al. Germline ETV6 mutations in familial thrombocytopenia and hematologic malignancy. Nat Genet 2015;47(2):180–5.
76. Hou HA, Kuo YY, Liu CY, et al. Distinct association between aberrant methylation of Wnt inhibitors and genetic alterations in acute myeloid leukaemia. Br J Cancer 2011;105(12):1927–33.
77. Wimmer K, Etzler J. Constitutional mismatch repair-deficiency syndrome: have we so far seen only the tip of an iceberg? Hum Genet 2008;124(2):105–22.
78. Locatelli F, Strahm B. How I treat myelodysplastic syndromes of childhood. Blood 2018;131(13):1406–14.
79. Madureira AB, Eapen M, Locatelli F, et al. Analysis of risk factors influencing outcome in children with myelodysplastic syndrome after unrelated cord blood transplantation. Leukemia 2011;25(3):449–54.
80. Glasser CL, Lee A, Eslin D, et al. Epigenetic combination therapy for children with secondary myelodysplastic syndrome (MDS)/acute myeloid leukemia (AML) and concurrent solid tumor relapse. J Pediatr Hematol Oncol 2017;39(7):560–4.
81. Inoue A, Kawakami C, Takitani K, et al. Azacitidine in the treatment of pediatric therapy-related myelodysplastic syndrome after allogeneic hematopoietic stem cell transplantation. J Pediatr Hematol Oncol 2014;36(5):e322–4.
82. Waespe N, Van Den Akker M, Klaassen RJ, et al. Response to treatment with azacitidine in children with advanced myelodysplastic syndrome prior to hematopoietic stem cell transplantation. Haematologica 2016;101(12):1508–15.